Breakthroughs in Smart Nursing With Generative AI

Suha Khalil Assayed
https://orcid.org/0000-0002-9924-0324
National Kaohsiung University of Science and Technology, Taiwan

Maha Atout
Philadelphia University, Jordan

Chin-Shiuh Shieh
National Kaohsiung University of Science and Technology, Taiwan

IGI Global
Scientific Publishing
Publishing Tomorrow's Research Today

Vice President of Editorial	Melissa Wagner
Director of Acquisitions	Mikaela Felty
Director of Book Development	Jocelynn Hessler
Production Manager	Mike Brehm
Cover Design	Jose Rosado

Published in the United States of America by
IGI Global Scientific Publishing
701 East Chocolate Avenue
Hershey, PA, 17033, USA
Tel: 717-533-8845 | Fax: 717-533-7115
Website: https://www.igi-global.com E-mail: cust@igi-global.com

Library of Congress Cataloging-in-Publication Data

LCCN: 2026003039 (CIP Data Pending)
ISBN13: 979-8-3373-8247-0
Isbn13Softcover: 979-8-3373-8248-7
EISBN13: 979-8-3373-8249-4

British Cataloguing in Publication Data
A Cataloguing in Publication record for this book is available from the British Library.

Table of Contents

Detailed Table of Contents

Healthcare professionals play an essential role in patient care, and ensuring the wellbeing of these professionals is essential to sustain a strong workforce. Yet, nurses face many challenges including employment shortages and heavy workloads, which could lead to higher error rates in clinical practice. At the same time, the rapid integration of AI and digital health technologies offers promising opportunities to enhance care quality and boost productivity, while also introducing new concerns such as data security and ethical risks. This chapter invites readers to explore the evolution of healthcare systems, starting from traditional, paper-based models to computerized and digital systems, and now toward AI-driven agentic health systems. It highlights the tools and practices for each era. along with the key opportunities and challenges in each stage, providing insightful perspectives on how AI technology is reshaping the future of healthcare. This chapter also illustrates some real-world examples highlighting the transformation of AI in nursing practice, by supporting clinical decision-making, enhancing patient monitoring, and ultimately improving the overall quality of healthcare delivery.

Generative AI in Clinical Documentation represents one of the most transformative intersections of machine intelligence and healthcare delivery, reconfiguring how clinicians record, interpret, and operationalise patient information in increasingly complex care environments. As global health systems grapple with rising administrative burdens, workforce shortages, and the escalating complexity of multimorbidity, generative AI functions not merely as a digital scribe but as an adaptive, context-aware partner that enhances the cognitive and operational capacity of clinical teams. At its core, generative AI leverages large-scale language models capable of parsing unstructured inputs—such as physician-patient conversations, fragmented notes across disparate electronic health record (EHR) environments, and evolving diagnostic narratives—to produce coherent, accurate, and contextually aligned documentation in real time. This shift from manual charting to dynamic, AI-assisted documentation not only minimises clerical load but also reshapes.

Communication failures between physicians and nurses are considered as one of the main contributors to to preventable patient harm, often resulting in delayed interventions and compromised care. While Electronic Health Records (EHRs) aim to improve data accessibility, they currently demand excessive time and cognitive resources, leading to clinician fatigue and reduced patient interaction. This chapter explores the capabilities of Generative AI (GenAI) in natural language processing and speech recognition to enhance clinical collaboration. We examine GenAI applications in real-time note generation, standardized handovers, and care plans to prevent ambiguity. Furthermore, this chapter proposes a human-supervised clinical documentation model emphasizing safety, transparency, and ethical use.

Preface

The rapid integration of AI and digital health technologies offers promising opportunities to enhance care quality and boost productivity among all healthcare professionals, including nurses, physicians, lab technicians, pharmacists, as well as others from allied health professions. For the nursing profession in particular, generative AI (GenAI) has great potential to enhance their work, reduce burnout, and improve patient care and outcomes. According to Rashidieranjbar et al. (2025), GenAI can revolutionize the healthcare profession by becoming an integral member within the medical staff.

In simple words, Generative AI (GenAI) is defined as a technology that has the ability to generate and create new, original content in response to user prompts. The generated content could be text, images, sound, video, and more.

Interestingly, Healthcare 5.0 represents smart AI technology designed to support nurses and other healthcare professionals in their daily work (Assayed et al., 2025). Rather than replacing their expertise, these technologies are designed to strengthen their medical and clinical skills, as well as enhance collaboration between nurses, physicians, patients, and health systems.

Additionally, predictive analytics used to monitor patient outcomes can add important value for nurses. These AI tools can analyze patient data in real time and accordingly alert early warning signs (Li et al., 2025). Therefore, when nurses are exposed to such AI tools in a supportive way, they feel more confident and can spend more time with their patients rather than long periods doing routine paperwork.

On the other hand, AI tools have the ability to increase work efficiency as well as team collaboration. On the theoretical side, healthcare managers should also promote innovative learning strategies by supporting the integration of AI tools into nursing education.

GenAI has inspired researchers and developers around the world to enhance education, particularly in adaptive and personalized learning (Georgieva-Tsaneva et al., 2024). As a result, medical education has significantly improved through new AI technologies and AI-powered simulations (Assayed & Maheshwari, 2023), which can enhance hands-on learning and clinical practice by using virtual patients and clinical simulations with smart AI tutoring systems rather than real people. Accordingly, nursing and medical students can improve their skills with confidence in a safe learning environment.

Interestingly, AI approaches in healthcare have developed to include not only GenAI, but also retrieval-augmented generation (RAG) and Agentic AI (Assayed, 2025), supporting more autonomous tasks such as interactive and multilingual chatbots that can perform multiple tasks to support patients.

Despite all the benefits and advantages of using GenAI in the medical domain, managers and administrators must ensure that all nurses and other healthcare staff are fully aware of the ethical implications and data-privacy considerations related to using AI tools (Momani, 2025). For example, managers and supervisors should educate healthcare staff regarding policies of confidentiality standards (Balogun et al., 2025).

This book aims to bring together nursing and medical students, educators, healthcare professionals including nurses and physicians, healthcare leaders, and technology developers to advance GenAI in healthcare, with a particular focus on nurses by improving their work experience, reducing burnout, and promoting well-being through the creation of a positive and healthy work environmen.

ORGANIZATION OF THE BOOK

The book is organized into 13 chapters, with a short summary of each provided below:

Chapter 1. This chapter explores the evolution of healthcare systems, starting from traditional, paper-based models to digital systems and AI-driven agentic health systems. It highlights the tools and practices for each era, along with the key opportunities and challenges in each stage, providing insightful perspectives on how AI technology is reshaping the future of healthcare. This chapter also illustrates some real-world examples highlighting the transformation of AI in nursing practice, by supporting clinical decision-making, enhancing patient monitoring, and ultimately improving the overall quality of healthcare delivery.

Chapter 2. This chapter examines the role of Generative AI in transforming clinical documentation within modern healthcare systems. It highlights how AI-driven language models can convert complex, unstructured clinical interactions into accurate, real-time medical records. The chapter emphasizes on the role of GenAI as an intelligent partner that enhances efficiency, accuracy, and care delivery in increasingly complex clinical environments

Chapter 3. This chapter explores the capabilities of Generative AI (GenAI) in natural language processing and speech recognition to enhance clinical collaboration. It examines GenAI applications in real-time note generation, standardized handovers, and care plans to prevent ambiguity. Furthermore, this chapter proposes a human-supervised clinical documentation model emphasizing safety, transparency, and ethical use.

Chapter 4. This chapter addresses the challenges of accurately diagnosing pneumonia in complex clinical settings. It introduces a hybrid fuzzy decision-making framework that combines FAHP and Fuzzy TOPSIS to evaluate key diagnostic criteria under uncertainty. The model helps prioritize clinical indicators such as symptoms, imaging, and laboratory findings using structured expert judgment. Overall, the chapter demonstrates how intelligent decision-support methods can improve diagnostic accuracy and clinical confidence.

Chapter 5. This paper explores how the Internet of Bodies (IoB) can support continuous observation, early prediction of health risks, and improved outcomes for patients, clinicians, and health systems. It shows how continuous streams of physiological, behavioral, and contextual data can be transformed into meaningful insights and risk signals that enable proactive, rather than reactive, care. The paper also examines key benefits, such as better chronic disease management and more personalized support, alongside major challenges related to privacy, security, equity, and usability.

Chapter 6. This chapter examines the uses of GenAI, in nursing emphasizing especially its ability to aid clinical decision-making improve risk assessment, automate patient documentation enhance ICU surveillance and produce precise prompt information that assists nurses in making quicker and safer choices at the bedside.

Chapter 7. This chapter talks about the merging of generative AI in nursing documentation systems, where it speaks about how these inventions will help in the accuracy of documentation, removing the administrative burden, as well as possibly potentially speed up clinical decision making.

Chapter 8. This chapter describes an experimental study for developing an affordable virtual nursing assistant by utilizing a neural network model to provide patients with immediate and effective answers to medical inquiries. The architecture of the proposed model starts with encoding the input of health enquiry into the embedding layer. Utilizing the MedQud dataset from Kaggle website, it includes 47,457 medical question-answer pairs covering questions about treatment, diagnosis and side effect During the execution phase, the performance metric shows a higher precision score compared to the recall and F1-score.

Chapter 9. This chapter explores the integration of AI technologies including machine learning, deep learning, natural language processing, and reinforcement learning within key hospital operational domains such as administrative workflows, staff scheduling, resource allocation, and performance optimization. It highlights how AI enhances patient flow, reduces delays, improves asset management, and supports real-time operational intelligence. The chapter also discusses challenges related to data privacy, bias, system interoperability, governance, and workforce acceptance.

Chapter 10. This chapter explores how Generative AI is transforming nursing practice by supporting clinical decisions, improving patient care, and streamlining workflows. It highlights applications such as predictive analytics, automated documentation, smart staffing, and remote patient monitoring. The chapter also addresses key challenges, including data quality, bias, and ethical considerations that require thoughtful implementation and training. Overall, it presents the future of nursing as a collaborative model where AI tools enhance, rather than replace, human expertise.

Chapter 11. This chapter examines how generative AI technologies support nurses in providing personalized, continuous and responsive care beyond traditional clinical settings. The chapter also explores AI driven patient engagement strategies that promote adherence, self-management and real time monitoring through conversational and remote care platforms. Ethical and practical challenges including data privacy, transparency, algorithmic bias, trust and equitable access are critically analyzed within a human centered design framework.

Chapter 12. This chapter examines the implications of generative artificial intelligence for advanced clinical nursing practice, with a focus on clinical judgement, professional education, leadership, and ethical governance. The chapter also explores how generative artificial intelligence is being integrated into healthcare systems and its potential role in supporting clinical reasoning, documentation, care coordination, and educational practice within advanced nursing roles. It evaluates as well both the opportunities and limitations of AI-enabled nursing practice. Particular attention is given to challenges related to automation bias, data governance, equity, and professional accountability, alongside the absence of nursing-specific regulatory guidance.

Chapter 13. This chapter examines how (AI) is transforming the nursing education and leadership by changing the roles and responsibilities of nurses' leaders and reshaping the way they design curricula. The chapter also highlights the opportunities of AI in nursing practice and how integrating AI tools can provide nursing students, nurses and clinicians with smarter solutions While AI offers opportunities to enhance nursing education, leadership efficiency and instructional support, it also raises challenges related to privacy, equity, and ethical issues related to AI health technologies.

Suha Khalil Assayed
National Kaohsiung University of Science and Technology, Taiwan & The British University in Dubai, UAE

REFERENCES

Assayed, S. K. (2025). *Transforming healthcare through generative and agentic AI: A systematic review.* In *Proceedings of the 10th International Conference on Information Technology Trends (ITT)* (pp. 124–129). IEEE. https://doi.org/DOI: 10.1109/ITT69610.2025.11352935

Assayed, S. K., & Maheshwari, S. (2023). *Agent-based simulation for university students' admission: Medical colleges in Jordanian universities.* Computer Science & Engineering [CSEIJ]. *International Journal (Toronto, Ont.), 13*(1).

Assayed, S. K., Shieh, C. S., & Gupta, S. K. (2025). Engineering intelligent healthcare systems: Understanding medical queries with AI and NLP. *Journal of Engineering and Applied Sciences (Asian Research Publishing Network), 72*(1), 212. DOI: 10.1186/s44147-025-00800-y

Balogun, A. Y., Metibemu, O. C., Olutimehin, A. T., Ajayi, A. J., Babarinde, D. C., & Olaniyi, O. O. (2025). The ethical and legal implications of shadow AI in sensitive industries: A focus on healthcare, finance and education. *Finance and Education (February 13, 2025).*

Georgieva-Tsaneva, G., Serbezova, I., & Beloeva, S. (2024). Application of virtual reality, artificial intelligence, and other innovative technologies in healthcare education (nursing and midwifery specialties): Challenges and strategies. *Education Sciences, 15*(1), 11. DOI: 10.3390/educsci15010011

Li, F., Wang, S., Gao, Z., Qing, M., Pan, S., Liu, Y., & Hu, C. (2025). Harnessing artificial intelligence in sepsis care: Advances in early detection, personalized treatment, and real-time monitoring. *Frontiers in Medicine, 11*, 1510792. DOI: 10.3389/fmed.2024.1510792 PMID: 39835096

Momani, A. (2025). Implications of Artificial Intelligence on Health Data Privacy and Confidentiality. *arXiv preprint arXiv:2501.01639.*

Rashidieranjbar, F., Farhadi, A., & Zamanifar, A. (2025). Revolutionizing Healthcare with Generative Artificial Intelligence Technologies. In Vajjhala, N. R., Roy, S. S., Taşcı, B., & Hoque Chowdhury, M. E. (Eds.), *Generative Artificial Intelligence (AI) Approaches for Industrial Applications. Information Systems Engineering and Management* (Vol. 24). Springer., DOI: 10.1007/978-3-031-76710-4_10

Acknowledgment

I'm very thankful to all my family and friends for their love and support, in particular, I would thank my parents, my husband, and my children. and this book would not have been possible without them.

I would also thank authors, reviewers, and contributors who participated in this book. Your expertise, dedication and commitment have played a crucial role in editing this book.

I also want to give a special thank you to the nursing community, for their compassion, and dedication that make a real difference in people's lives every day. You inspire us with your kindness and your commitment in providing the healthcare to keep enhancing healthcare through innovation and technology. Thank you for everything you do.

Suha Khalil Assayed
National Kaohsiung University of Science and Technology, Taiwan & The British University in Dubai, UAE

Chapter 1
Generative AI as the New Frontier in Healthcare:
From Traditional Health and Nursing Informatics to Next-Generation Agentic Systems

Suha Khalil Assayed
http://orcid.org/0000-0002-9924-0324
National Kaohsiung University of Science and Technology, Taiwan & The British University in Dubai, UAE

Maha Atout
Philadelphia University, Jordan

Muaath Ismail Alsufi
http://orcid.org/0009-0005-8564-7034
University of Jordan, Jordan

ABSTRACT

Healthcare professionals play an essential role in patient care, and ensuring the wellbeing of these professionals is essential to sustain a strong workforce. Yet, nurses face many challenges including employment shortages and heavy workloads, which could lead to higher error rates in clinical practice. At the same time, the rapid integration of AI and digital health technologies offers promising opportunities to enhance care quality and boost productivity, while also introducing new concerns such as data security and ethical risks. This chapter invites readers to explore the evolution of healthcare systems, starting from traditional, paper-based models to computerized and digital systems, and now toward AI-driven agentic health systems. It highlights the tools and practices for each era. along with the key opportunities

DOI: 10.4018/979-8-3373-8247-0.ch001

and challenges in each stage, providing insightful perspectives on how AI technology is reshaping the future of healthcare. This chapter also illustrates some real-world examples highlighting the transformation of AI in nursing practice, by supporting clinical decision-making, enhancing patient monitoring, and ultimately improving the overall quality of healthcare delivery.

1. INTRODUCTION

Healthcare professionals including nurses, physicians, lab technicians and others, are an essential part of the clinical workforce in delivering direct patient care (Norful et al., 2024). Therefore, supporting their wellbeing and reducing burnout plays an essential role in maintaining a strong healthcare workforce. According to a review study conducted by Scott-Marshall (2024), nurses face several challenges in their work, including staffing shortages, heavy workloads, and extended shifts which negatively affects their well-being and ultimately decrease the quality of patient care. Henceforth, researchers are inspired to find solutions to improve nurses' performances and to increase their satisfaction. A qualitative study was conducted by Paarima et al. (2024) on 213 nurses in three hospitals in Ghana to examine the impact of perceived organizational politics on job satisfaction and job stress among nurses, the results revealed that the more organizational politics nurses experience, the less satisfied they feel in their jobs. This behavior includes unfair treatment, inconsistent use of rules and policies, and others. When nurses become dissatisfied, their performance is negatively affected, leading to increased work errors.

Similarly, Galanis et al. (2023) examined the relationship between high levels of job burnout and low levels of job satisfaction among nurses and other healthcare workers after the COVID-19 pandemic. In their survey of 1760 healthcare workers, 91.1% of nurses experienced high levels of burnout. These results revealed that the nursing profession was an independent predictor of burnout and satisfaction. Additionally, many other demographic and job characteristics affected burnout and satisfaction rates among nurses, indicating that policy makers, organizations, and managers should adopt appropriate interventions to improve work conditions.

Interestingly, Hameed et al. (2024) reported that the intervention of digital health technology in healthcare can improve quality and productivity, however it raises other concerns such as security issues and other related challenges. Additionally, according to the World Health Organization (WHO), digital health technology is defined as "the field of knowledge and practice associated with the development and use of digital technologies to improve health", whereas, the WHO's Global Strategy on Digital Health 2020–2025 explains that digital health expands the concept of eHealth to include digital consumers and a wider range of smart and connected devices, incorporating various advanced digital technologies such as the Internet of Things (IoT), advanced computing, big data analytics, artificial intelligence which includes machine learning and robotics (World Health Organization, 2021).

This chapter aims to explore the different eras of healthcare, beginning with traditional systems, moving through computerized and digitalized health systems, and eventually reaching to AI-driven agentic systems. It also introduces readers to the key opportunities and challenges that describe each stage of this evolution.

2. TRADITIONAL HEALTHCARE SYSTEMS

Although we are now in the era of Industry 5, some clinics and hospitals are still using traditional healthcare systems. By "traditional" we refer to practices such as paper-based archiving and recording, manual communication processes between departments, and multiple decentralized systems. These approaches require physicians to spend more time communicating and coordinating with other clinical departments, as well as analyzing and interpreting historical patient data to make predictions. On the other side, the traditional diagnostic method, though generally reliable, depends heavily on the physician's experience and judgment, which can sometimes lead to inconsistencies and mistakes (Ajegbile et al., 2024).

In terms of nursing, much of their time is spent manually on writing and documenting vital signs and patient updates. Accordingly, this extra paperwork would take them away from direct patient care. For example, waiting for a paper file or searching for patient information during busy wards can slow treatment and adding more stress. As a result, nurses may feel overwhelmed as well as have less time to offer much-needed care to patients.

2.1 Tools and Practices

Within traditional healthcare, several methods and clinical practices are applied in different ways. Table 1 provides some details for each of these practices.

Table 1. Summarizes the tools and practices in traditional healthcare system

Tools & Practices	Description
Paper-based documents (Patients' records)	Physical documents including information about patients such as patient's medical history, treatment details and other related information. These records are usually stored in physical folders and within cabinets in archiving room.
Manual workflow processes	Coordination between other departments using memos is a traditional approach that depends heavily on human interaction as well as on physical documents.
Decentralized systems	In decentralized system, patient information is stored in disconnected different systems at different hospitals, clinics, labs, and pharmacies. All these entities have their own databases.
Manual analysis and diagnosis	This is related to a human expert reviewing patients' data and symptoms to come up with a decision.

2.2 Opportunities and Challenges

Despite the challenges from traditional healthcare, particularly decentralized processes to manual workflows, it has several strengths, especially its strong basis in real human interaction (Botrugno, 2019). This personal connection helps in building trust and accordingly supporting patients emotionally. Interestingly, Pan and Wang (2025), concluded in their study that paying more attention to patients' emotional needs and listening to their personal stories can enhance the patient care outcomes, and improve overall well-being as well as supporting the recovery process. For example, nurses usually take some time sitting close to patients, chatting through their worries before a surgery and offering some comfort that no system or device can replace. Similarly, in palliative care, nurses can tell when a patient is feeling uncomfortable and needs emotional support, or just wants someone close by (Moran et al., 2024). Such small moments of care can make a big difference in patients' comfort.

3. COMPUTERIZED AND DIGITALIZED HEALTH SYSTEMS

The digital health terminology is a broad term that refers to using information and communications technologies in medicine and other related health professions to manage illnesses and health risks as well as to promote wellness (Ronquillo et al., 2023). Moreover, it expands to include many components such as telehealth, electronic health record systems (EHS), capturing and retrieving patients' information electronically, computerized health systems and applications as well as the telecommunications networking infrastructure that connect the entire healthcare ecosystem (Abernethy et al., 2022).

In fact, over the past three decades, healthcare has experienced a remarkable digital transformation driven by the growing use of computerized systems (Gopal et al., 2019). While such technologies were not developed using artificial intelligence tools, they have laid the groundwork for intelligent and generative healthcare solutions.

3.1 Tools and Practices

Interestingly, Electronic Health Records (EHRs) and Electronic Medical Records (EMRs) have rapidly become the core of modern healthcare institutions (Bednorz et al. 2023; Adeniyi et al., 2024), such records include test results, doctors and all clinical notes, as well as patient histories in one place. Beside the EHRs and EMRs, other important digital tools have added more value to the healthcare system, such as medical X-ray imaging applications (Perez & Poletti 2022) which improve the storage and sharing of medical x-rays, while telehealth and mHealth apps (Chandrakar, 2024) have made care more accessible anywhere. Table 2 provides some of these tools along with a brief description of each.

Table 2. Summary of Main Digital Health Tools and Practices

Tool	Description
Electronic Health Records (EHRs) & Electronic Medical Records (EMRs)	Used as a centralized the patients electronic records such as patient histories, lab results, clinical notes and treatment plans.
Medical Imaging Systems	Storing and share diagnostic images.
Telehealth Services	Virtual and remote consultations.
Mobile Health (mHealth) Tools	Wearable devices for monitoring and tracking vitals and lifestyle behaviors.
Workflow Automation	ERP system for electronic prescribing, registration, payment systems and appointments.

3.2 Opportunities and Challenges

Digital and computerized health system provide many opportunities for improving healthcare, particularly in nursing practice. Electronic Health Records (EHRs) allow nurses to access patient information quickly, as well as improving quality of patient care (Adeniyi et al., 2024). Nurses would be able to monitor vital signs, and make informed decisions accordingly. Similarly, Telehealth and mobile health (mHealth) apps enable nurses to support patients remotely (Matlhaba, 2024;

Bakker et al., 2023). for enhancing follow-up care. Furthermore, the workflow automation tools, such as electronic prescribing and digital documentation can reduce the administrative burden and give nurses more time for direct patient interaction. Nevertheless, these systems might have some challenges, specifically in terms of ethical considerations and patients' data privacy. Accordingly, nurses need to have some training to use such systems effectively and efficiency. In addition, there is also concern that many medical devices which are connected to patients and healthcare provider could be easily accessed by other parties or hackers and lead to release of confidential patient information. For example, in 2024, the Synnovis cyberattack in southeast London showed how vulnerable the National Health Service (NHS) is to digital threats (Rajput et al., 2025). Many hospitals were affected, additionally, primary care was struggling with delayed tests, which caused many troubles and did quietly harm patient safety over time.

4. AI AND NEXT-GENERATION AGENTIC HEALTH SYSTEMS

As the development of AI has accelerated, many healthcare systems have shifted from relying mainly on Electronic Health Records (EHRs) to adopting smart AI applications. For example, AI is used to predict diseases through machine learning algorithms or to interpret X-rays (Knevel & Liao, 2023). Furthermore, Deep learning models have significantly improved the benefits regarding laboratory utilization, especially in handling large clinical blood results that are combined with other histological exams and genomic information. (Kothinti, 2024). According to van der Laak et al. (2021), deep learning models in histopathology particularly holds significant potential to improve medical diagnostics by enhancing the accuracy and efficiency while reducing clinician and nursing workload. Furthermore, Alowais et al. (2023) emphasized that integrating AI into healthcare is not limited only for disease predictions or clinical laboratory tests, but it can revolutionize personalized medicine and provide an effective virtual remote health assistants as well as supporting mental health care. Assayed et al. (2025) developed an AI model designed to classify a clinical query into different categories using a range of machine learning and deep learning algorithms, including Naïve Bayes, Logistic Regression, and the transformer-based BERT model. Recognizing user intent is a crucial step in building effective health-related question-answering (QA) systems, as it allows the system to correctly interpret medical inquiries and provide accurate, meaningful responses.

Interestingly, artificial intelligence is now participating in the operating room by transforming robotic surgery to be more precise, efficient, and safe. According to Iftikhar et al. (2024), AI-powered robotic tools can perform real-time image analysis and guide instrument movements which can enable surgeons and doctors to work with greater accuracy while reducing the exhaustion levels. Table 3 provides a summary of different AI tools that can be applied within the healthcare domain.

Table 3. provides a summary of key AI tools in the medical and healthcare domains.

AI Tool	Description
Machine Learning (ML) Algorithms	Predict diseases and outcomes such as stroke or heart disease risk prediction
Deep Learning (CNNs, LSTM, GPT, BERT)	Analyzing medical images (X-Ray) and using large datasets for analyzing patterns and predictions.
Natural Language Processing (NLP)	Analyzing and processing unstructured clinical documents and understanding patient enquiries, such as Chatbots and different virtual assistants,
AI within Robotic Surgery	Reducing the human error, enhance precision and accuracy with decreasing the exhaustion levels.
Chatbots and Virtual Assistants	Monitoring patients remotely and providing them with e-consultations using either text-text chatbots, or integrating voice conversations.

Beyond the traditional AI and GenAI applications, new agentic AI models have been applied in healthcare (Assayed, 2025a), particularly in clinical decision support as well as for diseases diagnostics, as traditional AI and ML models struggle with the dynamic healthcare settings (Karunanayake, 2025). Agentic AI, is defined as autonomous artificial intelligence systems that are capable of completing complex tasks and learning from their environment (Acharya et al., 2025), understanding context and making independant decisions without the need for human intervention (Pati, 2025). Interestingly, as stated by Acharya et al. (2025), the flexibility of Agentic AI allows it to respond differently even when situations look the same. For example, an agentic AI could adjust the way it evaluates patients as their symptoms change. If a patient's vital signs unexpectedly worsen, the AI can change its priorities and explore different treatment options that can best support the patient's health. Despite the benefits and effectiveness of using agentic AI, it is crucial to determine how these systems handle privacy and data security. Since these systems act more independently, even small misunderstandings of their goals can lead to mistakes or undesirable results (Broh et al., 2025), a phenomenon often referred to as "hallucinations" (Šekrst, 2025, Gosmar & Dahl, 2025). To mitigate these risks, the integration of Explainable AI (XAI) frameworks is essential. Unlike traditional deep learning models where decision pathways are unclear, Agentic AI using XAI frameworks would provide the reasoning (abnormal lab result, imaging abnormality, etc.) that lead to adjustment in the patient's management. This transparency allows healthcare professionals understand the rationale behind the agent's decision and to validate it against established medical protocols. (Bragazzi & Garbarino, 2024).

In summary, during the evolution of healthcare and nursing systems, from traditional approaches to agentic AI, different applications and models (see Figure 1) have been highlighted, showing various applications along with their associated opportunities and limitations. It is highly beneficial for all professionals, including nurses and other healthcare practitioners, to be aware of this evolution in order to understand its implications clearly.

Figure 1. Evolution of healthcare and nursing systems, the shift from traditional approaches to agentic AI applications.

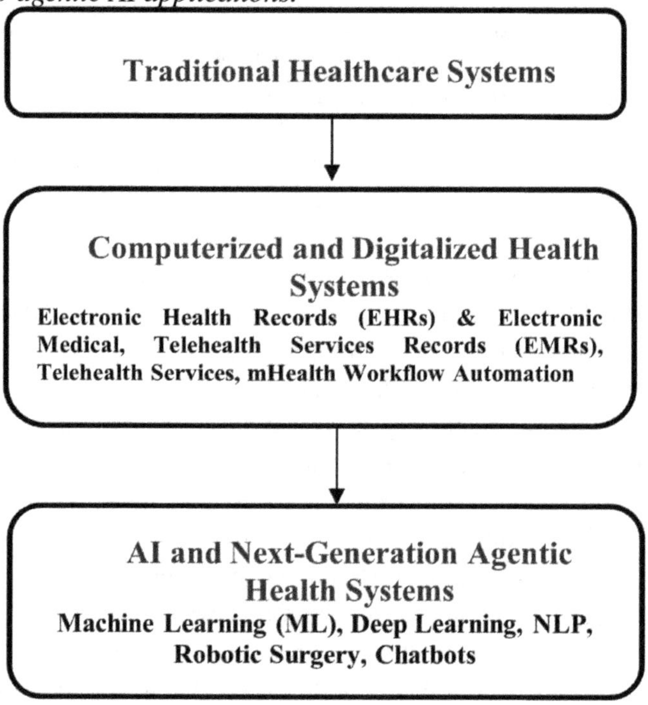

5. PRACTICAL CASE STUDIES ON AI ADOPTION IN NURSING CARE

There are several studies that have explored real case studies that integrated multiple AI tools and models to enhance nursing care. Seibert et al. (2021) studied a review by using 7016 publications and 704 full texts were screened, and 292 publications were included, the study combines literature on scenarios for applying the AI models and tools in nursing care settings, extracted from high standard databases such as PubMed, CINAHL, ACM Digital Library and IEEE. The findings in this review revealed that most papers used ML algorithms and the application and AI tools are focusing on imaging, monitoring and classification of activity, as well as care coordination and communication. In reference to the qualitative study conducted by Ramadan et al. (2024), which explored the perspectives of registered nurses in Saudi Arabia on AI adoption, the findings emphasize the need for tailored AI training and a clear ethical framework for nurses. Moreover, another study in Saudi Arabia involved 611 nurses from various educational hospitals to explore perceptions of AI-enabled wearable health technologies during the COVID-19 pandemic. These devices, enhanced by AI, support continuous monitoring, early diagnosis, and personalized care. Nurses generally viewed AI wearables positively, recognizing their potential to improve care and efficiency. The key concerns highlighted in this study included data accuracy and technical reliability (Alzghaibi, 2025). In Jordan, Almagharbeh (2025) examines the impact of artificial intelligence-based decision support systems on the operational processes of nurses in critical care units (CCU) by applying a study group of 112 registered nurses from hospitals in Jordan. The study focused on several features of nursing workflows, the employment of AI, encountered errors as well as the sufficiency of training and education. The results reveal that nurses report that AI can help them save more time, monitor patients better, and make effective clinical decisions, but they still struggle with limited training, and ongoing technical issues. Accordingly, this study highlights the important role of providing training programs for nurses within AI technologies and to maximize their use in critical care settings.

Additionally, Cho et al. (2022) applied natural language processing (NLP) to evaluate real-time medical records using the voice recognition-based AI (RMIS-AI) particularly in the emergency unit emergency department of a tertiary hospital in northwestern Seoul, South Korea. This voice recognition model transforms the nurses' spoken triage information into structured medical records using AI-NLP model called a Speech-to-Text model. Technically, this NLP model trained on 1,717 cases with high accuracy, however, it requires technical refinement before becoming a fully reliable alternative. In Turkey, Ergin et al. (2022) conducted a descriptive study involving 326 nurse managers who completed an online survey to examine their knowledge and attitudes toward AI and robot nurses using structured questionnaires. Results showed that 66.9% had previously heard of AI and robot-nurse concepts, and 67.2% believed robot nurses would benefit their career. However, 86.2% did not believe robots could replace human nurses. Overall, the findings indicate that nurse managers view AI and robotic technologies as supportive tools that can reduce workload but not as a replacement for human nursing care.

Interestingly, Rony et al. (2024) explored the opportunities of using AI to reduce the daily burdens faced by nurses such as automating the routing admin works, applying predictive models, and using virtual telemedicine for monitoring patients remotely. Accordingly, the healthcare entities can empower nurses to excel in their roles while supporting a more work-life balance.

Furthermore, to improve more the work-lift balance, Gerlach et al. (2025) conducted a qualitative study exploring nurse perspectives on AI-based shift scheduling in acute hospitals and home care services in Switzerland. By applying focus group interviews on 21 nurses and nurse leaders examining perceptions of fairness, transparency, and work-life balance in shift allocation. Participants stated that traditional scheduling usually lacked fairness and transparency, with significant dissatisfaction among permanent nursing staff, while temporary staff valued more flexibility. AI-based scheduling was perceived as promising for improving shift fairly and reducing the administrative burden, However, participants raised some concerns on emphasizing the need for human oversight to consider emotional and other factors that AI systems may overlook. In general, AI scheduling was perceived as a tool that could enhance fairness, transparency, and work-life balance if it's combined effectively with human supervision.

6. RECOMMENDATIONS FOR ADVANCING NURSING IN THE ERA OF AI

As healthcare systems evolve from traditional approaches to the AI and agentic models, all workers in healthcare occupations including nurses, physicians, lab technicians, admin staff, etc., must adapt to make best use of such technologies to improve patient care.

In fact, building AI literacy within the healthcare sector is essential now for everyone. It is also considered as one of the most important responsibilities of healthcare directors and decision-makers to ensure that staff receive good training and support to use AI effectively and successfully. In this section, multiples recommendations will be proposed from different perspectives, including advice aimed nurses personally as well as advice targeting health administrator and decision makers.

6.1. Recommendation for Nurses

Nurses should be able to use and exposed to different AI tools and generative AI (GenAI) for faster and simpler documentation. For example, GenAI tools like ChatGPT or Gemini and others, can be used to communicate with patients using different languages, these tools can translate instructions as we all as simplifying some of complex medical information (Genovese et al., 2024; Chen et al., 2024), and provide a clear explanation. This is especially important for nurses working in multicultural environments from different nationalities. With such GenAI tools, nurses can have compassionate communication with patients (Howcroft et al., 2025) using their language and ensuring that they fully understand their treatment as well their medications. Additionally, Evidence-Based GenAI tools like OpenEvidence and Hippocratic AI can be used for verifying medical decisions and reviewing the latest care guidelines. Such GenAI tools utilize Retrieval-Augmented Generation (RAG) to support every response with verified peer-reviewed literature (e.g., The Lancet, NEJM), which is vital for ensuring the reliability and trustworthiness of the information especially in the high-stakes healthcare setting.

On the other hand, utilizing predictive analytics to monitor patient outcomes can add significant value to nurses. These tools can analyze patient data in real time and highlight any early warning signs (Braun et al., 2022), so nurses can interfere immediately as well as providing more proactive care. Accordingly, when nurses are exposed to such AI tools in a supportive way, they feel more confident and can spend more time with their patients rather than spending long periods of time doing routine paperwork. Multiple studies examining the correlation between nursing workloads, stress, and patient outcomes (Alnawafleh, 2024; Babapour et al. 2022) show that when nurses are overwhelmed and stressed, the quality of patient care tends to decline. Therefore, nurse scheduling is a complex challenge (Renggli et al., 2025) within the healthcare domain due to its impacts on both patient care quality and nurse well-being. AI-based scheduling systems can significantly improve equality, transparency, and efficiency in nurse scheduling. Table 4 shows some of the recommendations for nurses in the Era of AI.

Table 4. Provides a summary of recommendations for nurses in in the Era of AI

	Recommendation	Details	References
1.	Exposure AI and GenAI tools & applications	Simplifying the documentation/ notes, translating instructions, communicating with patients using different languages, simplifying complex medical terms, as well as supporting compassionate care in multicultural environment.	Genovese et al., 2024; Chen et al., 2024; Howcroft et al., 2025
2.	Implementing predictive analytics	Monitoring and tracking the patient data in real time, highlighting any early warning signs which can be enabled to indicate any proactive interventions with supporting appropriate care accordingly.	Braun et al., 2022
3.	Supportive AI implementation-Admin Work	Increasing nurses' confidence by reducing routine paperwork and allowing more time for direct patients care.	Alnawafleh, 2024; Babapour et al., 2022
4.	AI-based nurse scheduling	Improves fairness, equality, transparency, and efficiency in scheduling, reducing stress and maintaining quality of patient care as well as enhancing nurse well-being.	Renggli et al., 2025

6.2. Recommendation for Healthcare Administrators

Several recent studies have highlighted the positive impact of AI in optimizing the administrative tasks and processes across different nursing and healthcare administration functions (Alenezi et al., 2024; Ali Mohamad et al., 2023). For example, the findings from a qualitative study conducted by Göktepe& Sarıköse (2025) after interviewing 22 nurse managers shows that integrating AI in healthcare play an essential role in patient flow management and workforce planning, as AI tools have the ability to minimize waste and increase work efficiency, mainly in archiving and inventory tracking as well as with team collaboration. On the theoretical side, managers and administrators in healthcare should promote and encourage innovative learning strategies by supporting the integration of AI tools into nursing education (Montejo et al., 2024). For example, they can include more hands-on activities and simulation-based training to enhance practical learning and provide opportunities for real-world applications.

However, besides all of these opportunities, managers should also ensure that all nurses and other healthcare staff are fully aware of the ethical implications and data-privacy considerations related to using AI tools (Shoghli et al., 2024; Nasir et al., 2024). For example, managers and supervisors should expose and educate healthcare staff regarding the policy of confidentiality standards (Haviana et al., 2025), potential risks of the bias of AI models in training the data (Oyeniran et al., 2022), and the importance of maintaining patient trust when integrating AI within the administrative workflows. Table 5 summarizes some of the main recommendations for managers on integrating artificial intelligence into nursing administration, highlighting opportunities and ethical and privacy safeguards.

Table 5. Summary of main recommendations for managers on integrating AI into Nursing Administration

Recommendation	Details	Refernces	Examples
Optimizing the Administrative Processes by Using AI	AI enhances efficiency and accuracy in administrative and nursing workflows.	Alenezi et al. (2024); Ali Mohamad et al. (2023)	Automating processes with effective workflow management and reducing workload.
Applying AI for Workforce Planning	Nurse managers' report AI as essential for managing patient flow, staff scheduling, and coordination.	Göktepe & Sarıköse (2025)	Improving staff allocation, improved patient movement, enhanced teamwork.
Improve the Resource Management by using AI Technology	AI reduces waste and improves archiving and inventory tracking.	Göktepe & Sarıköse (2025)	Real-time inventory systems with automated archiving, and reduced resource waste.

continued on following page

Table 5. Continued

Recommendation	Details	Refernces	Examples
Integrating AI in Nursing Education	Managers should support innovative learning strategies that include AI technologies.	Montejo et al. (2024)	Simulation-based learning, hands-on AI practice with real-world application training.
Educating Staff on Ethical and Privacy Considerations	Nurses must understand ethical guidelines and data-privacy issues tied to AI use.	Shoghli et al. (2024); Nasir et al. (2024)	Training on ethical using AI use, privacy policies, and responsible data handling.
Ensuring the Awareness of Confidentiality Standards	Staff should be trained on confidentiality rules when using AI tools.	Haviana et al. (2025)	Protecting patient data and confidentiality protocols, maintaining trust.
Addressing AI Bias and the fairness	Nurses should aware if the risks of bias in AI models such model training on limited or biased data.	Oyeniran et al. (2022)	Critical evaluation of AI output by identifying biased results, as well as safeguarding patient fairness.

7. CONCLUSIONS

Artificial intelligence has rapidly transformed this world, extending into various domains including education, finance, business, healthcare and more (Assayed, 2025b, Oyewole et al., 2024; Arinze et al., 2024).

In this chapter, we explored the evolution of healthcare systems, starting from traditional, paper-based models to computerized and digital health systems, and now towards AI-driven and agentic smart health systems. Each era has presented some different opportunities and challenges, offering valuable lessons for nurses, administrators as well as policymakers. To maximize the benefits of technology and AI, it is essential to integrate innovations thoughtfully, aligning them with the mission, vision, and cultural context of the country and health institution, while considering other local factors that may influence implementation. Since not all technologies advance at the same pace across different regions or healthcare settings, some challenges such as economic constraints, infrastructure limitations and the availability of internet access can influence the successful adoption of AI into healthcare systems. Moreover, political or regulatory factors can also hinder the successful adoption of AI and digital health solutions.

Accordingly, reflecting on past transitions and learning from each era, healthcare systems can strategically integrate AI and digital technologies to improve quality, efficiency as well as workforce wellbeing, while addressing the ethical, social, and practical challenges of modern AI healthcare applications.

REFERENCES

Abernethy, A., Adams, L., Barrett, M., Bechtel, C., Brennan, P., Butte, A., Faulkner, J., Fontaine, E., Friedhoff, S., Halamka, J., Howell, M., Johnson, K., Long, P., McGraw, D., Miller, R., Lee, P., Perlin, J., Rucker, D., Sandy, L., & Valdes, K. (2022). (2022). The Promise of Digital Health: Then, Now, and the Future. *NAM Perspectives*, *6*(22). Advance online publication. DOI: 10.31478/202206e

Acharya, D. B., Kuppan, K., & Divya, B. (2025). Agentic AI: Autonomous intelligence for complex goals—A comprehensive survey. *IEEE Access : Practical Innovations, Open Solutions*, *13*, 18912–18936. DOI: 10.1109/ACCESS.2025.3532853

Adeniyi, A. O., Arowoogun, J. O., Chidi, R., Okolo, C. A., & Babawarun, O. (2024). The impact of electronic health records on patient care and outcomes: A comprehensive review. *World Journal of Advanced Research and Reviews*, *21*(2), 1446–1455. DOI: 10.30574/wjarr.2024.21.2.0592

Adeniyi, A. O., Arowoogun, J. O., Chidi, R., Okolo, C. A., & Babawarun, O. (2024). The impact of electronic health records on patient care and outcomes: A comprehensive review. *World Journal of Advanced Research and Reviews*, *21*(2), 1446–1455. DOI: 10.30574/wjarr.2024.21.2.0592

Ajegbile, M. D., Olaboye, J. A., Maha, C. C., Igwama, G. T., & Abdul, S. (2024). The role of data-driven initiatives in enhancing healthcare delivery and patient retention. *World Journal of Biology Pharmacy and Health Sciences*, *19*(1), 234–242. DOI: 10.30574/wjbphs.2024.19.1.0435

Alenezi, A., Alshammari, M. H., & Ibrahim, I. A. (2024). Optimizing nursing Productivity: Exploring the role of Artificial Intelligence, Technology Integration, competencies, and Leadership. *Journal of Nursing Management*, *2024*(1), 8371068. DOI: 10.1155/2024/8371068

Ali Mohamad, T., Bastone, A., Bernhard, F., & Schiavone, F. (2023). How artificial intelligence impacts the competitive position of healthcare organizations. *Journal of Organizational Change Management*, *36*(8), 49–70. DOI: 10.1108/JOCM-03-2023-0057

Almagharbeh, W. T. (2025). The impact of AI-based decision support systems on nursing workflows in critical care units. *International Nursing Review*, *72*(2), e13011. DOI: 10.1111/inr.13011

Alnawafleh, K. A. (2024). The Impact of AI on Nursing Workload and Stress Levels in Critical Care Settings. *Pakistan Journal of Life and Social Sciences*, *22*(2), 8529–8542. DOI: 10.57239/PJLSS-2024-22.2.00643

Alowais, S. A., Alghamdi, S. S., Alsuhebany, N., Alqahtani, T., Alshaya, A. I., Almohareb, S. N., Aldairem, A., Alrashed, M., Bin Saleh, K., Badreldin, H. A., Al Yami, M. S., Al Harbi, S., & Albekairy, A. M. (2023). Revolutionizing healthcare: The role of artificial intelligence in clinical practice. *BMC Medical Education*, *23*(1), 689. DOI: 10.1186/s12909-023-04698-z

Alzghaibi, H. (2025). Nurses' perspectives on AI-Enabled wearable health technologies: Opportunities and challenges in clinical practice. *BMC Nursing*, *24*(1), 799. DOI: 10.1186/s12912-025-03343-y

Arinze, C. A., Izionworu, V. O., Isong, D., Daudu, C. D., & Adefemi, A. (2024). Integrating artificial intelligence into engineering processes for improved efficiency and safety in oil and gas operations. *Open Access Research Journal of Engineering and Technology*, *6*(1), 39–51. DOI: 10.53022/oarjet.2024.6.1.0012

Assayed, S. K. (2025a). *Transforming healthcare through generative and agentic AI: A systematic review.* In *Proceedings of the 10th International Conference on Information Technology Trends (ITT)* (pp. 124–129). IEEE. https://doi.org/DOI: 10.1109/ITT69610.2025.11352935

Assayed, S. K. (Ed.). (2025b). *Enhancing Student Support and Learning Through Conversational AI.* IGI Global. DOI: 10.4018/979-8-3373-3316-8

Assayed, S. K., Shieh, C. S., & Gupta, S. K. (2025). Engineering intelligent healthcare systems: Understanding medical queries with AI and NLP. *Journal of Engineering and Applied Sciences (Asian Research Publishing Network)*, *72*(1), 212. DOI: 10.1186/s44147-025-00800-y

Babapour, A. R., Gahassab-Mozaffari, N., & Fathnezhad-Kazemi, A. (2022). Nurses' job stress and its impact on quality of life and caring behaviors: A cross-sectional study. *BMC Nursing*, *21*(1), 75. DOI: 10.1186/s12912-022-00852-y

Bakker, C. J., Wyatt, T. H., Breth, M. C., Gao, G., Janeway, L. M., Lee, M. A., Martin, C. L., & Tiase, V. L. (2023). Nurses' roles in mHealth app development: Scoping review. *JMIR Nursing*, *6*, e46058. DOI: 10.2196/46058

Bednorz, A., Mak, J. K., Jylhävä, J., & Religa, D. (2023). Use of electronic medical records (EMR) in gerontology: Benefits, considerations and a promising future. *Clinical Interventions in Aging*, *18*, 2171–2183. DOI: 10.2147/CIA.S400887

Botrugno, C. (2019). Information technologies in healthcare: Enhancing or dehumanising doctor–patient interaction? *Health*, *25*(4), 475–493. DOI: 10.1177/1363459319891213

Bragazzi, N. L., & Garbarino, S. (2024). Toward Clinical Generative AI: Conceptual framework. *JMIR AI*, *3*, e55957. DOI: 10.2196/55957

Braun, E. J., Singh, S., Penlesky, A. C., Strong, E. A., Holt, J. M., Fletcher, K. E., Stadler, M. E., Nattinger, A. B., & Crotty, B. H. (2022). Nursing implications of an early warning system implemented to reduce adverse events: A qualitative study. *BMJ Quality & Safety*, *31*(10), 716–724. DOI: 10.1136/bmjqs-2021-014498

Chandrakar, M. (2024). Telehealth and digital tools enhancing healthcare access in rural systems. *Discover Public Health*, *21*(1), 144. DOI: 10.1186/s12982-024-00271-1

Chen, A., Liu, L., & Zhu, T. (2024). Advancing the democratization of generative artificial intelligence in healthcare: A narrative review. *Journal of Hospital Management and Health Policy*, *8*, 8. DOI: 10.21037/jhmhp-24-54

Cho, A., Min, I. K., Hong, S., Chung, H. S., Lee, H. S., & Kim, J. H. (2022). Effect of applying a real-time medical record input assistance system with voice artificial intelligence on triage task performance in the emergency department: Prospective interventional study. *JMIR Medical Informatics*, *10*(8), e39892. DOI: 10.2196/39892

Ergin, E., Karaarslan, D., Şahan, S., & Çınar Yücel, Ş. (2022). Artificial intelligence and robot nurses: from nurse managers' perspective: a descriptive cross-sectional study. *Journal of Nursing Management*, *30*(8), 3853–3862. DOI: 10.1111/jonm.13646

Galanis, P., Moisoglou, I., Katsiroumpa, A., Vraka, I., Siskou, O., Konstantakopoulou, O., Meimeti, E., & Kaitelidou, D. (2023). Increased Job Burnout and Reduced Job Satisfaction for Nurses Compared to Other Healthcare Workers after the COVID-19 Pandemic. *Nursing Reports*, *13*(3), 1090–1100. DOI: 10.3390/nursrep13030095

Genovese, A., Borna, S., Gomez-Cabello, C. A., Haider, S. A., Prabha, S., Forte, A. J., & Veenstra, B. R. (2024). Artificial intelligence in clinical settings: A systematic review of its role in language translation and interpretation. *Annals of Translational Medicine*, *12*(6), 117. DOI: 10.21037/atm-24-162

Gerlach, M., Renggli, F. J., Bieri, J. S., Sariyar, M., & Golz, C. (2025). Exploring nurse perspectives on AI-based shift scheduling for fairness, transparency, and work-life balance. *BMC Nursing*, *24*(1), 1161. DOI: 10.1186/s12912-025-03808-0

Göktepe, N., & Sarıköse, S. (2025). Perspectives and Experiences of Nurse Managers on the Impact of Artificial Intelligence on Nursing Work Environments and Managerial Processes: A Qualitative Study. *International Nursing Review*, *72*(2), e70043. DOI: 10.1111/inr.70043

Gopal, G., Suter-Crazzolara, C., Toldo, L., & Eberhardt, W. (2019). Digital transformation in healthcare–architectures of present and future information technologies. [CCLM]. *Clinical Chemistry and Laboratory Medicine*, *57*(3), 328–335. DOI: 10.1515/cclm-2018-0658

Gosmar, D., & Dahl, D. A. Hallucination mitigation using agentic ai natural language-based frameworks (2025). *arXiv preprint arXiv:2501.13946*. https://doi.org//arXiv.2501.13946DOI: 10.48550

Hameed, K., Naha, R., & Hameed, F. (2024). Digital transformation for sustainable health and well-being: A review and future research directions. *Discover Sustainability*, *5*(1), 104. DOI: 10.1007/s43621-024-00273-8

Haviana, E., Putriani, N. D., Novika, P. W., Pujadi, A., & Asfo, N. S. (2025). The Effect of Company Policy on Employee Compliance with the Implementation of AI to Maintain Company Data Security. [IJHESS]. *International Journal of Health, Economics, and Social Sciences*, *7*(1), 468–473.

Howcroft, A., Bennett-Weston, A., Khan, A., Griffiths, J., Gay, S., & Howick, J. (2025). AI chatbots versus human healthcare professionals: A systematic review and meta-analysis of empathy in patient care. *British Medical Bulletin*, *156*(1), ldaf017. Advance online publication. DOI: 10.1093/bmb/ldaf017

Karunanayake, N. (2025). Next-generation agentic AI for transforming healthcare. *Informatics and Health*, *2*(2), 73–83. DOI: 10.1016/j.infoh.2025.03.001

Knevel, R., & Liao, K. P. (2023). From real-world electronic health record data to real-world results using artificial intelligence. *Annals of the Rheumatic Diseases*, *82*(3), 306–311. DOI: 10.1136/ard-2022-222626

Kothinti, R. R.Rishi Reddy Kothinti. (2024). Deep learning in healthcare: Transforming disease diagnosis, personalized treatment, and clinical decision-making through AI-driven innovations. *World Journal of Advanced Research and Reviews*, *24*(2), 2841–2856. DOI: 10.30574/wjarr.2024.24.2.3435

Matlhaba, K. (2024). Telehealth and Remote Monitoring. In *Enhancing Clinical Competence of Graduate Nurses*. Springer., DOI: 10.1007/978-3-031-81407-5_13

Montejo, L., Fenton, A., & Davis, G. (2024). Artificial intelligence (AI) applications in healthcare and considerations for nursing education. *Nurse Education in Practice*, *80*, 104158. DOI: 10.1016/j.nepr.2024.104158

Moran, S., Bailey, M. E., & Doody, O. (2024). Role and contribution of the nurse in caring for patients with palliative care needs: A scoping review. *PLoS One*, *19*(8), e0307188. DOI: 10.1371/journal.pone.0307188

Nasir, S., Khan, R. A., & Bai, S. (2024). Ethical framework for harnessing the power of AI in healthcare and beyond. *IEEE Access : Practical Innovations, Open Solutions, 12*, 31014–31035. DOI: 10.1109/ACCESS.2024.3369912

Norful, A. A., Brewer, K. C., Cahir, K. M., & Dierkes, A. M. (2024). Individual and organizational factors influencing well-being and burnout amongst healthcare assistants: A systematic review. *International Journal of Nursing Studies Advances, 6*, 100187. DOI: 10.1016/j.ijnsa.2024.100187

Oyeniran, C. O., Adewusi, A. O., Adeleke, A. G., Akwawa, L. A., & Azubuko, C. F.Oyekunle Claudius OyeniranAdebunmi Okechukwu AdewusiAdams Gbolahan AdelekeLucy Anthony AkwawaChidimma Francisca Azubuko. (2022). Ethical AI: Addressing bias in machine learning models and software applications. *Computer Science & IT Research Journal, 3*(3), 115–126. DOI: 10.51594/csitrj.v3i3.1559

Oyewole, A. T., Adeoye, O. B., Addy, W. A., Okoye, C. C., Ofodile, O. C., & Ugochukwu, C. E.Adedoyin Tolulope OyewoleOmotayo Bukola AdeoyeWilhelmina Afua AddyChinwe Chinazo OkoyeOnyeka Chrisanctus OfodileChinonye Esther Ugochukwu. (2024). Promoting sustainability in finance with AI: A review of current practices and future potential. *World Journal of Advanced Research and Reviews, 21*(3), 590–607. DOI: 10.30574/wjarr.2024.21.3.0691

Paarima, Y., Kisinna, A. A., & Ofei, A. M. A. (2024). Perceived organizational politics: Implications for nurses' stress and job satisfaction. *International Journal of Africa Nursing Sciences, 20*, 100686. DOI: 10.1016/j.ijans.2024.100686

Pan, W. J., & Wang, S. F. (2025). Understanding patients' emotional needs to strengthen therapeutic relationships: A deep insight into narrative nursing. *World Journal of Psychiatry, 15*(3), 103093. DOI: 10.5498/wjp.v15.i3.103093

Pati, A. K. (2025). *Agentic AI: A Comprehensive Survey of Technologies, Applications, and Societal Implications*. IEEE., DOI: 10.1109/ACCESS.2025.3585609

Perez, A. M. M. M., & Poletti, M. E. (2022). Characterization of digital systems used in medical X-ray imaging. *Radiation Physics and Chemistry, 200*, 110307. DOI: 10.1016/j.radphyschem.2022.110307

Rajput, K., Darzi, A., & Ghafur, S. (2025). Overlooked and under-reported: The impact of cyberattacks on primary care in the UK National Health Service. *The Lancet. Digital Health, 7*(7), 100879. Advance online publication. DOI: 10.1016/j.landig.2025.100879

Ramadan, O. M. E., Alruwaili, M. M., Alruwaili, A. N., Elsehrawy, M. G., & Alanazi, S. (2024). Facilitators and barriers to AI adoption in nursing practice: A qualitative study of registered nurses' perspectives. *BMC Nursing*, *23*(1), 891. DOI: 10.1186/s12912-024-02571-y

Renggli, F. J., Gerlach, M., Bieri, J. S., Golz, C., & Sariyar, M. (2025). Integrating Nurse Preferences Into AI-Based Scheduling Systems: Qualitative Study. *JMIR Formative Research*, *9*(1), e67747. DOI: 10.2196/67747

Ronquillo, Y., Meyers, A., & Korvek, S. J. (2023, May 1). Digital health. In *StatPearls* [Internet]. StatPearls Publishing., Retrieved from https://www.ncbi.nlm.nih.gov/books/NBK470260/

Ronquillo, Y., Meyers, A., & Korvek, S. J. (2023, May 1). Digital health. In *StatPearls* [Internet]. StatPearls Publishing., Retrieved from https://www.ncbi.nlm.nih.gov/books/NBK470260/

Rony, M. K. K., Alrazeeni, D. M., Akter, F., Nesa, L., Das, D. C., Uddin, M. J., & Parvin, M. R. (2024). The role of artificial intelligence in enhancing nurses' work-life balance. *Journal of Medicine, Surgery, and Public Health*, *3*, 100135. DOI: 10.1016/j.glmedi.2024.100135

Scott-Marshall, H. K. (2024). Safe limits on work hours for the nursing profession: A rapid evidence review. *Frontiers in Global Women's Health*, *5*, 1455422. DOI: 10.3389/fgwh.2024.1455422

Seibert, K., Domhoff, D., Bruch, D., Schulte-Althoff, M., Fürstenau, D., Biessmann, F., & Wolf-Ostermann, K. (2021). Application scenarios for artificial intelligence in nursing care: Rapid review. *Journal of Medical Internet Research*, *23*(11), e26522. DOI: 10.2196/26522

Šekrst, K. (2025). Hallucinations. In *The Illusion Engine: The Quest for Machine Consciousness*. Springer., DOI: 10.1007/978-3-032-05562-0_12

Shoghli, A., Darvish, M., & Sadeghian, Y. (2024). Balancing innovation and privacy: Ethical challenges in AI-driven healthcare. *Journal of Research in Medical Sciences : the Official Journal of Isfahan University of Medical Sciences*, *4*(1), 1–11.

Van der Laak, J., Litjens, G., & Ciompi, F. (2021). Deep learning in histopathology: The path to the clinic. *Nature Medicine*, *27*(5), 775–784. DOI: 10.1038/s41591-021-01343-4

World Health Organization. (2021). *Global strategy on digital health 2020–2025*. World Health Organization.

Chapter 2

Generative AI Applications in Nursing Practice and Clinical Decision-Making

P. Selvakumar
http://orcid.org/0000-0002-3650-4548
Department of Science and Humanities, Nehru Institute of Technology, Coimbatore, India

R. Parthiban
http://orcid.org/0000-0002-3002-7648
IFET College of Engineering, India

T. C. Manjunath
http://orcid.org/0000-0003-2545-9160
Rajarajeswari College of Engineering, Bengaluru, India

S. Saradha
http://orcid.org/0009-0007-3572-4649
Thiagarajar College of Engineering, India

Syed Muqthadar Ali
http://orcid.org/0009-0007-0111-4092
CVR College of Engineering, India

K. K. Naresh
http://orcid.org/0009-0001-5795-0045
Padmashree Institute of Management and Sciences, India

ABSTRACT

Generative AI in Clinical Documentation represents one of the most transformative intersections of machine intelligence and healthcare delivery, reconfiguring how clinicians record, interpret, and operationalise patient information in increasingly complex care environments. As global health systems grapple with rising administrative burdens, workforce shortages, and the escalating complexity of multimorbidity, generative AI functions not merely as a digital scribe but as an adaptive, context-aware partner that enhances the cognitive and operational capacity of clinical teams. At its core, generative AI leverages large-scale language models capable of

DOI: 10.4018/979-8-3373-8247-0.ch002

parsing unstructured inputs—such as physician-patient conversations, fragmented notes across disparate electronic health record (EHR) environments, and evolving diagnostic narratives—to produce coherent, accurate, and contextually aligned documentation in real time. This shift from manual charting to dynamic, AI-assisted documentation not only minimises clerical load but also reshapes.

GENERATIVE AI IN CLINICAL DOCUMENTATION

Generative AI in Clinical Documentation represents one of the most transformative intersections of machine intelligence and healthcare delivery, reconfiguring how clinicians record, interpret, and operationalise patient information in increasingly complex care environments. As global health systems grapple with rising administrative burdens, workforce shortages, and the escalating complexity of multimorbidity, generative AI functions not merely as a digital scribe but as an adaptive, context-aware partner that enhances the cognitive and operational capacity of clinical teams. At its core, generative AI leverages large-scale language models capable of parsing unstructured inputs—such as physician-patient conversations, fragmented notes across disparate electronic health record (EHR) environments, and evolving diagnostic narratives—to produce coherent, accurate, and contextually aligned documentation in real time. This shift from manual charting to dynamic, AI-assisted documentation not only minimises clerical load but also reshapes the temporal and relational dynamics of clinical practice, enabling clinicians to redirect attention from screens to patients and thus reinforcing the humanistic core of care. The technology introduces a radical acceleration in documentation workflows by converting natural speech into structured templates, auto-populating assessment and plan fields, and generating differential diagnoses with evidence-linked reasoning. Furthermore, generative AI models trained on domain-specific corpora can capture subtle diagnostic cues—such as symptom clusters, risk factors, medication conflicts, and social determinants—that are frequently overlooked in hurried clinical settings.

This capacity strengthens diagnostic completeness and reduces variations in documentation quality across providers, departments, and shifts. At the system level, AI-generated documentation supports more accurate coding and billing, improved quality-of-care metrics, and enhanced audit readiness by ensuring that narratives are precise, time-stamped, and aligned with evolving regulatory standards. The benefits also extend to patient safety, as automated cross-checking mechanisms alert clinicians to drug allergies, guideline deviations, or potential errors before documentation is finalised. Such adaptability reduces friction with existing clinical routines and promotes higher adoption rates compared with earlier documentation technologies that were rigid, rule-based, or template-driven. As AI handles more routine documentation tasks, clinical training may shift toward higher-order reasoning, interpersonal communication, and ethical decision-making—domains that require human judgment. Looking ahead, the integration of generative AI into clinical documentation foreshadows a more proactive, predictive, and personalised healthcare ecosystem. Future systems may couple documentation with clinical decision-support engines capable of generating individualised care pathways, risk stratification profiles, and real-time recommendations aligned with clinical guidelines. Documentation may evolve into an interactive interface where clinicians can query patient narratives, visualise disease trajectories, or simulate treatment scenarios using conversational AI. The boundary between documentation and analytics will blur, as patient notes become structured inputs for population health monitoring, predictive modelling, and precision-medicine initiatives. As interoperability matures, AI-generated documentation will facilitate seamless data exchange across hospitals, insurers, pharmacies, and public-health agencies, strengthening longitudinal care continuity. At the same time, maintaining public trust will require transparent communication about how AI influences documentation, who retains control over clinical narratives, and how patient data is protected. Ultimately, generative AI in clinical documentation is not merely a technological upgrade but a systemic re-architecture of the informational backbone of healthcare. Its success will depend on collaborative governance among clinicians, technologists, ethicists, policymakers, and patients—ensuring that the future of documentation is not only efficient and intelligent but also equitable, trustworthy, and aligned with the fundamental ethos of medicine.

AI-DRIVEN CLINICAL DECISION SUPPORT SYSTEMS

AI-Driven Clinical Decision Support Systems (CDSS) represent a profound evolution in the architecture of modern healthcare, functioning as intelligent augmentation layers that enhance the precision, timeliness, and consistency of clinical decision-making across diverse care settings. Unlike traditional rule-based CDSS systems that largely rely on static guidelines, manually curated decision trees, and deterministic logic, AI-driven CDSS leverage machine learning, deep neural networks, natural language processing, and reinforcement learning to interpret complex, multimodal clinical data with unprecedented depth and nuance. These systems integrate structured information—such as laboratory values, physiological signals, medical histories, diagnostic codes, and medication lists—with unstructured inputs like clinician notes, radiology narratives, pathology reports, bedside observations, and even sensor-generated data from wearables or remote-monitoring devices (Elhaddad & Hamam, 2024). By fusing these heterogeneous streams, AI-enabled CDSS can generate probabilistic risk assessments, differential diagnoses, treatment plan suggestions, early-warning alerts, and personalised prognostic curves that reflect the dynamic reality of patient conditions rather than static snapshots captured during clinical encounters. A core advantage of AI-driven CDSS is their capacity to detect subtle patterns, nonlinear relationships, and temporal dynamics that exceed human cognitive limits, thereby supporting earlier identification of deteriorating conditions such as sepsis, cardiac arrhythmias, respiratory failure, and decompensating chronic disease. In acute care environments, these systems can continuously monitor vital signs, laboratory changes, and clinical events to trigger real-time alerts that support rapid response teams, reduce avoidable delays, and prevent escalation into critical states.

In chronic care, AI-driven CDSS facilitate precision-medicine interventions by stratifying patients according to long-term risk trajectories, behavioural patterns, environmental exposures, and genetic predispositions. The expansion of AI-driven CDSS also strengthens clinical workflows by embedding evidence-based recommendations directly into electronic health record (EHR) systems, enabling clinicians to access guideline-aligned insights at the point of care without interrupting patient interactions. These decision-support layers can automate routine cognitive tasks—such as medication reconciliation, dose adjustments, and radiologic triage—while assisting in more complex judgments like choosing optimal diagnostic pathways, evaluating therapy effectiveness, and identifying potential drug-drug interactions or contraindications (Comito C., et al, 2022). Natural language processing enriches these capabilities by extracting clinically relevant information from free-text notes, translating patient narratives into structured risk indicators, and synthesising information into concise, actionable summaries. AI-driven CDSS thus reframes the clinical decision process as an interactive, context-aware collaboration in which the system's recomputed suggestions evolve as new data points enter the patient's profile. The role of explainable AI becomes critical here, as transparent reasoning pathways—whether via feature-importance visualisation, model confidence intervals, counterfactual explanations, or narrative justifications—enable clinicians to validate AI outputs, understand causal drivers of recommendations, and integrate system insights into their professional judgment. This transparency also supports interdisciplinary communication, allowing specialists, generalists, pharmacists, nurses, and care coordinators to operate from a common informational foundation enriched by AI-translated signals.

The broader impact of AI-driven CDSS extends into organisational culture and health-system transformation. Hospitals adopting advanced AI systems often witness shifts in clinical roles, workforce skill requirements, and quality-assurance protocols. Medical education will increasingly incorporate AI literacy, emphasising competencies such as data interpretation, ethical reasoning, algorithmic oversight, and collaborative decision-making between clinicians and machine systems.

Health-system leadership must cultivate environments where AI introduction is paired with robust change-management initiatives, clear communication about system capabilities and limitations, and training programs that empower clinicians rather than intimidate them (Mohammed & Neravetla, 2024). At the same time, AI-driven CDSS can reduce systemic inefficiencies by standardising care pathways, decreasing diagnostic variability, enhancing coding accuracy, and contributing to better resource allocation through predictive demand modelling. For public health agencies, aggregated outputs from CDSS can inform epidemiological surveillance, early detection of outbreaks, and population-level risk assessments, provided that privacy and ethical constraints are rigorously upheld.

Looking to the future, AI-driven CDSS will likely evolve into proactive, omnipresent digital companions embedded throughout the care continuum. With the rise of multimodal models that integrate genomics, imaging, clinical notes, sensor streams, and environmental data, decision-support systems will gain the capacity to produce holistic, temporally dynamic patient representations that mirror real-world biological complexity. These systems may anticipate complications before they surface clinically, recommend preventive interventions, and even coordinate with automated care pathways or robotic systems to execute routine tasks (Ouanes & Farhah, 2024). As interoperability across health information exchanges improves, AI-driven CDSS could connect ambulatory, inpatient, home-care, and community settings into a seamless guidance ecosystem. Such a future demands careful stewardship to ensure that innovation does not compromise autonomy, equity, or the clinician-patient relationship. Ultimately, the emergence of AI-driven clinical decision support systems signals not merely a technological innovation but a paradigm shift in how medical knowledge is produced, operationalized, and democratized across healthcare systems—an evolution that holds the promise of more precise, responsive, ethical, and human-centered care if guided by thoughtful governance and sustained collaboration among clinicians, technologists, policymakers, and patients.

PERSONALISED CARE PLANS VIA GENERATIVE MODELS

Personalised Care Plans via Generative Models mark a transformative advance in the evolution of precision medicine, enabling healthcare systems to move from generalised, protocol-driven treatment strategies toward dynamic, patient-specific guidance that is continuously refined by real-time data, contextual understanding, and predictive intelligence. Generative AI—spanning large language models, generative probabilistic frameworks, variational autoencoders, diffusion models, and multimodal architectures—can synthesise vast, heterogeneous clinical inputs to create care plans that mirror the unique biological, behavioural, environmental, and psychosocial profile of each patient. Unlike traditional care-plan templates, which rely on coarse risk categories or linear guideline algorithms, generative models can create deeply individualized recommendations by integrating structured data such as laboratory trends, diagnosis codes, drug histories, imaging results, and genomic markers with unstructured or semi-structured sources like clinical notes, patient-reported outcomes, wearable-device signals, lifestyle indicators, social determinants of health, and even conversational inputs from telehealth interactions (Baig M M., et al, 2024). This capacity to interpret multidimensional and temporally dynamic data enables generative models to construct care pathways that adapt to evolving patient conditions—anticipating deterioration, adjusting medication regimens, personalising lifestyle guidance, and dynamically updating follow-up intervals based on probabilistic forecasts of symptom trajectories, comorbidity interactions, and treatment responses. Care plans generated in this manner no longer exist as static documents but function as living, learning frameworks that recalibrate as new information emerges, reflecting a paradigm in which medical guidance becomes both predictive and responsive.

The strengths of generative models extend beyond data synthesis to sophisticated personalisation of treatment strategies. By identifying patterns across massive patient populations, these models can suggest interventions most likely to be effective for individuals with similar phenotypic, genomic, or behavioural profiles, essentially enabling N-of-1 medicine at scale. For patients with chronic conditions—such as diabetes, cardiovascular disease, chronic kidney disease, asthma, or mental health disorders—generative models can outline care routines that optimally combine pharmacologic therapy, activity recommendations, nutritional guidance, remote monitoring schedules, early-warning marker thresholds, and behavioural nudges tailored to patient-level adherence patterns and socioeconomic constraints (Jiang F., et al, 2021). Multimodal generative architectures can integrate environmental exposures like pollution levels, climate data, or community-health indicators to refine risk estimates for conditions such as COPD exacerbations or asthma flare-ups. In oncology, generative models can support highly individualised treatment blueprints by synthesising tumour genomics, response biomarkers, radiomics signatures, immune profiling, prior therapy effects, and toxicity risk to outline chemotherapy regimens, immunotherapy strategies, dosing sequences, or trial-matching opportunities specifically aligned with each patient's biology. For surgical care, personalised plans may include prehabilitation pathways, predicted complication risks, anaesthesia optimisation, individualised postoperative monitoring schedules, and adaptive rehabilitation programs based on predicted recovery trajectories. In mental health, generative AI can help clinicians create integrated care plans that combine therapy modalities, relapse-prevention frameworks, psychoeducation, and digitally delivered behavioural interventions tailored to each person's psychological patterns, stress triggers, sleep cycles, and social support networks.

Within healthcare operations, generative models enhance care coordination by producing unified, cross-specialty plans that reconcile overlapping guidelines, reduce redundant testing, and identify conflicting medications or therapy recommendations across multi-provider networks. This is critical for patients with multimorbidity, where managing interactions between multiple care pathways can otherwise lead to fragmented, contradictory, or unsafe guidance. Generative AI can harmonise cardiology, endocrinology, psychiatry, and primary care recommendations into a single coherent plan, aligning all interventions with the patient's overarching health goals and risk profile. These integrated plans can also adapt to logistic barriers such as transportation limitations, financial constraints, pharmacy access, or caregiver availability—factors often overlooked in traditional care-plan development. By incorporating community-resource data, insurance coverage parameters, and social-service availability, generative models can propose realistic, actionable, and equitable care solutions that address structural barriers to adherence (Esteva A., et al, 2021). Bias poses another critical concern, as generative models trained on historically skewed datasets may unknowingly generate care plans that favor well-represented populations while underperforming for underserved groups. Bias could manifest in inappropriate risk scoring, unequal treatment recommendations, under-recognition of atypical symptoms, or reduced accuracy for marginalized communities. Ensuring fairness requires intentional dataset diversification, bias-detection metrics, harm-minimization protocols, and participatory design processes that incorporate perspectives from diverse patient populations.

Trust in generative AI will depend on explainability—clear articulation of why a care plan was recommended, which data points influenced decisions, and how the model weighed alternatives. Explainable AI techniques—such as feature attributions, causal reasoning summaries, counterfactual explorations, chain-of-thought rationales, and confidence intervals—must be embedded within the interface so clinicians can interrogate and understand outputs in a transparent, medically coherent manner (Sugapriya S., et al, 2026). Looking forward, the frontier of generative personalization points toward adaptive, lifelong care plans that evolve across the entire patient journey—from pre-disease prevention and early diagnosis to acute treatment, rehabilitation, chronic management, and end-of-life care. With advances in multimodal generative AI, care plans may integrate genomic individuality, microbiome signatures, proteomics, metabolomics, environmental exposures, psychosocial context, and digital phenotyping, offering genuinely holistic precision care. Models may forecast disease onset years before clinical symptoms emerge, recommend personalized preventive regimens, and simulate organ-level responses to treatment. As federated learning and privacy-preserving AI mature, personalized care models could benefit from population-level insights without compromising patient confidentiality. At scale, these innovations hold the potential to reduce health disparities, empower patients with more agency, improve chronic-disease outcomes, and create a healthcare system that is not only intelligent but deeply humane—one that sees each patient not as an average category but as a complex, dynamic individual whose care must be as unique as their lived experience.

PREDICTIVE ANALYTICS FOR EARLY DETERIORATION

Predictive analytics for early patient deterioration represents one of the most clinically transformative applications of artificial intelligence (AI) in contemporary healthcare, offering the potential to shift care delivery from reactive crisis management to proactive prevention. At its core, early-deterioration prediction leverages a spectrum of data—electronic health records (EHRs), vital signs, laboratory results, radiology findings, medication histories, streaming physiological signals, and increasingly patient-generated data—to detect subtle patterns that precede adverse events such as sepsis, cardiac arrest, respiratory failure, or unplanned ICU transfer (Uike D., et al, 2026). Traditional early warning systems, often based on threshold-based scoring rules such as MEWS, NEWS, or qSOFA, have provided partial support for clinicians but suffer from low sensitivity, inability to capture nonlinear physiological trajectories, and high false-alarm burdens that contribute to alert fatigue. In contrast, AI-driven predictive analytics can learn complex temporal signatures of instability, continuously update individualized risk profiles, and trigger early escalations of care that materially improve patient outcomes. As health systems worldwide grapple with rising acuity, staff shortages, and systemic pressure on emergency and critical care services, the ability to identify deterioration hours before overt clinical signs emerge is rapidly becoming a strategic imperative for ensuring safety, efficiency, and sustainability in care delivery.

Central to these predictive systems is the integration of machine learning models—ranging from tree-based ensembles and gradient boosting machines to recurrent neural networks, transformers, and multimodal architectures—that can synthesize high-dimensional clinical data. Time-series modelling, particularly through Long Short-Term Memory (LSTM) networks, Temporal Convolutional Networks (TCNs), and attention-based models, enables the capture of dynamic physiological changes that occur over minutes or hours (Mishra A., et al, 2025). These models are frequently trained on millions of patient encounters and billions of data points, allowing them to uncover prognostic indicators that humans cannot reliably perceive, such as micro-variability in heart rate, latent ventilation–perfusion mismatches, or early coagulation abnormalities. Increasingly, predictive deterioration systems incorporate multimodal inputs, fusing structured data with free-text clinical notes, imaging features, audio from patient assessments, and even genomic or biomarker signals. Natural language processing (NLP) models extract contextual cues from clinical narratives—such as expressions of clinician concern, subtle notations of altered mentation, or changes in functional status—that serve as early indicators of instability. Together, these innovations result in prediction models that are highly sensitive, adaptable, and capable of delivering continuous risk estimates rather than episodic assessments.

A pivotal strength of early-deterioration prediction is its capacity to support tiered escalation pathways. Instead of triggering broad emergency responses, risk scores can initiate graduated interventions such as increased monitoring frequency, rapid review by a critical-care outreach team, point-of-care diagnostics, or pre-emptive therapeutic adjustments. In many hospitals implementing such systems, deterioration alerts have been used to power automated care bundles—for example, early sepsis bundles that activate lactate testing, broad-spectrum antibiotics, and fluid resuscitation within a structured timeframe. Similarly, predictive analytics are increasingly integrated into remote monitoring programs, enabling hospital-at-home initiatives and chronic-care management programs to detect decompensation early and prevent emergency visits (Sullivan & Keim-Malpass, 2021). These capabilities are particularly valuable in resource-constrained settings, where limited critical-care capacity necessitates precise triage and early intervention to avoid preventable morbidity. Another major dimension of implementation involves the question of accountability. When predictive systems issue alerts that clinicians subsequently follow—or ignore—questions arise regarding liability, responsibility, and standards of care. Health organizations increasingly adopt "human-AI teaming" frameworks, positioning predictive analytics as decision-support rather than decision-making tools. Still, the growing reliance on algorithmic foresight raises the need for explicit protocols, legal clarity, and well-designed documentation structures that record how risk scores influenced clinical judgments. Simultaneously, there is a push for adaptive learning systems that continuously update based on new data, though real-time model updates pose regulatory challenges because of the need to maintain validation integrity. In response, many institutions adopt controlled update cycles, versioning strategies, and sandboxed testing environments before releasing model improvements into clinical workflows. Looking ahead, the future of early-deterioration prediction lies in the development of continuously learning, context-aware, and personalized systems (Ruiz V M., et al, 2022). Integration with digital twins—computational representations of patients that simulate physiological processes—may soon allow models not only to detect risk but also to test hypothetical interventions. Advances in edge computing and medical IoT will enable continuous analysis of streaming data from wearable sensors, smart hospital rooms, and implantable devices. Large multimodal models promise to unify data streams that were once siloed, while federated learning will allow institutions to collaborate on model improvement without sharing sensitive patient data. As healthcare systems advance toward vision-driven smart hospitals, predictive analytics will become a foundational layer that supports intelligent resource allocation, dynamic staffing, automated monitoring, and seamless integration between inpatient and outpatient care.

AI-ASSISTED TRIAGE IN EMERGENCY NURSING

AI-assisted triage in emergency nursing represents a transformative evolution in how frontline clinicians assess, prioritize, and manage patient care in high-pressure, resource-constrained environments. Emergency departments (EDs) worldwide face chronic challenges: overcrowding, prolonged wait times, rising patient acuity, staffing shortages, and escalating documentation burdens. Traditional triage models—often built around standardized scoring systems such as the Emergency Severity Index (ESI), the Canadian Triage and Acuity Scale (CTAS), and the Manchester Triage System (MTS)—have improved consistency but still rely heavily on subjective judgment, manual data interpretation, and episodic assessment. Artificial intelligence (AI), by contrast, introduces continuous, data-driven, and context-aware decision support capable of improving both accuracy and speed (Mann K D., et al, 2021). By analyzing vital signs, clinical histories, presenting symptoms, environmental factors, and increasingly patient-generated data, AI-driven triage tools help emergency nurses detect subtle signs of deterioration, predict risk trajectories, and allocate resources with unprecedented precision. Within minutes of patient arrival—sometimes even before physical arrival through pre-hospital data streams—AI systems can estimate disease severity, flag red-flag symptoms, and forecast the likelihood of critical events such as sepsis, stroke, myocardial infarction, and respiratory failure. As EDs struggle to balance safety, efficiency, and equity, AI-assisted triage is emerging as a cornerstone of modern emergency nursing practice, promising to improve patient flow, enhance clinical outcomes, and reduce cognitive burden on frontline staff. Importantly, AI-assisted triage does not replace the clinical expertise of emergency nurses; rather, it augments their ability to make informed, timely decisions under pressure. Emergency nursing practice is shaped by rapid situational awareness, holistic assessment, empathetic communication, and nuanced clinical reasoning—competencies that cannot be fully automated. However, AI enhances this practice by surfacing early warning signals that might be imperceptible to humans and by providing structured risk explanations that support evidence-based decision-making. For example, an AI model might indicate that a patient with seemingly mild symptoms is at elevated risk of sepsis based on subtle vital-sign variability combined with recent antibiotic exposure and immunocompromised status.

Figure 1. Generative AI applications in nursing practice

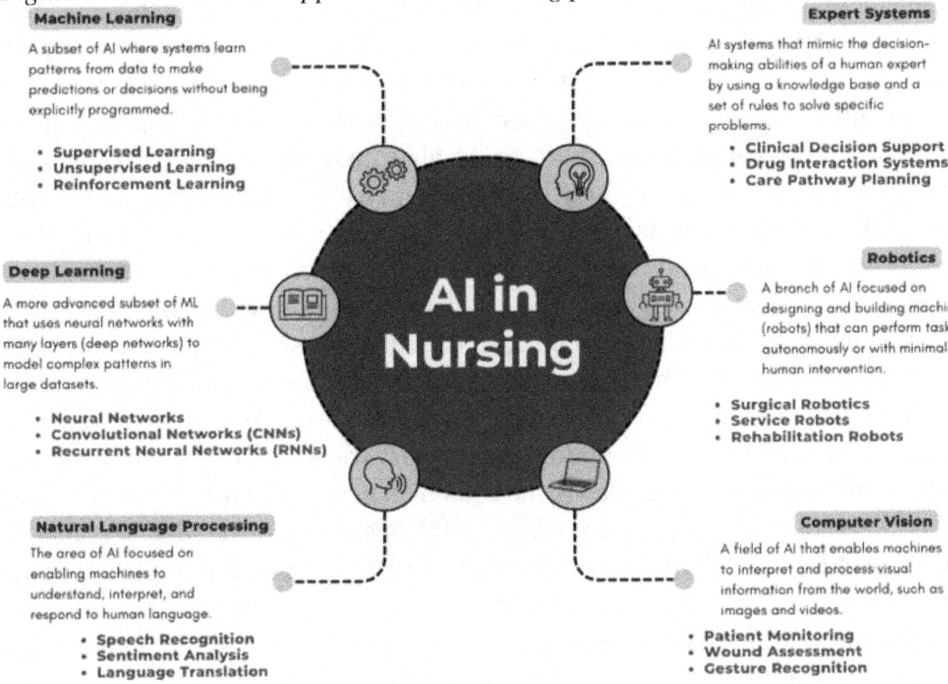

Nurses can use this signal to escalate care quickly, initiate sepsis protocols earlier, or request physician evaluation without delay. This synergy between human judgment and machine-driven insight exemplifies the emerging paradigm of "intelligence-supported nursing," where technology strengthens rather than replaces the clinician's role (Martinez V A., et al, 2022). However, implementing AI-assisted triage requires careful attention to sociotechnical factors, ethical principles, and clinical governance structures. Data quality remains a major challenge: incomplete documentation, missing vitals, inconsistent symptom descriptions, and noisy sensor readings can degrade model performance. Biases within training datasets—or within the healthcare system itself—may result in inaccurate prioritization for marginalized populations, including racial minorities, older adults, and individuals with atypical disease presentations. For example, if training data reflect historical underestimation of pain in certain groups, AI models may replicate those inequities. Additionally, differences in language, communication style, or cultural expression of symptoms may affect NLP-based triage tools. These concerns necessitate continuous auditing, bias-mitigation strategies, and inclusive dataset design. Regulatory frameworks are evolving to address these issues, emphasizing transparency, fairness, explainability, and accountable human oversight. Clinically, AI-based triage decisions must always remain advisory: ultimate responsibility lies with licensed nurses and physicians who contextualize algorithmic outputs within real-world patient presentations.

Another emerging dimension of AI-assisted triage is its use in prehospital and community settings. Ambulance teams equipped with AI-enhanced decision-support tools can perform early risk stratification en route to hospitals, transmitting live assessments to ED teams and enabling coordinated response planning. Wearables and home-monitoring devices linked to AI algorithms can detect early signs of acute deterioration among high-risk populations, enabling remote triage and early intervention before emergency conditions escalate. Tele-triage systems, enhanced by AI-driven symptom checkers and NLP-based conversational agents, enable nurses to safely manage patient inquiries, direct patients to appropriate levels of care, and reduce unnecessary ED visits (Fatai A., et al, 2025). These innovations extend the triage ecosystem beyond hospital walls and support more distributed, preventive models of acute-care delivery. The evaluation of AI-assisted triage systems requires rigorous methodology, ideally through multicenter trials, real-world observational studies, and continuous post-deployment monitoring. Performance metrics must extend beyond accuracy and AUC scores to include operational outcomes such as wait-time reduction, left-without-being-seen (LWBS) rates, resource utilisation patterns, and nurse satisfaction. Patient-centered outcomes—trust, perceived fairness, transparency, and cultural acceptability—are equally important. Hospitals must also monitor unintended consequences, such as over-reliance on algorithms, deskilling of clinical judgment, or new forms of cognitive burden created by frequent alerts or complex explanations. Feedback from frontline nurses is critical for iterative refinement, as they are the primary users and stewards of triage processes (Pawar P., et al, 2026). In essence, AI-assisted triage in emergency nursing represents not only a technological breakthrough but also a paradigm shift in how acute care is delivered, organized, and experienced. By fusing machine intelligence with human clinical expertise, AI transforms triage from a snapshot assessment into a dynamic, data-rich, continuously adaptive process. Its promise lies in a future where emergency departments are safer, more efficient, more equitable, and more resilient—where nurses spend less time battling documentation and operational bottlenecks and more time delivering high-quality, compassionate care. The path forward requires thoughtful design, ethical governance, and unwavering commitment to human-centred implementation, but the potential benefits are profound: earlier recognition of critical illness, more rational resource allocation, and ultimately, better outcomes for patients at their most vulnerable moments.

GENERATIVE AI FOR MEDICAL IMAGING INTERPRETATION

Generative artificial intelligence (AI) is rapidly redefining the landscape of medical imaging interpretation, reshaping diagnostic workflows, augmenting clinical decision-making, and expanding the capacity of health systems to detect, characterise, and monitor disease across diverse modalities. The field of radiology has long relied on the expert visual reasoning of radiologists who interpret complex patterns in X-rays, CT scans, MRI studies, ultrasound images, nuclear medicine scans, and pathology slides. While conventional machine-learning tools have supported imaging for years—through segmentation algorithms, CAD (computer-aided detection) systems, and pattern-recognition models—generative AI introduces an entirely new paradigm: models capable not only of analyzing existing images but also of producing new synthetic images, filling missing information, enhancing degraded scans, simulating disease progression, and generating pixel-level explanations (Selvakumar P., et al, 2026). Techniques such as generative adversarial networks (GANs), variational autoencoders (VAEs), diffusion models, and multimodal transformers enable the synthesis of highly realistic medical images with fine-grained anatomical precision. These capabilities have profound implications: from augmenting training datasets and reducing annotation burden to enabling more accurate diagnostic support in low-resource settings. As imaging volumes grow exponentially and radiology departments struggle with workforce shortages, generative AI is emerging as a critical tool to ensure timely, reliable, and high-quality imaging interpretation. Generative AI also enhances diagnostic image quality, enabling clearer visualization of anatomical structures and pathologic features. Traditional reconstruction methods in CT and MRI often involve trade-offs between scan time, radiation dose, contrast resolution, and image clarity.

Generative approaches can mitigate these limitations by reconstructing high-quality images from low-dose or accelerated scans. For example, diffusion and GAN-based super-resolution models can transform sparse or noisy MRI acquisitions into detailed images, reducing scan time for patients while preserving diagnostic accuracy. In CT imaging, generative denoising techniques allow clinicians to maintain low radiation exposure without compromising clarity (Abualruz H., et al, 2025). In ultrasound—which is highly operator-dependent—generative AI can stabilise image quality, interpolate missing data, and enhance boundary resolution. These improvements reduce diagnostic ambiguity, facilitate earlier disease detection, and support more confident clinical decision-making. For resource-limited or rural settings where high-end imaging equipment may not be available, generative enhancement models can dramatically improve the interpretability of scans produced by older or portable devices. Generative AI is also redefining report generation and radiology workflows. Modern vision-language models (VLMs), which integrate deep image encoders with large language models, can interpret imaging findings and produce coherent, structured radiology reports. These systems understand spatial relationships, recognise clinically relevant abnormalities, and translate visual insights into narrative descriptions aligned with reporting standards such as BI-RADS, PI-RADS, LI-RADS, and standardised lung nodule guidelines. Generative report systems can pre-populate impressions, highlight critical findings, and even compare current images with prior studies to track disease progression or treatment response. Radiologists maintain full oversight—verifying, editing, and approving the AI-generated content—but the automation significantly reduces dictation time and cognitive burden. In high-volume departments, where radiologists interpret hundreds of scans daily, generative report assistance improves consistency, reduces errors, and enables faster turnaround times.

Workflow integration remains a critical factor in the successful adoption of generative AI. For radiologists and imaging technologists, seamless EHR integration, PACS compatibility, and intuitive user interfaces are essential to prevent workflow fragmentation. Generative models must work unobtrusively in the background, providing image enhancement, risk scoring, and report drafting without disrupting existing diagnostic processes. Equally important is transparency; clinicians must be able to understand why a model produced a certain reconstruction, enhancement, or diagnostic suggestion. Explainable AI (XAI) techniques—such as attention maps, diffusion trajectory explanations, latent-space visualizations, and feature attribution—provide interpretability, allowing radiologists to critically evaluate AI outputs rather than blindly trusting automated results (Araouchi & Adda, 2025). Trust is paramount, especially in high-stakes scenarios such as detecting intracranial hemorrhage, diagnosing pulmonary embolism, or identifying malignant lesions. Moreover, generative AI may alter the professional identity and workflow of radiologists. While AI can reduce workload, eliminate repetitive tasks, and improve diagnostic consistency, concerns about over-automation or deskilling must be addressed. Radiology education must evolve to include computational imaging, generative model interpretation, AI ethics, and human-machine collaboration. Instead of replacing radiologists, generative AI will redefine the discipline—focusing human expertise on complex reasoning, ambiguous cases, interventional procedures, multidisciplinary discussions, and patient communication. This augmented-intelligence paradigm positions radiologists as supervisors of automated systems, ensuring that clinical judgment remains central. In essence, generative AI for medical imaging interpretation represents a profound evolution in how clinicians visualize disease, understand anatomy, and plan treatment (Rao V M., et al, 2025). By synthesizing, enhancing, interpreting, and predicting imaging data, generative AI amplifies human diagnostic capabilities while addressing structural challenges such as workforce shortages, variable image quality, and limited data availability. Its potential reaches far beyond incremental improvement: it promises a future where imaging is more equitable, more precise, more personalized, and more deeply integrated into the continuum of care. The path forward requires responsible development, rigorous validation, thoughtful regulation, and human-centered implementation—but the clinical and societal benefits are substantial. Generative AI stands not as a replacement for radiologists but as a transformative partner, augmenting expert interpretation and helping build a more efficient, intelligent, and patient-centered imaging ecosystem.

AI-POWERED REMOTE PATIENT MONITORING

AI-powered remote patient monitoring (RPM) represents one of the most transformative evolutions in modern healthcare, fundamentally reshaping how clinicians track health trajectories, anticipate clinical deterioration, and deliver proactive, patient-centred care beyond the boundaries of hospitals and clinics. At its core, AI-enabled RPM integrates wearable sensors, home-based diagnostic devices, ambient monitoring systems, and cloud-connected platforms that continuously collect physiological, behavioural, and contextual data from patients in real-world environments. These datasets—comprising heart rate variability, respiratory patterns, blood glucose fluctuations, sleep metrics, mobility trends, arrhythmia signatures, oxygen saturation, blood pressure patterns, and even subtle indicators such as voice changes or gait irregularities—are processed by machine learning models capable of extracting hidden patterns that human clinicians may not immediately recognise. The fundamental shift is from reactive care, where clinicians intervene only after symptoms worsen, to predictive and preventive care models where AI identifies deterioration hours, days, or even weeks earlier (Lee J O., et al, 2025). This paradigm has profound implications for chronic disease management, post-operative recovery, maternal health monitoring, geriatric care, and mental health support, enabling patients to receive continuous oversight without the burden of frequent hospital visits while giving clinicians unprecedented visibility into health dynamics that unfold outside clinical settings.

These micro-signals, once processed, can predict fluid overload or impending decompensation before symptomatic shortness of breath emerges. Similarly, in diabetes management, continuous glucose monitors paired with AI systems can forecast hyperglycemia or hypoglycemia events hours, enabling timely lifestyle adjustments or insulin titration. For patients with COPD, AI can detect worsening respiratory function through cough acoustics, inhaler usage patterns, and environmental exposures recorded via IoT-based air quality sensors. Such proactive alerts support early interventions, reduce emergency admissions, and improve long-term disease control by aligning treatment decisions with real-time physiological insights rather than lagging clinical assessments. AI-powered RPM also facilitates greater personalisation of care, tailoring interventions to each patient's unique behaviours, preferences, and daily routines. By integrating lifestyle data—from diet, activity levels, sleep quality, stress indices, and medication habits—with clinical metrics, AI systems create holistic digital health profiles that offer a deeper understanding of what drives each patient's health outcomes (Lang O., et al, 2024). In cardiac rehabilitation, for example, AI can monitor adherence to exercise regimens, identify periods of physiological strain, and adjust recommended intensity levels dynamically. In maternal health monitoring, AI can detect patterns in fetal heart rate, maternal blood pressure, and activity levels to flag early signs of hypertensive disorders or fetal distress. Mental health RPM systems use passive smartphone sensors and speech analytics to identify early signs of depression relapse, suicidal ideation, or mania based on changes in voice tone, movement, sleep rhythm, and social interaction patterns. AI-driven insights not only enhance medical outcomes but also improve patient engagement by delivering personalised nudges, educational prompts, or behaviour change recommendations aligned with the patient's health goals, literacy level, and readiness for change.

A significant contributor to the success of AI-powered RPM is its seamless integration with electronic health records (EHRs), clinical workflows, and decision support systems. When RPM data flows directly into clinician dashboards, AI can generate automated documentation, highlight trends, and correlate remote data with hospital-based diagnostics. Clinicians gain consolidated views of vital sign trajectories, symptom evolution, medication adherence, and algorithm-generated risk scores. Automated synthesis of remote data reduces cognitive load while ensuring that important clinical signals do not get buried in voluminous datasets (Huang J., et al, 2023). AI tools can suggest care plan modifications, recommend diagnostic tests, or flag medication adjustments, all while maintaining clinician oversight and accountability. In multidisciplinary care teams, integrated RPM data ensures synchronised decision-making between physicians, nurses, pharmacists, and care coordinators, fostering more cohesive and informed care delivery. Over time, the accumulation of RPM datasets also strengthens AI models, enabling continuous learning that refines prediction accuracy and clinical relevance. Looking ahead, the future of AI-powered remote patient monitoring promises an even deeper integration of real-time analytics, robotics, genomics, and precision medicine. Next-generation wearables will feature multimodal sensors capable of capturing biochemical markers, microfluidics-based diagnostics, continuous blood pressure measurements without cuffs, and non-invasive glucose monitoring.

AI models will increasingly incorporate genetic, proteomic, and microbiome data to create highly individualized health forecasts. Advances in edge computing will enable real-time AI inference directly on wearable devices, reducing latency and enhancing privacy by minimizing cloud transmission (Kaur H., et al, 2025). Voice-based monitoring systems may detect respiratory instability or cognitive decline via ambient microphones embedded in smart home ecosystems. Companion AI chatbots—integrated with RPM platforms—will offer personalised guidance, emotional support, and automated health coaching, further augmenting the continuity of care. Ultimately, AI-powered remote patient monitoring is poised to redefine healthcare as a distributed, anticipatory, and deeply personalised system where clinicians intervene not at the moment of crisis but at the earliest signs of deviation from wellness. By merging technology with compassionate, evidence-based clinical practice, AI-RPM strengthens the bridge between home and hospital, empowering individuals to live healthier lives while enabling health systems to deliver safer, smarter, and more sustainable care at scale.

SMART MEDICATION MANAGEMENT AND SAFETY CHECKS

Smart medication management and safety checks represent a pivotal transformation in contemporary healthcare, fundamentally redefining how medications are prescribed, dispensed, administered, and monitored across clinical and home-care environments. This transformation is driven by the convergence of digital health technologies, artificial intelligence (AI), Internet of Medical Things (IoMT) devices, automated dispensing systems, and advanced clinical decision support tools that collectively streamline medication workflows and significantly reduce preventable drug-related harm. Medication errors—ranging from incorrect dosages and omissions to harmful drug interactions and timing misalignments—remain one of the most persistent sources of patient morbidity and healthcare expenditure worldwide. Smart medication management seeks to address these challenges by introducing a multilayered, automated, and intelligence-enhanced ecosystem that ensures the right medication reaches the right patient at the right time and in the right dose (Islam M M., et al, 2023). Through this system, clinicians benefit from improved accuracy and efficiency, patients experience greater adherence and reduced adverse events, and healthcare institutions gain more dependable mechanisms for regulatory compliance, audit readiness, and quality assurance. As global populations age, chronic disease burdens rise, and polypharmacy becomes increasingly common, such smart systems form a cornerstone of safe, scalable, and sustainable medication management practices. At the foundation of smart medication management is AI-enhanced prescribing, wherein algorithms analyse clinical histories, laboratory values, genomic profiles, allergies, comorbidities, and medication lists to optimise drug selection and dosing. Unlike traditional prescribing, which depends heavily on clinician experience and memory, AI-supported prescribing systems offer real-time alerts for potential contraindications, drug–drug interactions, duplications, and renal- or hepatic-based dose adjustments.

Natural language processing (NLP) tools further assist clinicians by interpreting free-text notes, extracting relevant clinical details, and cross-checking them with medication protocols. These systems also incorporate evidence-based guidelines, formulary restrictions, and antimicrobial stewardship policies, ensuring adherence to best practices. Once medications reach the administration phase, smarter systems continue to uphold safety through automated protocols, AI-supported reminders, and sensor-driven error prevention mechanisms (Alwashmi M F., et al, 2021). Smart infusion pumps equipped with dose-error reduction systems (DERS) cross-check programmed dosages against clinical guidelines and institutional drug libraries, preventing common errors in rate, concentration, or unit entry. These pumps also integrate with EHRs to automatically document infusion start and stop times, eliminating manual charting inconsistencies and improving medication reconciliation accuracy. Wearable adherence devices—such as ingestible sensors, connected blister packs, and AI-enabled inhaler monitors—further enhance medication safety outside the hospital by ensuring patients follow prescribed regimens correctly. For chronic diseases like asthma, congestive heart failure, HIV, hypertension, or diabetes, small deviations in adherence can have significant clinical consequences; smart reminders, personalised dosing suggestions, and automated refill alerts improve treatment continuity and health outcomes. Ambient monitoring systems embedded in smart homes can detect patterns such as missed doses, unusual timing irregularities, or repeated access to PRN medications, alerting caregivers when deviations might signal cognitive decline, worsening symptoms, or adverse drug reactions.

Smart medication management also plays a crucial role in reducing the cognitive burden on healthcare providers, who face increasing workloads, documentation requirements, and patient complexity. AI-powered clinical decision support tools consolidate fragmented medication information, highlight safety-critical data, and automate repetitive tasks such as dose calculations, allergy checks, medication reconciliation, and chart review. In nursing workflows, these systems reduce the time spent double-checking orders, searching for missing medications, or resolving documentation discrepancies. Automated safety checks eliminate the need for manual verification of drug concentrations, pump settings, or infusion compatibility, freeing clinicians to focus on patient assessment and therapeutic engagement (Tsvetanov F., 2024). Moreover, when incorporated into interprofessional team structures, smart medication systems enhance communication among pharmacists, nurses, and physicians by synchronising medication lists, annotating alerts with meaningful explanations, and reducing misinterpretations stemming from illegible handwriting or incomplete orders. Ultimately, the harmonisation of medication data across the care continuum strengthens clinical efficiency, improves patient safety, and supports a culture of shared accountability. Looking toward the future, advances in AI, robotics, biosensing, and precision therapeutics promise to deepen the impact of smart medication management. Next-generation smart pill technologies may contain micro-sensors capable of capturing gastrointestinal pH, temperature, or motility, offering real-time pharmacokinetic insights.

Pharmacogenomic integration will become more routine, enabling dynamic dose adjustments and personalised therapeutic predictions embedded directly into e-prescribing platforms. Robotic dispensing units will grow more autonomous, capable of on-site sterile compounding, customised pill packaging, and 24/7 patient-facing medication pickup (Bates D W., et al, 2022). Augmented reality (AR) overlays may guide clinicians through medication preparation steps, reducing errors in complex compounding tasks. Ambient intelligence systems—powered by multi-modal sensors, AI cameras, and contextual reasoning engines—will continuously assess patient status and medication adherence in ways that blend seamlessly into everyday home environments. Meanwhile, healthcare organisations will gain powerful dashboards that visualise medication safety metrics, adherence patterns, and risk profiles at the population level, enabling performance improvement initiatives grounded in real-time, data-driven insights. Ultimately, smart medication management and safety checks embody a holistic, intelligent, and continuously learning ecosystem that enhances patient safety, empowers clinicians, optimises therapeutic outcomes, and bridges the gap between clinical science and everyday life. Through the combined strengths of automation, analytics, and empathetic clinical oversight, it stands poised to advance medication safety into a new era defined by precision, reliability, and human-centred innovation.

NATURAL LANGUAGE PROCESSING FOR EHR OPTIMIZATION

Natural Language Processing (NLP) has emerged as one of the most transformative technologies in modern healthcare informatics, particularly in its ability to optimise electronic health records (EHRs) by converting complex, unstructured clinical narratives into structured, interoperable, and actionable data. The rapid digitalisation of healthcare systems, propelled by EHR mandates, value-based care models, and data-driven clinical decision-making, has resulted in unprecedented documentation burdens for clinicians. Much of this burden stems from the sheer volume of unstructured text—progress notes, nursing assessments, operative reports, radiology impressions, discharge summaries, patient messages, and multidisciplinary care plans—that typically lacks standardisation, consistency, or ease of retrievability. NLP technologies address these challenges by enabling systems to "read," interpret, and meaningfully reorganise clinical text, thereby improving the overall efficiency, accuracy, and usability of EHRs across clinical, administrative, and research contexts (Márquez Fosser S., et al, 2021). By leveraging techniques such as named-entity recognition, syntactic parsing, semantic role labelling, topic modelling, sentiment analysis, and transformer-based contextual embeddings, NLP enhances data capture, reduces documentation time, supports clinical decision-making, and enables secondary use of data. These capabilities directly contribute to reducing clinician burnout, improving patient safety, and advancing the quality of care delivered within complex health ecosystems.

A second major dimension of NLP-driven EHR optimisation involves reducing cognitive load and documentation time for clinicians. Over the past decade, providers have increasingly reported feelings of documentation fatigue due to rigid EHR templates, excessive data entry requirements, and redundancy in clinical workflows. NLP mitigates these burdens through ambient listening tools, dictation-to-structure systems, automated summarisation engines, and intelligent note-generation features integrated directly into the EHR interface. For instance, advanced NLP models can transcribe clinician-patient conversations in real time, identify clinically relevant concepts, and insert them into the appropriate sections of the visit note—history of present illness, review of systems, physical examination findings, assessment, and plan—while allowing clinicians to validate and edit the content before finalising it (Peddisetti V., et al, 2024). This functionality reduces after-hours charting ("pyjama time"), enhances real-time documentation accuracy, and allows clinicians to maintain rapport and eye contact with patients rather than focusing on keyboards and screens. Beyond dictation and transcription, NLP-enabled summarisation tools can generate concise handoff briefs, discharge instructions, and progress-note synopses, eliminating repetitive work and ensuring consistency across care teams. Automated detection of redundant or irrelevant text also contributes to cleaner, more readable notes.

Beyond day-to-day clinical operations, NLP plays a vital role in accelerating medical research by enabling secondary use of EHR data. Traditional research workflows depend on manually curated datasets, which are time-consuming to build and often limited in scope. NLP techniques can quickly extract research-relevant variables from millions of clinical notes, enabling large-scale retrospective studies, real-world evidence generation, and clinical-trial matching. For example, NLP can identify phenotype characteristics for genomic studies, detect rare adverse events from speciality department notes, or classify patient subgroups based on disease progression patterns (Negro-Calduch E., et al, 2021). By reducing the time researchers spend extracting variables and cleaning data, NLP accelerates hypothesis development, cohort identification, and statistical analysis. Moreover, NLP enables automated de-identification of clinical text to protect patient privacy while allowing datasets to be shared ethically for research collaborations. These capabilities position NLP as a cornerstone technology for modern clinical data science and population-health analytics. Looking ahead, the future of NLP-driven EHR optimisation is poised to become more advanced, contextualised, and proactive as generative AI models grow in sophistication. Large language models (LLMs) fine-tuned on clinical corpora are increasingly capable of producing coherent, clinically accurate summaries, generating patient-friendly explanations, and engaging in interactive documentation dialogues with clinicians. These models will enable EHR interfaces that feel more conversational, intuitive, and intelligent, drastically reducing manual documentation while improving narrative richness and clinical fidelity. Multimodal integration of NLP with imaging, biosensor data, and genomic profiles will create holistic patient representations that support precision-medicine applications (Ashburner J M., et al, 2022). Additionally, ongoing advances in explainability and uncertainty quantification will enhance clinicians' trust in NLP-derived recommendations. As healthcare systems evolve toward integrated, learning-health frameworks, NLP will serve as a foundational infrastructure that continuously extracts insights, improves care delivery, and supports real-time learning from clinical practice. When thoughtfully designed, ethically governed, and responsibly deployed, NLP has the power to transform EHRs from static documentation platforms into dynamic, intelligent systems that elevate clinical practice, amplify human expertise, and strengthen the patient-provider relationship.

REAL-TIME CLINICAL ALERTING WITH GENERATIVE MODELS

Real-time clinical alerting with generative models represents a significant advancement in modern healthcare informatics, leveraging the capabilities of generative artificial intelligence (AI) to provide proactive, context-aware, and adaptive decision support at the point of care. Traditional clinical alerting systems—such as early warning scores, rule-based notifications, or threshold-based triggers—have historically suffered from limitations including alert fatigue, limited contextual awareness, rigid logic, and delayed response times. In contrast, generative models possess the capacity to synthesise heterogeneous clinical data streams, interpret complex temporal patterns, and generate alerts that are not only timely but also nuanced, personalised, and actionable (Thatoi P., et al, 2023). By integrating electronic health records (EHRs), continuous monitoring devices, laboratory data, imaging findings, and patient-reported inputs, generative models can anticipate adverse events, detect early signs of physiological deterioration, and recommend specific interventions tailored to the individual patient's clinical trajectory. This approach transforms clinical alerting from a reactive, static process into a dynamic, predictive, and intelligence-enhanced system that enhances patient safety, optimises clinician workflows, and supports evidence-based interventions. Using probabilistic modelling and sequence prediction, these AI systems can forecast potential deterioration events—such as sepsis, respiratory failure, acute kidney injury, or arrhythmias—minutes to hours before they reach clinically critical thresholds. By generating context-aware alerts that reflect predicted probabilities and potential clinical outcomes, generative models enable proactive interventions that can reduce morbidity, prevent ICU transfers, and improve patient outcomes. Another transformative aspect of generative model-based alerting is its ability to provide actionable recommendations alongside notifications (Lee K., et al, 2024). Alerts that simply flag abnormal values or risk thresholds often leave clinicians uncertain about next steps, contributing to cognitive overload. Generative AI systems, however, can produce interpretive narratives, suggested diagnostic pathways, or treatment options informed by up-to-date clinical guidelines, institutional protocols, and patient-specific parameters. For instance, in a patient showing early signs of sepsis, a generative alert could provide an explanation of the contributing risk factors, recommend immediate laboratory tests, suggest empiric antimicrobial therapy, and prioritise interventions in line with hospital policy. By combining prediction with context-specific action guidance, generative models shift alerting systems from passive notification tools to active clinical partners that enhance situational awareness and decision-making efficiency.

The predictive power of generative models is further amplified by their ability to continuously learn from incoming data. Unlike static rule-based systems, these models can update predictions in near real-time as new vital signs, lab results, medication adjustments, and clinical observations are recorded. Continuous learning allows the model to refine its understanding of patient-specific baselines, detect deviations from expected recovery trajectories, and adjust alert thresholds dynamically. Over time, the system develops personalised predictive profiles for individual patients, improving sensitivity and specificity for adverse event detection (Biswas & Talukdar, 2024). This personalisation is particularly valuable for patients with complex comorbidities, polypharmacy, or atypical physiological responses, where traditional alert systems often underperform due to rigid standardisation. Despite the numerous advantages, the deployment of generative models in real-time clinical alerting presents significant ethical, technical, and operational challenges. Model transparency and explainability are critical to ensure clinician trust and prevent over-reliance on AI-generated alerts. Generative models can occasionally produce plausible yet inaccurate outputs, a phenomenon known as "hallucination," which may compromise patient safety if not properly monitored. Rigorous validation, continuous monitoring, and human-in-the-loop oversight are therefore essential. Bias in training data—such as underrepresentation of certain patient populations—can lead to inequitable alerting performance, necessitating careful dataset curation, fairness auditing, and adaptive learning mechanisms. Furthermore, integration into existing clinical workflows requires careful change management, user training, and usability testing to ensure that alerts enhance rather than hinder clinical efficiency (Vaccari I., et al, 2021). Looking ahead, the evolution of generative models in real-time clinical alerting is likely to incorporate multimodal learning, combining electronic health records, continuous monitoring signals, genomics, imaging, and patient-reported outcomes. This will enable even more precise prediction of adverse events, tailored intervention guidance, and early detection of rare but high-risk clinical scenarios. Advances in federated learning and privacy-preserving AI will facilitate cross-institutional model training without compromising patient confidentiality, expanding the generalizability and robustness of alerting systems. Integration with virtual assistants, augmented reality, and mobile platforms will further streamline alert delivery, ensuring that predictive insights are actionable, timely, and seamlessly embedded into clinical decision-making. As healthcare systems continue to adopt data-driven approaches, real-time clinical alerting with generative models has the potential to transform patient safety, enhance workflow efficiency, and support a proactive, anticipatory model of care that significantly reduces adverse events and improves clinical outcomes.

CONCLUSION

The integration of generative artificial intelligence (AI) into nursing practice and clinical decision-making marks a pivotal transformation in the healthcare landscape—one that redefines not only how care is delivered but also how it is conceptualised, coordinated, and continuously improved. As demonstrated across the domains of clinical documentation, decision support systems, personalised care planning, predictive analytics, and emergency triage, generative AI is no longer a speculative innovation but a tangible force reshaping the informational, operational, and ethical foundations of modern nursing. In parallel, AI-driven Clinical Decision Support Systems (CDSS) offer a profound augmentation of clinical reasoning. These systems transcend the limitations of traditional rule-based models by leveraging deep learning, natural language processing, and multimodal data fusion to generate probabilistic risk assessments, differential diagnoses, and personalised treatment recommendations. Whether in acute care settings—where early detection of sepsis or cardiac arrhythmias can be life-saving—or in chronic disease management, where long-term risk trajectories guide precision interventions, AI-driven CDSS empower clinicians with insights that are both timely and deeply contextual. The emphasis on explainable AI ensures that these systems remain transparent and trustworthy, enabling clinicians to validate recommendations and integrate them into their professional judgment with confidence. Predictive analytics for early deterioration further exemplifies the proactive potential of AI in nursing. By continuously analysing time-series data from EHRs, vital signs, and clinical notes, AI models can detect subtle physiological changes that precede adverse events, enabling timely escalations of care. These systems support tiered intervention strategies, reduce alert fatigue, and enhance resource allocation—critical benefits in overstretched healthcare environments. Moreover, the integration of predictive analytics into remote monitoring and hospital-at-home programs extends the reach of nursing care beyond institutional walls, fostering a more distributed and preventive model of healthcare delivery. Despite these transformative benefits, the deployment of generative AI in nursing practice must be guided by rigorous ethical governance, inclusive design, and collaborative stewardship. Bias in training data, opacity in model reasoning, and disparities in access to AI-enhanced tools pose significant risks to equity and trust. Ensuring fairness requires intentional dataset diversification, harm-minimisation protocols, and participatory design processes that incorporate the voices of diverse patient populations and frontline clinicians. Transparency about how AI influences care decisions, who retains control over clinical narratives, and how patient data is protected will be essential to maintaining public trust. Looking ahead, the convergence of generative AI with emerging technologies such as digital twins, edge computing, federated learning, and multimodal modelling promises to further expand the horizons of nursing practice. Documentation may become an interactive interface for querying patient narratives and simulating treatment scenarios. Decision-support systems may anticipate complications before they surface clinically. Personalised care plans may evolve into lifelong, adaptive frameworks that guide patients from prevention to end-of-life care. Predictive analytics may power intelligent staffing and resource allocation in smart hospitals. Triage systems may extend into community settings, enabling distributed acute-care networks.

REFERENCES

Abualruz, H., Yasin, I., Sabra, M A A., & Abunab, H. Y. (2025). The role of artificial intelligence in enhancing triage decisions in healthcare settings: A systematic review. . *Applied Nursing Research*, *62*, 151576. DOI: 10.1016/j.apnr.2025.152024

Alwashmi, M. F., Hawboldt, J., Davis, E., Marra, C., & Gamble, J. M. (2021). "The use of digital health technologies for remote monitoring in chronic disease management: An overview." Frontiers in Public Health, Volume 9. *Article*, *652456*, 1–10. DOI: 10.3389/fpubh.2021.652456

Araouchi, Z., & Adda, M. (2025). A Comprehensive Literature Review on AI-Assisted Multimodal Triage Systems for Health Centers. . *Procedia Computer Science*, *250*, 311–318. DOI: 10.1016/j.procs.2025.03.029

Ashburner, J. M., Chang, Y., Wang, X., Khurshid, S., Anderson, C. D., Dahal, K., Weisenfeld, D., Cai, T., Liao, K. P., Wagholikar, K. B., Murphy, S. N., Atlas, S. J., Lubitz, S. A., & Singer, D. E. (2022). Natural language processing to improve prediction of incident atrial fibrillation using electronic health records. . *Journal of the American Heart Association*, *11*(15), e023123. DOI: 10.1161/JAHA.122.026014

Baig, M. M., Hobson, C., GholamHosseini, H., Ullah, E., & Afifi, S. (2024). Generative AI in improving personalized patient care plans: Opportunities and barriers towards its wider adoption. . *Applied Sciences (Basel, Switzerland)*, *14*(23), 9876. DOI: 10.3390/app142310899

Bates, D. W., Cheng, H. Y., Cheung, N. T., Jew, R., Mir, F., Tamblyn, R., & Li, Y.-C. (2022). 'Improving smart medication management': An online expert discussion. . *BMJ Health & Care Informatics*, *29*(1), e100345. Advance online publication. DOI: 10.1136/bmjhci-2021-100540

Biswas, A., & Talukdar, W. (2024). "Enhancing Clinical Documentation with Synthetic Data: Leveraging Generative Models for Improved Accuracy." arXiv preprint arXiv:2406.06569. DOI: /arXiv.2406.06569.DOI: 10.48550

Comito, C., Falcone, D., & Forestiero, A. (2022). AI-driven clinical decision support: Enhancing disease diagnosis exploiting patients similarity. . *IEEE Access : Practical Innovations, Open Solutions*, *10*, 123456–123469. DOI: 10.1109/ACCESS.2022.3142100

Elhaddad, M., & Hamam, S. (2024). AI-driven clinical decision support systems: An ongoing pursuit of potential. . *Cureus*, *16*, e12345. DOI: 10.7759/cureus.57728

Esteva, A., Robicquet, A., Ramsundar, B., Kuleshov, V., DePristo, M., Chou, K., Cui, C., Corrado, G., Thrun, S., & Dean, J. (2021). A guide to deep learning in healthcare. *Nature Medicine*, *27*(7), 1129–1145. DOI: 10.1038/s41591-021-01312-x

Fatai, A., Sattayarom, C., Laochai, W., & Faksook, E. (2025). Effectiveness of AI-assisted ESI triage on accuracy and selected outcomes in emergency nursing: A systematic review.. *Journal of Emergency Nursing: JEN*, *51*, 45–54. DOI: 10.1016/j.jen.2024.10.003

Huang, J., Neill, L., Wittbrodt, M., Melnick, D., Klug, M., Thompson, M., Bailitz, J., Loftus, T., Malik, S., Phull, A., Weston, V., Heller, J. A., & Etemadi, M. (2023). Generative artificial intelligence for chest radiograph interpretation in the emergency department. . *JAMA Network Open*, *6*(10), e2312345. DOI: 10.1001/jamanetworkopen.2023.36100

Islam, M. M., Maddison, R., Talukder, A., & Kamal, A. H. M. (2023). "Artificial intelligence in remote patient monitoring: A systematic review." Sensors, Volume 23, Issue 3. *Article*, *1234*, 1–20. DOI: 10.3390/s23031234

Jiang, F., Jiang, Y., Zhi, H., Dong, Y., Li, H., Ma, S., Wang, Y., Dong, Q., Shen, H., & Wang, Y. (2021). Artificial intelligence in healthcare: Past, present and future. *Stroke and Vascular Neurology*, *6*(3), 230–243. DOI: 10.1136/svn-2020-000101

Kaur, H., Selvakumar, P., Haashni, S., Anute, N., Sharma, M., & Manjunath, T. C. (2025). Representations in developing thinking regarding probabilities in higher education. In Anastasiadou, S., & Seremeti, L. (Eds.), *Modes of representation in developing statistical thinking in education* (pp. 89–118). IGI Global Scientific Publishing. , DOI: 10.4018/979-8-3693-9934-7.ch006

Lang, O., Yaya-Stupp, D., Traynis, I., & Cole-Lewis, H. (2024). Using generative AI to investigate medical imagery models and datasets.. *The Lancet. Digital Health*, *6*, e354–e366. DOI: 10.1016/S2589-7500(24)00017-9

Lee, J. O., Zhou, H. Y., Berzin, T. M., Sodickson, D. K., & Rajpurkar, P. (2025). Multimodal generative AI for interpreting 3D medical images and videos. . *NPJ Digital Medicine*, *8*(1), 45–57. DOI: 10.1038/s41746-025-01649-4

Lee, K., Liu, Z., Mai, Y., Jun, T., Ma, M., Wang, T., Ai, L., Calay, E., Oh, W., Stolovitzky, G., Schadt, E., & Wang, X. (2024). Optimizing clinical trial eligibility design using natural language processing models and real-world data: Algorithm development and validation. . *JMIR AI*, *5*, e34567. DOI: 10.2196/50800

Mann, K. D., Good, N. M., Fatehi, F., Khanna, S., Campbell, V., Conway, R., Sullivan, C., Staib, A., Joyce, C., & Cook, D. (2021). Predicting patient deterioration: A review of tools in the digital hospital setting. . *Journal of Medical Internet Research, 23*(9), e23456. DOI: 10.2196/28209

Márquez Fosser, S., Mahmoud, N., Habib, B., & Weir, D. L. (2021). Smart about medications (SAM): A digital solution to enhance medication management following hospital discharge. . *Journal of the American Medical Informatics Association : JAMIA, 28*, 2105–2112. DOI: 10.1093/jamia/ocab095

Martinez, V. A., Betts, R. K., Scruth, E. A., Buckley, J. D., Cadiz, V. R., Bertrand, L. D., Paulson, S. S., Dummett, B. A., Abhyankar, S. S., Reyes, V. M., Hatton, J. R., Sulit, R., & Liu, V. X. (2022). The Kaiser Permanente Northern California Advance Alert Monitor Program: An automated early warning system for adults at risk for in-hospital clinical deterioration. . *Joint Commission Journal on Quality and Patient Safety, 48*(8), 61–69. DOI: 10.1016/j.jcjq.2022.05.005

Mishra, A., Majumder, A., Kommineni, D., & Joseph, C. A. (2025). Role of generative artificial intelligence in personalized medicine: A systematic review. . *Cureus, 17*, e14567. DOI: 10.7759/cureus.82310

Mohammed, A. S., & Neravetla, A. R. (2024). "Understanding the impact of AI-driven clinical decision support systems." *15th IEEE International Conference on Healthcare Informatics*, pages 456-462. DOI: .DOI: 10.1109/ICCCNT61001.2024.10726136

Negro-Calduch, E., Azzopardi-Muscat, N., Krishnamurthy, R. S., & Novillo-Ortiz, D. (2021). Technological progress in electronic health record system optimization: Systematic review of systematic literature reviews. . *International Journal of Medical Informatics, 151*, 104467. DOI: 10.1016/j.ijmedinf.2021.104507

Ouanes, K., & Farhah, N. (2024). Effectiveness of artificial intelligence (AI) in clinical decision support systems and care delivery. . *Journal of Medical Systems, 48*(1), 56. Advance online publication. DOI: 10.1007/s10916-024-02098-4

Pawar, P., Anute, N., Tripathi, S., Ahluwalia, G. K., & Kalshetti, P. (2026). AI and its importance in the development of luxury consumption. In Vale, V. (Ed.), *Multidisciplinary approach to luxury consumption and AI* (pp. 1–34). IGI Global Scientific Publishing. , DOI: 10.4018/979-8-3693-8422-0.ch001

Peddisetti, V., Kandregula, P. K., & John, J. A. (2024). Smart medication management: Enhancing medication adherence with an IoT-based pill dispenser and smart cup. . *IEEE Journal of Biomedical and Health Informatics, 28*, 2950–2958. DOI: 10.1109/JBHI.2024.3456789

Rao, V. M., Hla, M., Moor, M., Adithan, S., Kwak, S., Topol, E. J., & Rajpurkar, P. (2025). Multimodal generative AI for medical image interpretation. . *Nature*, *610*(8056), 62–70. DOI: 10.1038/s41586-025-08675-y

Ruiz, V. M., Goldsmith, M. P., Shi, L., Simpao, A. F., Gálvez, J. A., Naim, M. Y., Nadkarni, V., Gaynor, J. W., & Tsui, F. R. (2022). Early prediction of clinical deterioration using data-driven machine-learning modeling of electronic health records. . *The Journal of Thoracic and Cardiovascular Surgery*, *164*(1), 1083–1091. DOI: 10.1016/j.jtcvs.2021.10.060

Selvakumar, P., & Haashni, S. SudhaAnanthi G, Manjunath T C, (2026). "Cybernetic systems thinking: Foundations for organizational adaptability." In L. Tsvasman (Ed.), Cybernetic leadership for sustainable innovation, IGI Global Scientific Publishing, 99-124. DOI: .DOI: 10.4018/979-8-3373-2484-5.ch004

Sugapriya, S., Garg, S., Mahalle, A., Yewale, A. U., & Manjunath, T. C. (2026). Medical imaging and radiology: AI-powered diagnostics. In Ather, D., Mun, N., Jain, S., Jain, V., & Kukreja, V. (Eds.), *Applied AI and computational intelligence in diagnostics and decision-making* (pp. 191–218). IGI Global Scientific Publishing. , DOI: 10.4018/979-8-3373-3311-3.ch008

Sullivan, B. A., & Keim-Malpass, J. (2021). BARRIERS to early detection of deterioration in hospitalized infants using predictive analytics. . *Hospital Pediatrics*, *11*(9), 897–903. DOI: 10.1542/hpeds.2020-004382

Thatoi, P., Choudhary, R., & Shiwlani, A. (2023). Natural language processing (NLP) in the extraction of clinical information from electronic health records (EHRs) for cancer prognosis. . *International Journal of Medical Informatics*, *169*, 104957. DOI: 10.1016/j.ijmedinf.2022.104957

Tsvetanov, F. (2024). "Integrating AI technologies into remote monitoring patient systems." Engineering Proceedings, Volume 45, pages not available. DOI: .DOI: 10.3390/engproc2024070054

Uike, D., Sugapriya, S., Kaur, M., Mahalle, A., Dhule, N., & Manjunath, T. C. (2026). Drug discovery and optimization with AI. In Ather, D., Mun, N., Jain, S., Jain, V., & Kukreja, V. (Eds.), *Applied AI and computational intelligence in diagnostics and decision-making* (pp. 379–404). IGI Global Scientific Publishing. , DOI: 10.4018/979-8-3373-3311-3.ch014

Vaccari, I., Orani, V., Paglialonga, A., Cambiaso, E., & Giusto, D. D. (2021). A generative adversarial network (GAN) technique for internet of medical things data. . *Sensors (Basel)*, *21*(11), 3456. DOI: 10.3390/s21113726

Chapter 3
Generative AI for Clinical Communication, Healthcare Worker Wellbeing, and Patient Care

Muaath I. Alsufi
http://orcid.org/0009-0005-8564-7034
University of Jordan, Jordan

Sana Alsayed
http://orcid.org/0009-0002-1419-219X
Philadelphia University, Jordan

Muthafar Alsufi
University of Jordan, Jordan

Fares A. Qtaishat
University of Jordan, Jordan

ABSTRACT

Communication failures between physicians and nurses are considered as one of the main contributors to to preventable patient harm, often resulting in delayed interventions and compromised care. While Electronic Health Records (EHRs) aim to improve data accessibility, they currently demand excessive time and cognitive resources, leading to clinician fatigue and reduced patient interaction. This chapter explores the capabilities of Generative AI (GenAI) in natural language

DOI: 10.4018/979-8-3373-8247-0.ch003

processing and speech recognition to enhance clinical collaboration. We examine GenAI applications in real-time note generation, standardized handovers, and care plans to prevent ambiguity. Furthermore, this chapter proposes a human-supervised clinical documentation model emphasizing safety, transparency, and ethical use. By reducing administrative burdens, GenAI functions as a collaborative partner that enables professionals to prioritize patient care, representing a vital evolution in team-based healthcare

1. INTRODUCTION

Communication failures between physicians and nurses are considered as one of the main contributors to preventable patient harm and serious safety events in hospitals and clinical centers, which usually resulting in medical misinterpretations, delayed interventions, as well as compromised care (Umberfield et al., 2019; Watson & Wu, 2023). Despite the advancements in electronic health records (EHRs), clinical documentation still requires excessive time and cognitive resources, which complicates and reduces the opportunities for patient care (Gaffney et al., 2022a). The emerging capabilities of generative artificial intelligence in natural language processing (NLP), speech & voice recognition, and related text generation present great potential for enhancing collaboration and improving the reliability of clinical and medical cooperation.

The relationship between nurses and physicians is essential in terms of diagnosis, treatment, monitoring, and escalation of care. However, the complexity of the healthcare environment can make the communication subject to error. However, research has shown that both doctors and nurses demonstrating the positive attitudes toward their collaboration, which is essential for preserving the safety and quality in patient care (Gregoriou et al., 2025). Electronic health records were intended to update documentation as well as to improve data accessibility. Moreover, EHRs have been associated with clinician and medical fatigue and dissatisfaction, as healthcare workers spend significant time interacting with screens rather than patients and other healthcare staff. (Gaffney et al., 2022b; Gesner et al., 2022). Communication's failures in healthcare are frequently caused by documentation gaps, such as missing setting, unclear wording, and information overload (Orenstein et al., 2019).

Therefore, this chapter explores the role of generative AI as a communication tool across physician–nurse teams, by examining the applications in real-time note generation, standardized handovers, care plans, preventing ambiguity, and supporting shared clinical reasoning. By exploring current research, we propose a human-supervised clinical documentation AI model that emphasises safety, transparency, and ethical use. While AI cannot replace professional judgment, it can function as a collaboration partner by reducing the administrative burden, enhancing care, and enabling physicians to spend more time with patients. In doing so, generative AI represents the next evolution in team-based healthcare.

2. GENERATIVE AI IN CLINICAL NOTE TAKING AND DOCUMENTATION

Real Time Speech to Clinical Notes

The clinical documentation plays an essential role for patient safety, legal accountability, as well as for professional communication. Nevertheless, that it has become one of the primary causes of inefficiency in this era of healthcare (Alobayli et al., 2023; Olakotan et al., 2025) and the Electronic Health Records were intended to centralize data and modernise clinical documentation away from physical note-taking. Instead, they considerably increased the administrative burden on healthcare providers which leads that clinicians spending more time on entering data with less caring for patients. Interestingly, research highlights that EHR workload as a significantly linked to the clinician burnout, with documentation tasks frequently spilling over into personal time (Alobayli et al., 2023). Furthermore, the traditional manual entry is largely retrospective, relying on memory recall after the clinical encounter has ended, which increases the susceptibility to omission errors and loss of critical information. Consequently, there is a significant need to transition from labor-intensive manual entry to automated documentation solutions that return the focus to the patient interaction.

Furthermore, Large language models (LLMs) are capable of transforming physician and patient speech into standardized clinical documentation have demonstrated improvements in accuracy and time savings. Recent literature shows that nurses spend up to 35% of shift time documenting care, AI assisted tools can reduce redundancy and improve clarity during handoffs. Specifically, AI-models can convert bedside conversation into formatted admission notes and discharge summaries. These systems can also analyse reported symptoms and medical history to generate a differential diagnosis. Finally, such AI tools are capable of identifying missing or inconsistent data throughout a patients notes such as in allergies and incorrect doses to prompt clinicians to correct critical information. (Lee et al., 2024; Perkins et al., 2024; Watson et al., 2025.).

Reducing Ambiguity and Standardizing Clinical Language

Effective professional collaboration in the healthcare system relies heavily on the precision of shared clinical language. however, semantic variability remains a barrier to safe patient care. Although physicians and nurses treat the same patients, their documentation often reflects their distinct training and terminologies, this creates potential misunderstanding in medical records. Clinical documents are characterized by frequent use of abbreviations and simplifications of complex medical terms, for example, the abbreviation of "MS" in the EHR indicates that Multiple Sclerosis, a serious autoimmune neurological condition, or it could refer as well to the Mitral Stenosis, a valvular heart disease requiring an entirely different management approach. In other contexts, "MS" may indicate Morphine Sulfate, a high-risk medication where misinterpretation could result in dosing errors, respiratory depression, or regulatory noncompliance. It is also frequently used to denote the Mental Status, particularly in emergency or inpatient notes, or Musculoskeletal when describing the physical examination findings. These lack of the standardization is particularly hazardous during transitions of care, where subjective descriptions, treatments, and tests can be misinterpreted or overlooked by the receiving team. Research indicates that documentation discrepancies are frequent causes of adverse safety events and preventable harm (Tariq & Sharma, 2025).

Besides of that, AI tools have the potential to serve as the suitable solution to any ambiguity or variability in language, AI tools can detect the use of abbreviations in unclear contexts and prompt lengthened explanations where necessary. Additionally, such tools can detect vague phrases such as ("continue as before", "mobile with assistance") and suggest precise alternatives ("Moves 10 m with assistance using a walker") (Sung et al., 2024). Ambiguity is a known risk factor in drug dose errors and post-operative care failures. Physicians and nurses often use different terms to describe similar findings (e.g. "altered consciousness" vs. "confused and disoriented"), LLM models trained on professional terminology could translate any vague words into standardised words without altering the text's original meaning (Stallinga et al., 2015).

Structured Handover Summaries

Indeed, the clinical handovers the transfer of professional responsibility for some or all aspects of care for a patient to another healthcare professional, including both physicians and nurses, are one of the most high-stakes moments in a patient's treatment process. However, they are often where communication errors occur (Eggins & Slade, 2015). Even with the help of EHRs, trying to condense days of labs, vitals, and nursing notes into a quick update is a massive mental task that is prone to human error. When important details about a patient's progress are omitted, the incoming team loses vital input, leading to delayed treatments and safety risks. Therfore, this way can automate the way of sharing the information as a crucial step in making hospital transitions safer for all to be involved (Assayed, 2025; Delardes et al., 2020; Tataei et al., 2023).

However, tools using such as the generative AI can automatically generate handover summaries using standardized frameworks (SBAR, IPASS, SOAP). Though, studies show that standardized handovers reduce preventable ICU complications and readmissions (Genes et al., 2025). Indeed, leveraging such Large Language Models can instantly synthesize the EHR data into these structured formats, since AI relieves the heavy cognitive burden on clinicians particularly. Furthermore, recent literature indicates that LLM-generated drafts can match or exceed the quality of physician-written notes in terms of conciseness and coherence, are significantly reducing the time required for documentation (Van Veen et al., 2024). Such systems allow clinicians to focus on verifying critical details rather than manual gathering, thereby ensuring a more complete and unbiased transfer of information.

According to Bhuyan et al. (2025) Generative AI can enhance the following:

- Highlight trends (vitals, labs, fluid balance)
- Prioritize risk alerts (delirium risk, aspiration, fall risk)
- Generate summaries for specific clinicians (e.g., “brief for surgeon,” “brief for night nurse”)

Figure 1. Overview of Generative AI-Enhanced Clinical Handover Process

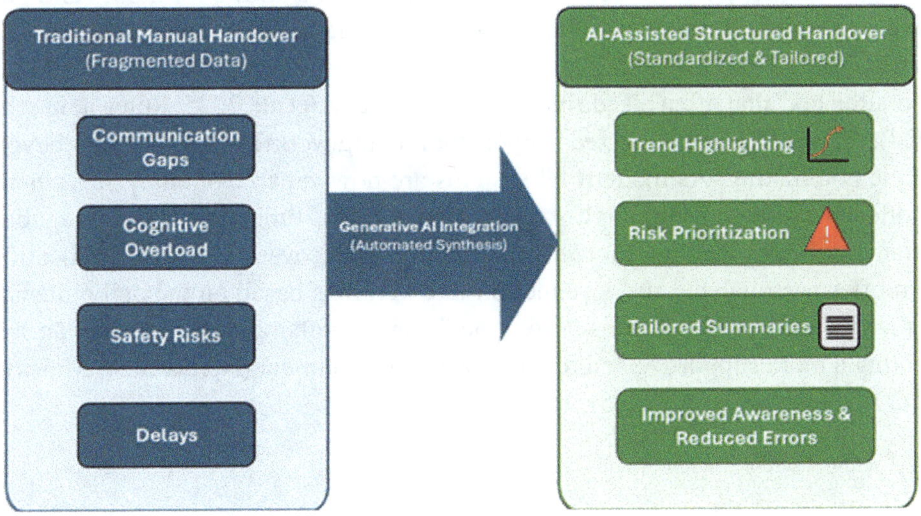

AI as a Second Listener

On the other hand, during the medical clinical round in hospitals, the GenAI can be used as well to transcribe the decisions into simple language for patient communication. Since, possible outputs can include the following, clinical plan summaries, task lists for nursing care plans, as well as automated handover notes. Such systems can reduce the risk of lost verbal orders or misremembered conversations. Furthermore, GenAI can utilise different modalities such as laboratory results, imaging data, and patient histories, combining them into coherent summaries (Bienefeld et al., 2024).

Interestingly, that beyond just taking notes, this model acts as a vital safety net during the critical environment of clinical rounds. In these moments, multi-professional teams often make rapid decisions, and verbal orders can easily be missed or misheard in the noise of a busy hospital. GenAI can continuously monitor and double check these interactions, flagging when a medication change or a new lab request hasn't been logged in the system. However, taking the role as a neutral observer, the AI ensures that the physician and nurse records are perfectly aligned, and that no crucial information is lost during a busy shift (Topaz et al., 2025; Tu et al., 2025).

3. BENEFITS TO STAFF WELLBEING, PATIENT CARE, AND HEALTHCARE WORKFLOW

One of the most main benefits of generative AI (GenAI) is the potential to combat the epidemic of burnout currently that affect the medical and nursing professions. The implementation of ambient AI could scribe and lead to a decrease in clinician exhaustion and therefore a boost in performance.. This allows for nurses and physicians to finish their documentation before leaving the hospital. Restoring such personal time is vital for long-term career sustainability and reducing the "documentation tax" that often bleeds into family life (Lukac et al., 2025; Rotenstein et al., 2024). AI can offer a specialized support for nursing workflows which goes beyond simple note-taking. As modern AI systems are now capable of analyzing nursing workloads and identifying high-stress patterns in real-time, helping charge nurses manage staffing schedules more effectively to prevent overload. Some applications even offer personalized stress-reduction interventions based on the daily intensity of the shift. As providing this "safety net" for the nursing team, the AI can help creating a more supportive and resilient work environment (Nematollahi Maleki et al., 2025; Renggli et al., 2025).

Patient Care

AI models and algorithms can translate the difficult medical technical words into plain language in real-time, with ensuring patients actually understand their diagnoses as well as treatment plans before they leave the hospital. This improved communication can directly correlate with higher patient satisfaction and better adherence to medication schedules, as patients feel like active, informed participants in their own care rather than passive recipients. Besides of that, some studies show that patients feel more "heard" when AI is used, and clinicians report a renewed sense of purpose. By acting as a digital partner for routine tasks, AI allows healthcare workers to return to the human-focused care they were trained to provide. (Almotairi et al., 2024; Olson et al., 2025). Besides of that a conversational AI (Assayed et al., 2025) can work as an assistant to patients if they need any further information or to repeat any medical advices to them.

Improved Patient Safety

In fact, the patient safety and wellbeing is one of the main pillars of healthcare, yet medical errors remain as a leading cause of morbidity and mortality globally. As the communication failures as well as information mismanagement are one of the primary causes of these adverse events. In a complex medical environment, where care involves multidisciplinary teams, the accuracy of the clinical record serves as the primary source of patient information ensuring continuity of care. When documentation is incomplete, delayed, or inaccurate, patient safety is at stake. Consequently, the integration of AI into documentation practices is a critical patient safety intervention designed to ensure that the right information reaches the right clinician at the right time (Alder, 2026; Hosseinzadegan et al., 2025).

Moreover, depending on such systems with technology alone cannot correct safety flaws; it must be integrated into existing workflows without introducing new forms of error, such as "automation bias", defined that clinicians and healthcare team all relying more on AI-generated outputs without sufficient evidence (Connolly et al., 2017). Furthermore, trust is a critical issue too, if clinicians perceive that AI as opaque or unreliable, clinicians and healthcare systems will avoid these systems, negating potential safety gains. Therefore, institutional strategies must focus on ensuring that staff are not only trained on how to use these tools but also educated on the limitations of generative models and the necessity of maintaining rigorous human oversight (Tun et al., 2025).

Reduced Cognitive Load and Administrative Burden

From a cognitive perspective, the generative AI can reduce as well the multitasking required during a patient encounter. Usually, doctors must listen to the patient to perform a physical exam, and mentally format a clinical note, which leads to significant cognitive fatigue. AI acts as an always-on second listener, allowing the clinician to feel more secure knowing that there is always a 3rd party that can remind him of any important details. This reduction in cognitive load not only prevents errors but also leaves the provider with more mental energy for complex diagnostic and problem solving (Hudson et al., 2025).

Moreover, the cognitive load theory suggests that reducing insignificant information increases mental capacity for complex reasoning. By offloading text generation using LLM clinical note management that clinicians can focus more into mental effort to patients, while maintaining clinical notes with increased efficiency and accuracy (Asgari et al., 2024; J. Han et al., 2024).

Improved Continuity of Care

AI-supported documentation can enhance the continuity of care by producing standardized and structured summaries that remain consistent across clinical settings. By reducing variability in terminology and documentation style, these tools mitigate information gaps during transitions, support accurate situational awareness for receiving teams, and contribute to safer and more coordinated patient management (Biswas & Talukdar, 2024).

Furthermore, the literature highlights the capacity of generative models to address and summarise longitudinal patient history, combining years of labs, specialist notes, and imaging into coherent and relevant clinical notes. This capability is crucial for patients with complex, chronic conditions, where the patient's history is often obscured by the large volume of EHR data. By automating the generation of high-fidelity discharge summaries and transfer notes, AI ensures that critical follow-up actions are explicitly flagged rather than buried in unstructured text, directly addressing the communication failures that traditionally lead to medication errors and preventable readmissions (Foad et al., 2026.).

Healthcare Workflow

Interestingly, on a systemic level, generative AI has the ability to smooth out many of the friction points in a hospital operation. For example, AI is well suited to deal with the boring administrative task of physician and nurse scheduling, modern AI agents can efficiently output the most efficient work schedules for resident and nursing teams and automatically optimise the schedule according to individual needs, predictive intelligence can also anticipate bottlenecks before they happen and automatically adjust nursing staff schedules based on the predicted severity of incoming patients, AI agents can also trigger room cleaning alerts the moment a discharge summary is drafted (Almagharbeh et al., 2025; Biot et al., 2026). By connecting departments like the lab, pharmacy, and nursing units into a single, automated intelligence model, AI reduces the constant back and forth of phone calls and manual follow-ups that typically slow down care. This model ensures that the right resources are in the right place at the right time, creating a more fluid environment where the healthcare team can focus on clinical decision-making rather than logistics (Poon et al., 2025).

4. ETHICAL, LEGAL, AND PRACTICAL IMPLEMENTATION CHALLENGES

In fact, the integration of GenAI tools within the clinical workflows could present a gap in deploying that preceded the regulation, since many healthcare workers report that using AI tools in their clinical practice could create an environment that AI algorithms are deployed in highly risk without adequate safety network.. Additionally, institutions must also protect patient privacy against always-on surveillance (Colasacco & Born, 2024; Templin et al., 2024), as well as maintaining equitable standards for patients when training data remains biased against underrepresented populations (Alderman et al., 2025; Chinta et al., 2025). To address these issues demands a fundamental evaluation of professional accountability and the human-in-the-loop doctrine to bridge the divide between innovation and patient safety (Nouis et al., 2025).

Hallucinations and Fabrication Risks

In fact, that foundation of medical decisions is the reliability of the clinical record, particularly when the physician working on a patient's history, they would operate under the assumption that the documented allergies, medication dosages as well as past diagnoses are factually accurate, as errors in documentation usually arise due to fatigue, memory lapses, or typos. In the study 2025, AI-driven clinical decision tools revealed hallucination rates ranging from 50% to 82%, with the risk increasing significantly when using shorter prompts (Omar et al., 2025).. The integration of generative AI introduces a fundamentally different type of risk. Unlike a human who makes mistakes, Large Language Models function as probabilistic engines, where they predict the next plausible word rather than verifying truth. This difference means that LLM models remain vulnerable to "confidently wrong" outputs. However, without the validation, hallucinated diagnoses could be dangerously included within the notes, especially in healthcare settings. This supports the case for a human-supervised model, where AI suggests but does not finalize.(Khurram Shahzad Warraich et al., 2025)

Privacy and Surveillance

The digitization of the health records are usually carried a security risk, however the deployment of AI listening tools can introduce as well a new level of surveillance into the exam room. Since, collecting continuous audio data from bedside interactions transforms a private consultation into a recorded digital record. However, the environment raises serious in HIPAA/GDPR, especially during such sensitive moments. This shift requires a re-evaluation for patient consent, as the convenience of automated scribing must not compromise the patient trust to private care (Blease, 2024; Wilcox et al., 2023). A 2025 survey indicates that while 48% of patients expect AI note-taking to positively impact their visit if it allows their doctor to focus on them, 39% and 15% of these patients expressed concerns about the documentation accuracy as well the privacy respectively (Leiserowitz et al., 2025).

Policies must define the following:

- When recording is allowed
- How long data is stored
- Who owns derivative content

Equity, Algorithmic Bias, and Accountability

Finally, the deployment of AI in healthcare couldn't be separated from the broader ethical frameworks of justice and accountability. Medical ethics is traditionally based on the concept of individual professional liability, the idea that a specific clinician is responsible for their decisions. However, as care becomes increasingly algorithmic, these lines of responsibility begin to blur. According to a recent survey, in the public's mind: 58% of patients believe the physician is responsible for medical errors caused by AI, whereas 22% believe the AI software developer should be liable for data breaches (Khullar et al., 2021). Additionally, a 2025 survey of clinicians found that 89% had no formal training on the legal implications of AI, and confidence in compliance was critically low (Alanazi, 2025).

However, the AI in clinical documentation and decision-support systems can introduce ethical and legal considerations. Since, models can be trained on datasets from specific populations that could reflect cultural or clinical biases, potentially leading to biased misinterpretation for patient narratives. For example, some AI models have failed to accurately analyse dermatological conditions in darker skin tones due to unrepresentative training datasets (Hasanzadeh et al., 2025). So, the degree of liability of such tools must be defined, and whether the responsibility is on the clinician, the institution that deploys the system, or the technology developer. These concerns highlight the need for transparent models, bias mitigation strategies, as well as regulatory frameworks that outline the responsibility in AI-assisted clinical decision-making (Aquino, 2023; Weiner et al., 2025).

5. PROPOSED FRAMEWORK FOR RESPONSIBLE DEPLOYMENT

In this section, we proposed a framework for deploying an effective GenAI within the clinical documentation. A systematic review that conducted by Han et al. (2025) reports that out of 65 trials, only 71% reported improvement of AI-based clinicians compared with other unassisted clinicians. Therefore, the core of this framework relies on "human-in-the-loop" oversight, AI-generated drafts must be reviewed and approved by the responsible clinician. The framework also includes transparency protocols to mitigate the risks of generative AI, such as hallucinations and automation bias. Recent literature shows that Large Language Models (LLMs) can significantly reduce administrative burdens, however they must function as assistive tools rather than autonomous agents, meaning that clinicians must verify AI output to maintain accountability (Khude & Shende, 2025; Oei et al., 2025). This process is critical to counter automation bias, where clinicians might over-rely on sensible but incorrect AI suggestions. This transparency not only helps regulation, but also creates a feedback that helps organizations to identify model drift (Falco et al., 2021; Stirbu et al., 2023)

As AI tools become embedded in clinical workflows, physicians, nurses, and health staff must complete joint training to understand the model's limitations and confidence scoring (Jha et al., 2025). Khan (2025) discussed that without structured instruction, healthcare professionals risk over-reliance and clinical skill loss Therefore, this framework promotes a culture where staff are encouraged to challenge AI-generated outputs without fear of reprisal. Furthermore, ethical safeguards such as data minimization are used, by using the least amount of patient data necessary for the task, the system would automatically strips non-essential patient identifiers before data enters the prompt window, ensuring that the AI processes only the clinical context necessary for the task (Hallaj et al., 2025; Yadav et al., 2023), which is essential to align with evolving digital ethics and privacy standards.

Principle	Implementation
Human-in-the-loop misunderstanding	AI drafts → Clinician approve
Transparency	Audit log of edits
Interprofessional training	Joint AI literacy curricula
Ethics & privacy	Data minimization
Fail-safe culture	AI is assistive, not authoritative

Figure 2. A framework that shows integrating the five main key principles.

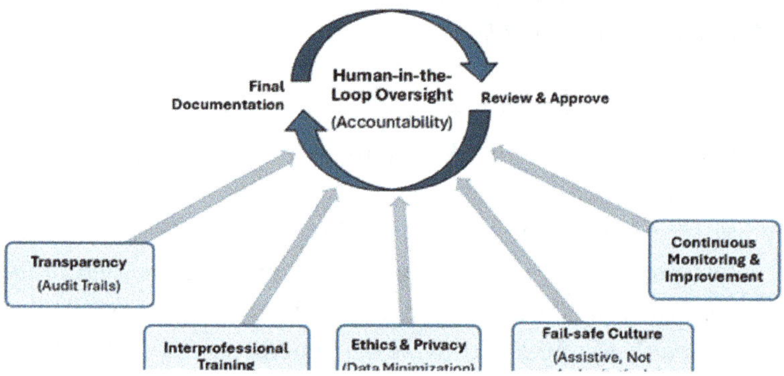

To summarise this section, the above proposed framework emphasizes on transparency, inter-professional competency, ethical safeguards as well as a fail-safe culture as important factors for responsible AI deployment. Also it shows the shared AI training reduces variability, strengthens communication, and builds mutual understanding of system capabilities and limitations. Besides the role of privacy and data-minimization practices with emerging digital ethical standards. Central to the framework is the principle that AI remains assistive, rather than replacing clinical expertise and team-based judgment. This framework can promote the collaborative and accountable approach that integrates technology while preserving patient-focused values.

6. FUTURE DIRECTIONS

Emotionally Intelligent AI

AI has an important role on the Sentiment detection (Assayed et al., 2023) and behaviours such as frustration, fear, or uncertainty in patient communication. However, detecting such signs could enhance psychological safety as well as alerting the clinicians to patient distress, that might allowing them for intervention from psychiatry if needed.

Predictive Collaboration Tools

Integrating the AI tools within health applications could enhance the physiologic trends, as well as documenting the clinical concern to identify early deterioration patterns and automatically alert the clinical team in recommending possible treatment. Such tools could expect risky outcomes before they occur allowing for earlier intervention.

AI-Generated Shared Care Maps

GenAI can produce a clear narrative documentation that can be updated in real time. These representations would align it as well with the team members to understand and discuss patient status and plans.

REFERENCES

Alanazi, A. (2025). Assessing Clinicians' Legal Concerns and the Need for a Regulatory Framework for AI in Healthcare: A Mixed-Methods Study. *Health Care*, *13*(13), 1487. DOI: 10.3390/healthcare13131487 PMID: 40648512

Alder, S. (2026, January 2). Effects of Poor Communication in Healthcare—2026 Update. *The HIPAA Journal*. https://www.hipaajournal.com/effects-of-poor-communication-in-healthcare/

Alderman, J. E., Palmer, J., Laws, E., McCradden, M. D., Ordish, J., Ghassemi, M., Pfohl, S. R., Rostamzadeh, N., Cole-Lewis, H., Glocker, B., Calvert, M., Pollard, T. J., Gill, J., Gath, J., Adebajo, A., Beng, J., Leung, C. H., Kuku, S., Farmer, L.-A., & Liu, X. (2025). Tackling algorithmic bias and promoting transparency in health datasets: The STANDING Together consensus recommendations. *The Lancet. Digital Health*, *7*(1), e64–e88. DOI: 10.1016/S2589-7500(24)00224-3 PMID: 39701919

Almagharbeh, W. T., Alfanash, H. A., Alnawafleh, K. A., Alasmari, A. A., Alsaraireh, F. A., Dreidi, M. M., & Nashwan, A. J. (2025). Application of artificial intelligence in nursing practice: A qualitative study of Jordanian nurses' perspectives. *BMC Nursing*, *24*(1), 92. DOI: 10.1186/s12912-024-02658-6 PMID: 39863852

Almotairi, M. A., Alotaibi, A. S. M., Alharbi, K. F. N., Alqarni, A. M. G., Alshammari, M. S. F., Alqasir, M. A., Alshammari, F. N. S., Alrowaily, S. A. T., Bellen, A. C., Alsoaib, A., Alraggas, T. M., Alojairi, A. A., Alessa, N. H., Alrabeeah, R. T., Alshehri, W. D., & Alqahtani, S. T. A. (2024). Nursing Documentation as a Foundation of Safe, Ethical, and Accountable Care: A Systematic Review. *Journal of Angiotherapy*, *8*(5), 1–13. DOI: 10.25163/angiotherapy.8510497

Alobayli, F., O'Connor, S., Holloway, A., & Cresswell, K. (2023). Electronic Health Record Stress and Burnout Among Clinicians in Hospital Settings: A Systematic Review. *Digital Health*, *9*, 20552076231220241. DOI: 10.1177/20552076231220241 PMID: 38130797

Aquino, Y. S. J. (2023). Making decisions: Bias in artificial intelligence and data-driven diagnostic tools. *Australian Journal of General Practice*, *52*(7), 439–442. DOI: 10.31128/AJGP-12-22-6630 PMID: 37423238

Asgari, E., Kaur, J., Nuredini, G., Balloch, J., Taylor, A. M., Sebire, N., Robinson, R., Peters, C., Sridharan, S., & Pimenta, D. (2024). Impact of Electronic Health Record Use on Cognitive Load and Burnout Among Clinicians: Narrative Review. *JMIR Medical Informatics*, *12*(1), e55499. DOI: 10.2196/55499 PMID: 38607672

Assayed, S., Shaalan, K., Al-Sayed, S., & Alkhatib, M. (2023). Psychological emotion recognition of students using machine learning based chatbot. [IJAIA]. *International Journal of Artificial Intelligence & Applications*, *14*(2), 29–39. DOI: 10.5121/ijaia.2023.14203

Assayed, S. K. (2025). *Transforming healthcare through generative and agentic AI: A systematic review*. In *Proceedings of the 10th International Conference on Information Technology Trends (ITT)* (pp. 124–129). IEEE. https://doi.org/DOI: 10.1109/ITT69610.2025.11352935

Assayed, S. K., Shieh, C. S., & Gupta, S. K. (2025). Engineering intelligent healthcare systems: Understanding medical queries with AI and NLP. *Journal of Engineering and Applied Sciences (Asian Research Publishing Network)*, *72*(1), 212. DOI: 10.1186/s44147-025-00800-y

Bhuyan, S. S., Sateesh, V., Mukul, N., Galvankar, A., Mahmood, A., Nauman, M., Rai, A., Bordoloi, K., Basu, U., & Samuel, J. (2025). Generative Artificial Intelligence Use in Healthcare: Opportunities for Clinical Excellence and Administrative Efficiency. *Journal of Medical Systems*, *49*(1), 10. DOI: 10.1007/s10916-024-02136-1 PMID: 39820845

Bienefeld, N., Keller, E., & Grote, G. (2024). Human-AI Teaming in Critical Care: A Comparative Analysis of Data Scientists' and Clinicians' Perspectives on AI Augmentation and Automation. *Journal of Medical Internet Research*, *26*, e50130. DOI: 10.2196/50130 PMID: 39038285

Biot, C., Tabbuso, T., & Marechal, Y. (2026). Artificial Intelligence for Hospital Scheduling: A Simple, Reproducible, and Effective Model. *Cureus*, *18*(1), e101412. DOI: 10.7759/cureus.101412 PMID: 41536626

Biswas, A., & Talukdar, W. (2024). Intelligent Clinical Documentation: Harnessing Generative AI for Patient-Centric Clinical Note Generation. *International Journal of Innovative Science and Research Technology (IJISRT)*, 994–1008. DOI: 10.38124/ijisrt/IJISRT24MAY1483

Blease, C. (2024). Open AI meets open notes: Surveillance capitalism, patient privacy and online record access. *Journal of Medical Ethics*, *50*(2), 84–89. DOI: 10.1136/jme-2023-109574 PMID: 38050159

Chinta, S. V., Wang, Z., Palikhe, A., Zhang, X., Kashif, A., Smith, M. A., Liu, J., & Zhang, W. (2025). AI-driven healthcare: A review on ensuring fairness and mitigating bias. *PLOS Digital Health*, *4*(5), e0000864. DOI: 10.1371/journal.pdig.0000864 PMID: 40392801

Colasacco, C. J., & Born, H. L. (2024). A Case of Artificial Intelligence Chatbot Hallucination. *JAMA Otolaryngology-Head & Neck Surgery, 150*(6), 457–458. DOI: 10.1001/jamaoto.2024.0428 PMID: 38635259

Connolly, F., Byrne, D., Lydon, S., Walsh, C., & O'Connor, P. (2017). Barriers and facilitators related to the implementation of a physiological track and trigger system: A systematic review of the qualitative evidence. *International Journal for Quality in Health Care : Journal of the International Society for Quality in Health Care, 29*(8), 973–980. DOI: 10.1093/intqhc/mzx148 PMID: 29177409

Delardes, B., McLeod, L., Chakraborty, S., & Bowles, K.-A. (2020). What is the effect of electronic clinical handovers on patient outcomes? A systematic review. *Health Informatics Journal, 26*(4), 2422–2434. DOI: 10.1177/1460458220905162 PMID: 32114869

Eggins, S., & Slade, D. (2015). Communication in Clinical Handover: Improving the Safety and Quality of the Patient Experience. *Journal of Public Health Research, 4*(3), 666. DOI: 10.4081/jphr.2015.666 PMID: 26753165

Falco, G., Shneiderman, B., Badger, J., Carrier, R., Dahbura, A., Danks, D., Eling, M., Goodloe, A., Gupta, J., Hart, C., Jirotka, M., Johnson, H., LaPointe, C., Llorens, A. J., Mackworth, A. K., Maple, C., Pálsson, S. E., Pasquale, F., Winfield, A., & Yeong, Z. K. (2021). Governing AI safety through independent audits. *Nature Machine Intelligence, 3*(7), 566–571. DOI: 10.1038/s42256-021-00370-7

Foad, N. C., Lippert, J., & Lippert, W. C. (2026, January 1). (n.d.). Bridging Inpatient and Outpatient Care: A Scoping Review on Discharge Summary Documentation Timeliness and Quality. *Journal of Brown Hospital Medicine, 5*(1), 151812. DOI: 10.56305/001c.151812 PMID: 41488445

Gaffney, A., Woolhandler, S., Cai, C., Bor, D., Himmelstein, J., McCormick, D., & Himmelstein, D. U. (2022a). Medical Documentation Burden Among US Office-Based Physicians in 2019: A National Study. *JAMA Internal Medicine, 182*(5), 564–566. DOI: 10.1001/jamainternmed.2022.0372 PMID: 35344006

Gaffney, A., Woolhandler, S., Cai, C., Bor, D., Himmelstein, J., McCormick, D., & Himmelstein, D. U. (2022b). Medical Documentation Burden Among US Office-Based Physicians in 2019: A National Study. *JAMA Internal Medicine, 182*(5), 564–566. DOI: 10.1001/jamainternmed.2022.0372 PMID: 35344006

Genes, N., Simon, G., Koziatek, C., Kim, J. G., Woo, K., Dahn, C., Chan, L., & Wiesenfeld, B. (2025). Generative Artificial Intelligence Summaries to Facilitate Emergency Department Handoff. *Applied Clinical Informatics, 16*(04), 1185–1191. DOI: 10.1055/a-2681-5008 PMID: 40795949

Gesner, E., Dykes, P. C., Zhang, L., & Gazarian, P. (2022). Documentation Burden in Nursing and Its Role in Clinician Burnout Syndrome. *Applied Clinical Informatics, 13*(05), 983–990. DOI: 10.1055/s-0042-1757157 PMID: 36261113

Gregoriou, P. L., Charalambous, A., Rousou, E., Papastavrou, E., & Merkouris, A. (2025). Attitudes of Physicians and Nurses Toward Interprofessional Collaboration: A Systematic Literature Review. *Materia Socio-Medica, 37*(1), 64–73. DOI: 10.5455/msm.2025.37.64-73 PMID: 40098756

Hallaj, S., Heinke, A., Kalaw, F. G. P., Gim, N., Blazes, M., Owen, J., Dysinger, E., Benton, E. S., Cordier, B. A., Evans, N. G., Li-Pook-Than, J., Snyder, M. P., Nebeker, C., Zangwill, L. M., Baxter, S. L., McWeeney, S., Lee, C. S., Lee, A. Y., & Patel, B. (2025). Navigating open data sharing and privacy in the age of clinical AI research: From reidentification to pseudo-reidentification. *EClinicalMedicine, 91*, 103729. DOI: 10.1016/j.eclinm.2025.103729 PMID: 41542222

Han, J., Park, J., Huh, J., Oh, U., Do, J., & Kim, D. (2024). AscleAI: A LLM-based Clinical Note Management System for Enhancing Clinician Productivity. *Extended Abstracts of the CHI Conference on Human Factors in Computing Systems, CHI EA '24*, 1–7. DOI: 10.1145/3613905.3650784

Han, R., Acosta, J. N., Shakeri, Z., Ioannidis, J. P. A., Topol, E. J., & Rajpurkar, P. (2024). Randomised controlled trials evaluating artificial intelligence in clinical practice: A scoping review. *The Lancet. Digital Health, 6*(5), e367–e373. DOI: 10.1016/S2589-7500(24)00047-5 PMID: 38670745

Hasanzadeh, F., Josephson, C. B., Waters, G., Adedinsewo, D., Azizi, Z., & White, J. A. (2025). Bias recognition and mitigation strategies in artificial intelligence healthcare applications. *NPJ Digital Medicine, 8*(1), 154. DOI: 10.1038/s41746-025-01503-7 PMID: 40069303

Hosseinzadegan, F., Salamatbakhsh, M., Salehzadeh, M., Nournezhad, H., & Mohammadpour, Y. (2025). Hospital errors and their consequences among healthcare professionals a: Descriptive correlational investigation. *Annals of Medicine and Surgery (London), 87*(7), 4026–4033. DOI: 10.1097/MS9.0000000000003280 PMID: 40852022

Hudson, T. J., Albrecht, M., Smith, T. R., Ator, G. A., Thompson, J. A., Shah, T., & Shanks, D. (2025). Impact of Ambient Artificial Intelligence Documentation on Cognitive Load. *Mayo Clinic Proceedings. Digital Health, 3*(1), 100193. DOI: 10.1016/j.mcpdig.2024.100193 PMID: 40206994

Jha, D., Durak, G., Sharma, V., Keles, E., Cicek, V., Zhang, Z., Srivastava, A., Rauniyar, A., Hagos, D. H., Tomar, N. K., Miller, F. H., Topcu, A., Yazidi, A., Håkegård, J. E., & Bagci, U. (2025). A Conceptual Framework for Applying Ethical Principles of AI to Medical Practice. *Bioengineering (Basel, Switzerland)*, *12*(2), 180. DOI: 10.3390/bioengineering12020180 PMID: 40001699

Khan, F. A. (2025). AI in clinical diagnostics: Is overreliance eroding clinical expertise? *PLOS Digital Health*, *4*(8), e0000959. DOI: 10.1371/journal.pdig.0000959 PMID: 40758655

Khude, H., & Shende, P. (2025). AI-driven clinical decision support systems: Revolutionizing medication selection and personalized drug therapy. *Advances in Integrative Medicine*, *12*(4), 100529. DOI: 10.1016/j.aimed.2025.100529

Khullar, D., Casalino, L. P., Qian, Y., Lu, Y., Chang, E., & Aneja, S. (2021). Public vs physician views of liability for artificial intelligence in health care. *Journal of the American Medical Informatics Association : JAMIA*, *28*(7), 1574–1577. DOI: 10.1093/jamia/ocab055 PMID: 33871009

Khurram Shahzad Warraich, M., Usman, H., Zakir, S., & Mehboob, M. (2025). Ethical Governance of artificial intelligence Hallucinations in legal practice. *Social Sciences Spectrum*, *4*(2), 603–615. DOI: 10.71085/sss.04.02.297

Lee, C., Vogt, K. A., & Kumar, S. (2024). Prospects for AI clinical summarization to reduce the burden of patient chart review. *Frontiers in Digital Health*, *6*, 1475092. Advance online publication. DOI: 10.3389/fdgth.2024.1475092 PMID: 39575412

Leiserowitz, G., Mansfield, J., MacDonald, S., & Jost, M. (2025). Patient Attitudes Toward Ambient Voice Technology: Preimplementation Patient Survey in an Academic Medical Center. *JMIR Medical Informatics*, *13*(1), e77901. DOI: 10.2196/77901 PMID: 41308194

Lukac, P. J., Turner, W., Vangala, S., Chin, A. T., Khalili, J., Shih, Y.-C. T., Sarkisian, C., Cheng, E. M., & Mafi, J. N. (2025). Ambient AI Scribes in Clinical Practice: A Randomized Trial. *NEJM AI*, *2*(12), AIoa2501000. DOI: 10.1056/AIoa2501000

Nematollahi Maleki, R., Shahbazi, S., Hosseinzadeh, M., Ghafourifard, M., Gholizad Gougjehyaran, H., & Faravan, A. (2025). Artificial intelligence-assisted nursing care: A concept analysis using Walker and Avant approach. *BMC Nursing*, *24*(1), 1175. DOI: 10.1186/s12912-025-03818-y PMID: 40993699

Nouis, S. C., Uren, V., & Jariwala, S. (2025). Evaluating accountability, transparency, and bias in AI-assisted healthcare decision- making: A qualitative study of healthcare professionals' perspectives in the UK. *BMC Medical Ethics*, *26*(1), 89. DOI: 10.1186/s12910-025-01243-z PMID: 40629303

Oei, S. P., Bakkes, T. H. G. F., Mischi, M., Bouwman, R. A., van Sloun, R. J. G., & Turco, S. (2025). Artificial intelligence in clinical decision support and the prediction of adverse events. *Frontiers in Digital Health*, *7*, 1403047. DOI: 10.3389/fdgth.2025.1403047 PMID: 40520218

Olakotan, O., Samuriwo, R., Ismaila, H., & Atiku, S. (2025). Usability Challenges in Electronic Health Records: Impact on Documentation Burden and Clinical Workflow: A Scoping Review. *Journal of Evaluation in Clinical Practice*, *31*(4), e70189. DOI: 10.1111/jep.70189 PMID: 40581989

Olson, K. D., Meeker, D., Troup, M., Barker, T. D., Nguyen, V. H., Manders, J. B., Stults, C. D., Jones, V. G., Shah, S. D., Shah, T., & Schwamm, L. H. (2025). Use of Ambient AI Scribes to Reduce Administrative Burden and Professional Burnout. *JAMA Network Open*, *8*(10), e2534976. DOI: 10.1001/jamanetworkopen.2025.34976 PMID: 41037268

Omar, M., Sorin, V., Collins, J. D., Reich, D., Freeman, R., Gavin, N., Charney, A., Stump, L., Bragazzi, N. L., Nadkarni, G. N., & Klang, E. (2025). Multi-model assurance analysis showing large language models are highly vulnerable to adversarial hallucination attacks during clinical decision support. *Communications Medicine*, *5*(1), 330. DOI: 10.1038/s43856-025-01021-3 PMID: 40753316

Orenstein, E. W., Ferro, D. F., Bonafide, C. P., Landrigan, C. P., Gillespie, S., & Muthu, N. (2019). Hidden health IT hazards: A qualitative analysis of clinically meaningful documentation discrepancies at transfer out of the pediatric intensive care unit. *JAMIA Open*, *2*(3), 392–398. DOI: 10.1093/jamiaopen/ooz026 PMID: 31984372

Perkins, S. W., Muste, J. C., Alam, T., & Singh, R. P. (2024). Improving Clinical Documentation with Artificial Intelligence: A Systematic Review. *Perspectives in Health Information Management*, *21*(2), 1d. PMID: 40134899

Poon, E. G., Lemak, C. H., Rojas, J. C., Guptill, J., & Classen, D. (2025). Adoption of artificial intelligence in healthcare: Survey of health system priorities, successes, and challenges. *Journal of the American Medical Informatics Association : JAMIA*, *32*(7), 1093–1100. DOI: 10.1093/jamia/ocaf065 PMID: 40323320

Renggli, F. J., Gerlach, M., Bieri, J. S., Golz, C., & Sariyar, M. (2025). Integrating Nurse Preferences Into AI-Based Scheduling Systems: Qualitative Study. *JMIR Formative Research*, *9*(1), e67747. DOI: 10.2196/67747 PMID: 40466089

Rotenstein, L., Melnick, E. R., Iannaccone, C., Zhang, J., Mugal, A., Lipsitz, S. R., Healey, M. J., Holland, C., Snyder, R., Sinsky, C. A., Ting, D., & Bates, D. W. (2024). Virtual Scribes and Physician Time Spent on Electronic Health Records. *JAMA Network Open*, *7*(5), e2413140. DOI: 10.1001/jamanetworkopen.2024.13140 PMID: 38787556

Stallinga, H. A., Ten Napel, H., Jansen, G. J., Geertzen, J. H., De Vries Robbé, P. F., & Roodbol, P. F. (2015). Does language ambiguity in clinical practice justify the introduction of standard terminology? An integrative review. *Journal of Clinical Nursing*, *24*(3–4), 344–352. DOI: 10.1111/jocn.12624 PMID: 24813851

Stirbu, V., Granlund, T., & Mikkonen, T. (2023). Continuous design control for machine learning in certified medical systems. *Software Quality Journal*, *31*(2), 307–333. DOI: 10.1007/s11219-022-09601-5

Sung, S.-F., Hu, Y.-H., & Chen, C.-Y. (2024). Disambiguating Clinical Abbreviations by One-to-All Classification: Algorithm Development and Validation Study. *JMIR Medical Informatics*, *12*(1), e56955. DOI: 10.2196/56955 PMID: 39352715

Tariq, R. A., & Sharma, S. (2025). Inappropriate Medical Abbreviations. In *StatPearls*. StatPearls Publishing., https://www.ncbi.nlm.nih.gov/books/NBK519006/

Tataei, A., Rahimi, B., Afshar, H. L., Alinejad, V., Jafarizadeh, H., & Parizad, N. (2023). The effects of electronic nursing handover on patient safety in the general (non-COVID-19) and COVID-19 intensive care units: A quasi-experimental study. *BMC Health Services Research*, *23*(1), 527. DOI: 10.1186/s12913-023-09502-8 PMID: 37221502

Templin, T., Perez, M. W., Sylvia, S., Leek, J., & Sinnott-Armstrong, N. (2024). Addressing 6 challenges in generative AI for digital health: A scoping review. *PLOS Digital Health*, *3*(5), e0000503. DOI: 10.1371/journal.pdig.0000503 PMID: 38781686

Topaz, M., Peltonen, L. M., & Zhang, Z. (2025). Beyond human ears: Navigating the uncharted risks of AI scribes in clinical practice. *NPJ Digital Medicine*, *8*(1), 569. DOI: 10.1038/s41746-025-01895-6 PMID: 40993221

Tu, T., Schaekermann, M., Palepu, A., Saab, K., Freyberg, J., Tanno, R., Wang, A., Li, B., Amin, M., Cheng, Y., Vedadi, E., Tomasev, N., Azizi, S., Singhal, K., Hou, L., Webson, A., Kulkarni, K., Mahdavi, S. S., Semturs, C., & Natarajan, V. (2025). Towards conversational diagnostic artificial intelligence. *Nature, 642*(8067), 442–450. DOI: 10.1038/s41586-025-08866-7 PMID: 40205050

Tun, H. M., Rahman, H. A., Naing, L., & Malik, O. A. (2025). Trust in Artificial Intelligence–Based Clinical Decision Support Systems Among Health Care Workers: Systematic Review. *Journal of Medical Internet Research, 27*(1), e69678. DOI: 10.2196/69678 PMID: 40772775

Umberfield, E., Ghaferi, A. A., Krein, S. L., & Manojlovich, M. (2019). Using Incident Reports to Assess Communication Failures and Patient Outcomes. *Joint Commission Journal on Quality and Patient Safety, 45*(6), 406–413. DOI: 10.1016/j.jcjq.2019.02.006 PMID: 30935883

Van Veen, D., Van Uden, C., Blankemeier, L., Delbrouck, J.-B., Aali, A., Bluethgen, C., Pareek, A., Polacin, M., Reis, E. P., Seehofnerová, A., Rohatgi, N., Hosamani, P., Collins, W., Ahuja, N., Langlotz, C. P., Hom, J., Gatidis, S., Pauly, J., & Chaudhari, A. S. (2024). Adapted large language models can outperform medical experts in clinical text summarization. *Nature Medicine, 30*(4), 1134–1142. DOI: 10.1038/s41591-024-02855-5 PMID: 38413730

Watson, A. L., Bond, C., Aveyard, H., Smith, G. D., & Jackson, D. (n.d.). Generative AI at the Bedside: An Integrative Review of Applications and Implications in Clinical Nursing Practice. *Journal of Clinical Nursing, n/a*(n/a). DOI: 10.1111/jocn.70151

Watson, B. M., & Wu, X. I. (2023). Sentinel Events and Miscommunication What do we know in 2021: A Language and Social Psychology Framework. *Health Communication, 38*(9), 1770–1779. DOI: 10.1080/10410236.2022.2031451 PMID: 35209746

Weiner, E. B., Dankwa-Mullan, I., Nelson, W. A., & Hassanpour, S. (2025). Ethical challenges and evolving strategies in the integration of artificial intelligence into clinical practice. *PLOS Digital Health, 4*(4), e0000810. DOI: 10.1371/journal.pdig.0000810 PMID: 40198594

Wilcox, L., Brewer, R., & Diaz, F. (2023). AI Consent Futures: A Case Study on Voice Data Collection with Clinicians. *Proc. ACM Hum.-Comput. Interact., 7*(CSCW2), 316:1-316:30. DOI: 10.1145/3610107

Yadav, N., Pandey, S., Gupta, A., Dudani, P., Gupta, S., & Rangarajan, K. (2023). Data Privacy in Healthcare: In the Era of Artificial Intelligence. *Indian Dermatology Online Journal, 14*(6), 788–792. DOI: 10.4103/idoj.idoj_543_23 PMID: 38099022

Chapter 4
Hybrid Fuzzy MCDM Method for Pneumonia Diagnosis

Sekar Kidambi Raju
http://orcid.org/0000-0003-4300-2041
School of Computing, SASTRA University, Thanjavur, India

Sathiamoorthy Gopalan
http://orcid.org/0000-0001-8899-2240
Department of Maths, SASHE, SASTRA University, Thanjavur, India

Raj Anand Sundaramoorthy
School of Computing, SASTRA University, Thanjavur, India

Ganesh Karthikeyan Varadarajan
http://orcid.org/0009-0000-6982-716X
School of Computing, SASTRA University, Thanjavur, India

Muthusamy Periyasamy
Paavai Engineering College, Namakkal, India

ABSTRACT

Diagnostic accuracy and efficiency of pneumonia remain one of the major challenges in clinical decision-making due to the diverse symptoms, variable patient response to treatment, and ambiguous medical data. In order to overcome those problems, this chapter presents a hybrid fuzzy Multi-Criteria Decision-Making (MCDM) framework that determines Fuzzy Analytical Hierarchy Process (FAHP) alongside Fuzzy Technique for Order Preference by Similarity to Ideal Solution (Fuzzy TOPSIS). Our innovative methodology analysis of key diagnosis criteria on shortness of

DOI: 10.4018/979-8-3373-8247-0.ch004

breath, chest X-ray, blood, sputum culture, and immunization status on the uncertainty basis through hesitant assessment and linguistic assessment. FAHP is used to calculate the weights of trustworthy criteria through paired comparisons, which are fuzzy and attempt to achieve consensus among two or more decision makers. Fuzzy TOPSIS, in its turn, ranks the diagnosis options in terms of proximity to the ideal profile of the physician. The hybrid method utilizes the capabilities of FAHP and Fuzzy TOPSIS to enhance the robustness, reduce the ambiguity in the clinical judgment of the physician, and streamline the prioritization of the diagnosis to doctors. Particularly, experimental examination indicates that the integrated model offers consistent, clarified, and probable decisions aiding in diagnosing pneumonia. The chapter proves fuzzy MCDM as having a potential to develop the intelligent healthcare system, particularly when medical information is vague and incomplete.

1. INTRODUCTION

Pneumonia is a severe health issue in the world that is characterized by the inflammation of the lung parenchyma, which is linked to a high morbidity and mortality rate (Sun et al., 2022). Proper and timely diagnosis is a fundamental component of effective management of pneumonia, and traditional forms of diagnostic testing, including laboratory results, chest x-rays, and physical examination, may be subjective and changeable (Wang et al., 2024). New approaches to the enhancement of diagnostic accuracy have been taken in the recent developments of decision-making processes. One such development is the fuzzy TOPSIS (Technique of the Order of Preference by the Similitude to Ideal Solution) model. This model deals with the ambiguity and imprecision that are common features of medical data through the application of fuzzy logic (Pramanik et al., 2022). Fuzzy TOPSIS is an effective model when solving diagnostic problems in complex conditions whereby appropriate data might not necessarily be readily available. It develops the ordinary TOPSIS method by incorporating fuzzy sets. The fuzzy TOPSIS model provides a systematic way of ranking diagnostic decisions by considering the alternatives according to their proximity to the optimal answer. This method comes in particularly useful in medical diagnostics, when multiple criteria have to be combined and assessed in ambiguous conditions, e.g., symptoms, test results, and imaging data. The fuzzy TOPSIS model is a more developed and reliable diagnostic system that considers the variation of patient information and clinical assessment. In this paper, the author will discuss the use of the fuzzy TOPSIS model in the diagnosis of pneumonia. Our suggestion is a holistic framework that combines different parameters of diagnosis into a common decision-making process. We plan to show how the fuzzy TOPSIS model can enhance the accuracy of the diagnostic process, compare it to the existing approaches, and comment on how the model can be applied to clinical practice. Serious health problems, such as acute respiratory infections, such as pneumonia, that cause inflammation of the lung tissue have the same high morbidity and mortality rates all over the world. Treatment and patient management of pneumonia would require accurate diagnosis, which is still a challenging diagnostic procedure. Traditional methods of diagnosis, such as laboratory, chest radiography, and clinical tests, may suffer a lack of sensitivity and specificity and may often be subjective in interpretation (Ayan & Ünver, 2019). Clinical assessment involves the assessment of symptoms that can be confused with other respiratory diseases, e.g., fever, dyspnea, and cough, which might result in a misinterpretation of the diagnosis. Although chest radiography is a widely used technique, it may fail to detect early or uncharacteristic cases of pneumonia, and its effectiveness can be limited. To respond to these challenges, more individuals are drawn to adopt advanced methods of decision-making in order to enhance the accuracy of the diagnosis. The fuzzy Technique of Order of Preference by Similarity to the Ideal Solution (TOPSIS) model is one of the techniques that has been shown to be promising in the process of dealing with complex and uncertain data. This model, which is an extension of the conventional TOPSIS model, includes fuzzy logic to deal with the imprecision and vagueness that are very common in medical data (Ali et al., 2024).

The fuzzy TOPSIS model, however, evaluates the diagnostic possibilities by computing the distance between them and the optimum solution. This approach integrates a range of criteria, such as the imaging data, test results, and clinical symptoms, in a broad framework that will allow a more flexible and subtle evaluation. Fuzzy logic is a source of uncertainty management. Moreover, the fuzzy TOPSIS model is specifically the best model to be applied to medical diagnostics in cases where data can be imprecise or incomplete. The reason is that it is able to work with various types of data input, such as qualitative decisions and quantitative values. Fuzzy TOPSIS gives the opportunity to enhance the diagnostic results and make informed clinical decisions by integrating numerous diagnostic features within a single, unified model.

1.1 Novelty

The originality of the study consists in the fact that it has the first application of the Hesitant Fuzzy FAHP-TOPSIS model to the estimation and ranking of the different types of pneumonia on the basis of a combination of multi-medical factors that include shortness of breath, chest X-ray outcome, and immunization coverage. It is not similar to the traditional methods since, although the techniques require the use of fixed or single-value criteria weight, this study integrates hesitant fuzzy logic into the FAHP to enable the determination of the weight dynamically so as to accommodate the intrinsic uncertainty and variation of medical decisions. The fact that the TOPSIS ranking is used increases the capacity of the model to give a complete analysis on the types of pneumonia in terms of the relative proximity of each alternative to the optimal solution. Moreover, the use of the Jaccard similarity index to confirm the agreement of decision-makers is an addition that provides some credence and objectivity to this study, which is sometimes unmatched by similar methods of the validity of the consensus. It is rather a holistic method, where pneumonia treatment is prioritized on the basis of the closeness coefficients and the combination of multiple aspects of decision-making, which is a much better approach than traditional methods that could not take uncertainty and change of decision-makers into account.

2. RELATED WORK

MCDM that was applied in the comparison of various treatment techniques of AMH is given. The sequential neutralization method was most preferred. In the tests conducted on lime-based neutralization, Fe metal concentration was decreased to 1 mg/L at pH 4, 1 mg/L at pH 7 (Cu, Zn, Ni), and 1 mg/L at pH 10 (Mn, Cd). The best method in this wastewater seemed to be the sequential neutralization (Štirbanović et al., 2021). The issue of selecting the optimal COVID-19 treatment is addressed through the implementation of a multi-criteria decision-making framework using PHFS to address the issue of ambiguity. Treatment options are considered in three options and compared with ten criteria: antibacterial medication and plasma therapy, vaccination, and quarantine/in-house isolation (Ali et al., 2024). The Fuzzy AHP-TOPSIS algorithm is used to choose the optimum color treatment process using a carbon-based adsorbent, using all the top-ranked parameters, including accessibility, reuse, and adsorption capacity. Powder-activated carbon was more effective in the removal of the color than other forms of adsorbents (Azari et al., 2022). TOPSIS-case-based reasoning (CBR) and goal programming to solve the dose optimization problem in prostate cancer treatment. Making use of the TOPSIS-CBR hybrid method enables the system to consume the experience of oncologists and subsequently modulate the dose plans retrieved using a goal programming model by trading off opposed criteria (Malekpoor et al., 2022). Mammograms are processed in order to identify abnormal areas and isolate characteristics such as morphology, texture, and histograms. These characteristics are then relied on to propose solutions that present an issue of multi-criteria decision-making. The options among the treatments are then ranked using the TOPSIS method, which takes these features and the views of the experts into consideration (Basu et al., 2020). Bayesian TOPSIS, or B-TOPSIS, is a strategy to modify a traditional TOPSIS model by a probabilistic aggregation strategy of multiple decision-makers. The defining difference between B-TOPSIS and standard TOPSIS is in the fact that it is not as sensitive to outliers given that it employs a hierarchical Bayesian model rather than the simplistic aggregation strategy of the traditional TOPSIS (Li et al., 2022). . Use of fuzzy TOPSIS to achieve the optimal choice of treatment of GERD. Four out of four treatment options, including antacids, histamine blockers, proton pump inhibitors (PPIs), and prokinetics, were considered in this study based on cost, efficacy, and safety factors. PPIs were ranked the best choice of treatments with the closest coefficient (Ci) to GERD, having a Ci of 0.642, and antacids were ranked last with a Ci of 0.33 (Terry et al., 2024). Other decision-making methods that are multi-criteria are TOPSIS-AHP and TOPSIS-COV. Both compare closed-loop recycling as the solution with the best environmental, economic, and social criteria in PET waste management. The performance indicators (i.e., cost and photochemical oxidant potential) in both methods have shown a variation; however, it was more in AHP, as it prioritizes cost, as the decision-makers of the company desire to save their cost (Al-Thani et al., 2022).

The TOPSIS, water management of mango under the regulated deficit irrigation at maturity, and medium fertilization treatment in the Southwest of China increase water use efficiency, quality, and yield of the fruit by 10.1 and 35.6, respectively (Liu et al., 2021). The TOPSIS technique changed to the uncertain environment, in which the distance measures are substituted by interval-valued Pythagorean fuzzy (IVPF) sets, and Pearson-like Pearson-type IVPF correlation coefficients are to be used to establish the extent of association and proximity of the alternatives to the ideal solutions. This is due to the fact that a new correlation-based closeness coefficient is derived to resolve more MCDA problems (Ho et al., 2020). Case-based reasoning (CBR) and TOPSIS of optimal dose planning in the treatment of prostate cancer. These will entail the application of multi-criteria decision-making in estimating the similar cases through the experience of the past cases of oncologists that have been captured to prescribe the most appropriate dose plan (Malekpoor et al., 2017). . The Taguchi-neural networks-fuzzy best-worst method (FBWM)-TOPSIS joint method of optimizing the selection at the power plants considering the environmental, social, economic, and technical factors has been employed. There are five power plants developed in comparison, and these are gas, steam, combined cycle, wind, and hydroelectric power plants. The computations of design combinations were performed through the Taguchi method, which was founded on the estimates of the signal-to-noise ratios in addition to the calculation of other data through the neural networks (Omrani et al., 2018). Heat and electrical power are supplied to homes, greenhouses, and health centers using the integrated AHP-TOPSIS model in the Simav IGES system. Designing the best option in the combination of energy, exergy, and economic approaches, i.e., maximum residential heating (16311 homes), maximum greenhouse (631449 m^2), and minimum power generation (41153 kWh) (Arslan et al., 2021). The strategy will make the process of decision-making easier, as it will provide a chance to consider alternatives. DOE-TOPSIS does not necessitate full re-examination in case a few alternatives are introduced or eliminated, but this will a bit undermine the accuracy. The DOE-TOPSIS approach has a lot to do with flexibility as compared to the traditional TOPSIS (Sabaghi et al., 2015). To address the drawbacks of fuzzy and intuitionistic fuzzy sets when it comes to decision-making, a new measure of knowledge of picture fuzzy sets is outlined. The justification of the measure suggested here is supported with the numerical examples in a bid to demonstrate its superiority over the other methods. Moreover, a new accuracy measure of PIF sets is developed using the new knowledge measure to ensure that the issues concerning the pattern identification can be solved effectively. The above accuracy measure has been utilized in the modified VIKOR approach in solving a multi-criteria decision-making problem (Dinesh & Kumar, 2024).

2.1 Research gap

The existing gap in the traditional approaches toward the evaluation criteria of pneumonia treatment, constant or single-value weights, without considering the inherent uncertainty of the medical judgment, has been determined. In addition, the methods employed ought to be suitable to carry out consensus validation, and the obtained findings are not so confident. The novelty study gap is the following: Hesitant Fuzzy FAHP-TOPSIS ensures the dynamism of weight changes according to hesitant fuzzy logic. The Jaccard similarity index is used in doing consensus validity, and this ensures a better validity of the model. In addition, the approach that considers the relative closeness to an optimal solution offers a much more detailed analysis of the treatment of pneumonia by far exceeding the parameters that the classic approaches may have limitations.

3. PROPOSED METHODOLOGY

The study utilizes FAHP and TOPSIS as tools to assess the major types of pneumonia: bacterial, viral, mycoplasma, fungal, and aspiration pneumonia by looking at five variables such as the history of the patient, including Shortness of Breath, Chest X-Rays, Blood Tests, Sputum Cultures, and Vaccination History. The weights of these variables are determined by FAHP and the closeness coefficient for TOPSIS to each pneumonia type was calculated using TOPSIS. There were three decision-makers who provided input on how best to assess the model. Jaccard Similarity was the similarity measure used for evaluating results from the study. The authors of the study indicated that using this model to assess pneumonia diagnosis has the potential to improve decision-making among healthcare providers; through a collaborative decision-making process, the patient can directly benefit from the decisions being made.

The combination of Fuzzy Analytical Hierarchy Process (FAHP) and TOPSIS is used to evaluate and rank several pneumonia versions based on a set of parameters. The equations of FAHP and TOPSIS are presented here. Fuzzy Analytical Hierarchical Process (FAHP). The weight for the criteria of FAHP can be calculated using the following equation. The pairwise comparison matrix A is constructed from the fuzzy numbers, and the eigenvector provides the criterion weights.

$$B = \begin{bmatrix} 1 & \widetilde{b}_{12} & \widetilde{b}_{13} & \cdots \widetilde{b}_{1n} \\ \frac{1}{\widetilde{b}_{12}} & 1 & \widetilde{b}_{23} & \cdots \widetilde{b}_{2n} \\ \vdots & \vdots & \vdots & \cdots \vdots \\ \frac{1}{\widetilde{b}_{1n}} & \frac{1}{\widetilde{b}_{2n}} & \frac{1}{\widetilde{b}_{2n}} & \cdot \quad \cdots 1 \end{bmatrix} \tag{1}$$

B is the fuzzy pairwise comparison matrix. $\widetilde{b}_{ij}$. is the fuzzy comparison value of criterion i and criterion j. The values in the bottom half are inverse of those in the top half since $\widetilde{b}_{ij} = \frac{1}{b_{ji}}$ in a consistent AHP matrix. All the elements of the diagonal are 1 since the comparison of any criterion with itself is necessarily 1.

Figure 1. Architectural Diagram

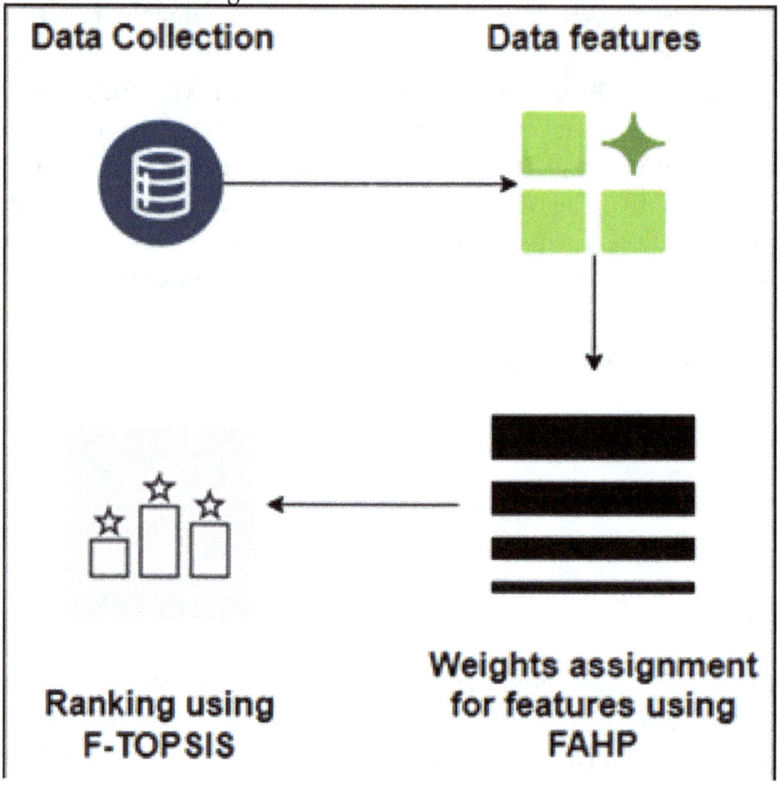

Figure 1 shows the overall architectural diagram for the FAHP with the Fuzzy TOPSIS model in MCDM for ranking pneumonia disease.

$$W = \frac{\overline{w}_i}{\sum_{i=1}^{n} \overline{w}_i} \tag{2}$$

Weight Calculation in fuzzy priority weight vector $\overline{w}_i = (\overline{w}_1, \overline{w}_2, \ldots, \overline{w}_n)$ similar equations The fuzzy eigenvector id of the matrix is used to compute weight calculation in equation 2. The fuzzy priority weight vector is obtained through normalization of the fuzzy eigenvector of B matrix. The weights of the various criteria can then be rounded to sharp values using one of the defuzzification methods, e.g. centroid method. TOPSIS will be applied to rank the various types of pneumonia based on the performance scores and the FAHP criterion weights. In order to normalize the choice matrix, the decision matrix, X R_{ij} in equation 3, is normalized, and the value Y_{ij} is the original value of the i th type of pneumonia in relation to the jth criterion.

$$R_{ij} = \frac{Y_{ij}}{\sqrt{\sum_{i=1}^{m} . Y_{ij}^2}} \quad (3)$$

FAHP obtains the weights W_j multiplied by the normalized matrix. V_{ij} equation 4 is the weighted normalized value of the ith type of pneumonia in the jth criterion

$$V_{ij} = R_{ij} \times W_j \quad (4)$$

Equations 5 and 6 of this paper can be used to determine what is known as the Positive Ideal Solution (PIS) and the Negative Ideal Solution (NIS). The PIS represents how closely an alternative is to achieving the highest possible level of desirability in terms of a defined criterion in a given situation, while the NIS reflects the lowest value that can be attained on that same scale when weighed against the worst possible outcome associated with the same alternative option. As a result, if we evaluate all the alternatives based upon these criteria, we would want to select the one that has the least distance from the PIS and the largest distance from the NIS.

Positive ideal solution A^+:

$$A^+ = \left(max\ V_{ij}\ if\, j\ is\ a\ benefit\ criterion\right) \quad (5)$$

Negative ideal solution A^-:

$$A^- = \left(min\ V_{ij}\ if\, j\ is\ a\ benefit\ criterion\right) \quad (6)$$

Calculate the positive distance ideal solution $D_i^+$and, the formulas are

$$D_i^+ = \sqrt{\sum_{j=1}^{n} (V_{ij} - A_j^+)^2} \quad (7)$$

$$D_i^- = \sqrt{\sum_{j=1}^{n} (V_{ij} - A_j^-)^2} \quad (8)$$

Closeness coefficient Cc of each alternative (pneumonia type) is obtained by applying equation 9, where Cc_i denotes the proximity of the ith pneumonia type to the ideal one. The closer the coefficient of closeness, the closer the pneumonia type is to the ideal solution, which implies that the former should be addressed initially.

$$Cc_i = \frac{D_i^-}{D_i^+ + D_i^-} \tag{9}$$

4. RESULTS AND DISCUSSION

Table 1. 5-Point Scale

Term	Fuzzy Number
Very Low - VL	1.0,1.0,3.0
Low - L	1.0,3.0,5.0
Medium - M	3.0,5.0,7.0
High - H	5.0,7.0,9.0
Very High - VH	7.0,7.0,9.0

Table 1 presents the fuzzy numbers that are allocated to the qualitative terms applied in making decisions or conducting an evaluation. Regarding every term, there is a fuzzy number expressed by triangular fuzzy sets (a, b, c) that are associated with the terms Very Low, Low, Medium, High, and Very High, respectively. These numbers come in handy to model uncertainty since they give a range of possible values rather than set numbers.

Table 2. Decision Maker-1 with their values

Diseases	SoB	CXrR	BTR	SC	IS
Bacterial Pneumonia (BP)	H	H	L	VH	VH
Viral Pneumonia (VP)	VH	VL	L	H	H
Mycoplasma Pneumonia (MP)	M	H	VH	M	VH
Fungal Pneumonia (FP)	L	VH	H	VH	VH
Aspiration Pneumonia (AP)	VL	VH	L	VL	VH

Legend: Shortness of Breath - *SoB*, Chest X-ray Results – *CXrR*, Blood Test Results - *BTR*, Sputum Culture - *SC*, Immunization Status – *IS*

Table 3. Decision Maker-2 with their values

Diseases	SoB	CXrR	BTR	SC	IS
Bacterial Pneumonia (BP)	L	L	M	M	VL
Viral Pneumonia (VP)	VL	H	H	VL	L
Mycoplasma Pneumonia (MP)	VH	VL	L	M	M
Fungal Pneumonia (FP)	M	L	M	VH	H
Aspiration Pneumonia (AP)	M	VH	VH	H	VH

Table 4. Decision Maker-3 with their values

Diseases	SoB	CXrR	BTR	SC	IS
Bacterial Pneumonia (BP)	VL	VL	M	L	VH
Viral Pneumonia (VP)	L	H	VL	H	VH
Mycoplasma Pneumonia (MP)	L	VH	H	VH	VH
Fungal Pneumonia (FP)	H	H	VH	VH	H
Aspiration Pneumonia (AP)	M	VH	VH	VL	L

The initial assessment of the various categories of pneumonia was completed by Decision Maker 1, Decision Maker 2, and Decision Maker 3, as shown in Table 2, Table 3, and Table 4, respectively. To determine the five types of pneumonia (e.g., tube, e.g., bacterial pneumonia, viral pneumonia, fungal pneumonia, and aspiration pneumonia), a panel of decision makers uses five evaluation criteria, which include shortness of breath, chest X-ray results, blood test results, sputum culture, and immunization status. Each of the panel members has evaluated their ratings through misleading language (i.e., "High," "Medium," "Very Low") on all five criteria to describe their rating. These three tables should not be interpreted as constraints on how a panel member will interpret their criteria but rather as a guideline that uses their opinion (with some degree of subjectivity and ambiguity).

Table 5. Convert into Fuzzy Values in Decision Maker-1

Diseases	SoB	CXrR	BTR	SC	IS
Bacterial Pneumonia (BP)	5.0, 7.0, 9.0	5.0, 7.0, 9.0	1.0, 3.0, 5.0	7.0, 7.0, 9.0	7.0, 7.0, 9.0
Viral Pneumonia (VP)	7.0, 7.0, 9.0	1.0, 1.0, 3.0	1.0, 3.0, 5.0	5.0, 7.0, 9.0	5.0, 7.0, 9.0
Mycoplasma Pneumonia (MP)	3.0, 5.0, 7.0	5.0, 7.0, 9.0	7.0, 7.0, 9.0	3.0, 5.0, 7.0	7.0, 7.0, 9.0
Fungal Pneumonia (FP)	1.0, 3.0, 5.0	7.0, 7.0, 9.0	5.0, 7.0, 9.0	7.0, 7.0, 9.0	7.0, 7.0, 9.0
Aspiration Pneumonia (AP)	1.0, 1.0, 3.0	7.0, 7.0, 9.0	1.0, 3.0, 5.0	1.0, 1.0, 3.0	7.0, 7.0, 9.0

Table 6. Convert into Fuzzy Values in Decision Maker-2

Diseases	SoB	CXrR	BTR	SC	IS
Bacterial Pneumonia (BP)	1.0, 3.0, 5.0	1.0, 3.0, 5.0	3.0, 5.0, 7.0	3.0, 5.0, 7.0	1.0, 1.0, 3.0
Viral Pneumonia (VP)	1.0, 1.0, 3.0	5.0, 7.0, 9.0	5.0, 7.0, 9.0	1.0, 1.0, 3.0	1.0, 3.0, 5.0
Mycoplasma Pneumonia (MP)	7.0, 7.0, 9.0	1.0, 1.0, 3.0	1.0, 3.0, 5.0	3.0, 5.0, 7.0	3.0, 5.0, 7.0
Fungal Pneumonia (FP)	3.0, 5.0, 7.0	1.0, 3.0, 5.0	3.0, 5.0, 7.0	7.0, 7.0, 9.0	5.0, 7.0, 9.0
Aspiration Pneumonia (AP)	3.0, 5.0, 7.0	7.0, 7.0, 9.0	7.0, 7.0, 9.0	5.0, 7.0, 9.0	7.0, 7.0, 9.0

Table 7. Convert into Fuzzy Values in Decision Maker-3

Diseases	SoB	CXrR	BTR	SC	IS
Bacterial Pneumonia (BP)	1.0, 1.0, 3.0	1.0, 1.0, 3.0	3.0, 5.0, 7.0	1.0, 3.0, 5.0	7.0, 7.0, 9.0
Viral Pneumonia (VP)	1.0, 3.0, 5.0	5.0, 7.0, 9.0	1.0, 1.0, 3.0	5.0, 7.0, 9.0	7.0, 7.0, 9.0
Mycoplasma Pneumonia (MP)	1.0, 3.0, 5.0	7.0, 7.0, 9.0	5.0, 7.0, 9.0	7.0, 7.0, 9.0	7.0, 7.0, 9.0
Fungal Pneumonia (FP)	5.0, 7.0, 9.0	5.0, 7.0, 9.0	7.0, 7.0, 9.0	7.0, 7.0, 9.0	5.0, 7.0, 9.0
Aspiration Pneumonia (AP)	3.0, 5.0, 7.0	7.0, 7.0, 9.0	7.0, 7.0, 9.0	1.0, 1.0, 3.0	1.0, 3.0, 5.0

In the case of Decision Makers 1, 2, and 3, Table 5, Table 6, and Table 7 present the translation of the language assessments in fuzzy numbers. The fuzzy value of (5, 7, 9) may represent a high rating. Such fuzzy numbers are used to denote the membership in a fuzzy collection. The process that lies behind these tables involves converting the qualitative assessments care of the numerical fuzzy sets in a manner that would enable the data to be mathematically operated under the FAHP-TOPSIS framework.

Table 8. Combined Decision Matrix

Diseases	SoB	CXrR	BTR	SC	IS
Bacterial Pneumonia (BP)	1.0, 3.67, 9.0	1.0, 3.67, 9.0	1.0, 4.33, 7.0	1.0, 5.0, 9.0	1.0, 5.0, 9.0
Viral Pneumonia (VP)	1.0, 3.67, 9.0	1.0, 5.0, 9.0	1.0, 3.67, 9.0	1.0, 5.0, 9.0	1.0, 5.67, 9.0
Mycoplasma Pneumonia (MP)	1.0, 5.0, 9.0	1.0, 5.0, 9.0	1.0, 5.67, 9.0	3.0, 5.67, 9.0	3.0, 6.33, 9.0
Fungal Pneumonia (FP)	1.0, 5.0, 9.0	1.0, 5.67, 9.0	3.0, 6.33, 9.0	7.0, 7.0, 9.0	5.0, 7.0, 9.0
Aspiration Pneumonia (AP)	1.0, 3.67, 7.0	7.0, 7.0, 9.0	1.0, 5.67, 9.0	1.0, 3.0, 9.0	1.0, 5.67, 9.0

Table 9. Combined Decision Matrix with weights

	Beneficial	Beneficial	Beneficial	Beneficial	Non-Beneficial
Weight	5.0, 7.0, 9.0	3.0, 5.0, 7.0	1.0, 3.0, 5.0	1.0, 1.0, 3.0	7.0, 7.0, 9.0

Diseases	SoB	CXrR	BTR	SC	IS
Bacterial Pneumonia (BP)	0.11, 0.41, 1.0	0.11, 0.41, 1.0	0.11, 0.48, 0.78	0.11, 0.56, 1.0	0.11, 0.20, 1.0
Viral Pneumonia (VP)	0.11, 0.41, 1.0	0.11, 0.56, 1.0	0.11, 0.41, 1.0	0.11, 0.56, 1.0	0.11, 0.18, 1.0
Mycoplasma Pneumonia (MP)	0.11, 0.56, 1.0	0.11, 0.56, 1.0	0.11, 0.63, 1.0	0.33, 0.63, 1.0	0.11, 0.16, 0.33
Fungal Pneumonia (FP)	0.11, 0.56, 1.0	0.11, 0.63, 1.0	0.33, 0.70, 1.0	0.78, 0.78, 1.0	0.11, 0.14, 0.20
Aspiration Pneumonia (AP)	0.11, 0.41, 1.0	0.78, 0.78, 1.0	0.11, 0.63, 1.0	0.11, 0.33, 1.0	0.11, 0.18, 1.0

Table 8 combines a fuzzy value decision matrix of all decision-makers and a normalization of their fuzzy values for the decision of each type of pneumonia based on the five criteria. The fuzzy ratings of all the decision-makers are merged into one and normalized so that they can be easily compared. Table 9 is utilized as a basis for computing the TOPSIS (Technique for Order of Preference by Similarity to Ideal Solution), whereby these normalized matrices now carry weights. The weights represent the relative importance of the different criteria, as determined through the FAHP procedure (Fuzzy Analytic Hierarchy Process). The weighted matrix is then utilized to calculate the distance between the best and worst solutions according to the data in these decision matrices. These weights indicate how each criterion was rated by each decision maker and indicate its importance in relation to all of the information gathered through the process of diagnosing pneumonia.

Table 10. Normalize the Fuzzy Decision Matrix

Diseases	SoB	CXrR	BTR	SC	IS
Bacterial Pneumonia (BP)	0.11, 0.41, 1.0	0.11, 0.41, 1.0	0.11, 0.48, 0.78	0.11, 0.56, 1.0	0.11, 0.20, 1.0
Viral Pneumonia (VP)	0.11, 0.41, 1.0	0.11, 0.56, 1.0	0.11, 0.41, 1.0	0.11, 0.56, 1.0	0.11, 0.18, 1.0
Mycoplasma Pneumonia (MP)	0.11, 0.56, 1.0	0.11, 0.56, 1.0	0.11, 0.63, 1.0	0.33, 0.63, 1.0	0.11, 0.16, 0.33

continued on following page

Table 10. Continued

Diseases	SoB	CXrR	BTR	SC	IS
Fungal Pneumonia (FP)	0.11, 0.56, 1.0	0.11, 0.63, 1.0	0.33, 0.70, 1.0	0.78, 0.78, 1.0	0.11, 0.14, 0.20
Aspiration Pneumonia (AP)	0.11, 0.41, 1.0	0.78, 0.78, 1.0	0.11, 0.63, 1.0	0.11, 0.33, 1.0	0.11, 0.18, 1.0

Table 11. Compute the weight

Diseases	SoB	CXrR	BTR	SC	IS
Bacterial Pneumonia (BP)	0.550, 2.871, 9.001	0.330, 2.051, 7.001	0.110, 1.441, 3.901	0.110, 0.561, 3.001	0.770, 1.401, 9.001
Viral Pneumonia (VP)	0.551, 2.872, 9.002	0.331, 2.801, 7.002	0.111, 1.231, 5.001	0.111, 0.562, 3.002	0.771, 1.261, 9.002
Mycoplasma Pneumonia (MP)	0.552, 3.921, 9.003	0.332, 2.802, 7.003	0.112, 1.891, 5.002	0.332, 0.631, 3.003	0.772, 1.121, 2.971
Fungal Pneumonia (FP)	0.553, 3.922, 9.004	0.333, 3.151, 7.004	0.333, 2.101, 5.003	0.781, 0.781, 3.004	0.773, 0.981, 1.801
Aspiration Pneumonia (AP)	0.554, 2.873, 9.005	2.341, 3.901, 7.005	0.113, 1.892, 5.004	0.113, 0.331, 3.005	0.113, 1.261, 9.006
A★ (FPIS)	0.555, 3.923, 9.006	2.342, 3.151, 7.006	0.334, 2.101, 5.005	0.782, 0.782, 3.006	0.774, 1.402, 9.007
A^- (FNIS)	0.556, 2.874, 9.007	0.334, 2.052, 7.007	0.114, 1.232, 3.902	0.114, 0.332, 3.007	0.114, 0.982, 1.802

Table 12. Fuzzy Positive ideal solution and Fuzzy Negative ideal solution (Distance Positive)

Diseases	SoB	CXrR	BTR	SC	IS
Bacterial Pneumonia (BP)	0.611	1.321	0.751	0.411	0.001
Viral Pneumonia (VP)	0.612	1.181	0.521	0.412	0.081
Mycoplasma Pneumonia (MP)	0.002	1.182	0.171	0.271	3.601
Fungal Pneumonia (FP)	0.003	1.161	0.002	0.002	4.161
Aspiration Pneumonia (AP)	0.003	1.571	0.741	0.003	0.161

Table 13. Fuzzy Positive ideal solution and Fuzzy Negative ideal solution (Distance Negative)

Diseases	SoB	CXrR	BTR	SC	IS
Bacterial Pneumonia (BP)	0.001	0.002	0.211	0.271	4.181
Viral Pneumonia (VP)	0.002	0.431	0.631	0.272	2.711
Mycoplasma Pneumonia (MP)	0.601	0.432	0.661	0.212	4.172
Fungal Pneumonia (FP)	0.602	0.632	0.811	0.461	0.771
Aspiration Pneumonia (AP)	0.003	1.571	0.741	0.003	0.161

Table 14. Total Distance of Positive and Negative

Diseases	D	D^-
Bacterial Pneumonia (BP)	3.531	2.921
Viral Pneumonia (VP)	4.351	2.271
Mycoplasma Pneumonia (MP)	2.031	3.671
Fungal Pneumonia (FP)	3.071	4.611
Aspiration Pneumonia (AP)	6.541	3.911

Table 15. Calculating Cci

Diseases	D	D^-	CC
Bacterial Pneumonia (BP)	3.091	4.661	3.871
Viral Pneumonia (VP)	2.801	4.041	2.281
Mycoplasma Pneumonia (MP)	5.221	6.071	5.641
Fungal Pneumonia (FP)	5.321	3.271	4.281
Aspiration Pneumonia (AP)	2.161	2.471	2.311

Table 16. Final Ranking

Diseases	Cci	Ranks
Bacterial Pneumonia (BP)	3.871	3
Viral Pneumonia (VP)	2.281	5
Mycoplasma Pneumonia (MP)	5.643	1

continued on following page

Table 16. Continued

Diseases	Cci	Ranks
Fungal Pneumonia (FP)	4.282	2
Aspiration Pneumonia (AP)	2.312	4

The distributions between every type of pneumonia and the positive ideal solution (PIS) and negative ideal solution (NIS) are represented in Table 10 and Table 11. The tables are aimed at calculating the distance between each variant of pneumonia and the best (PIS) and worst outcomes (NIS). The distance between the nodes is then used to compute the proximity coefficient.

Table 12 and Table 13 provide the proximity coefficients for each type of pneumonia to measure how closely these bacteria are to being ideal candidates for treatment. The proximity coefficients play a key role in ranking the types of pneumonia in terms of their proximity to an ideal pneumonia type. CCI values can be found in Table 15, which indicates how far the bacteria are away and, therefore, the order that they should be treated in. Table 16 gives our experimental data on how we ranked the bacteria to be treated and gives physicians vital information as to what types of pneumonia to treat first.

5. CONCLUSION

The overall findings of this study show that the combination of fuzzy sets, FAHP, and TOPSIS allowed comparisons of the various types of pneumonia and a subjective evaluation of the decision makers to make an accurate classification. The processes outlined in this study provided an avenue to convert qualitative data to fuzzy values. The application of the multi-criteria framework allowed for addressing the uncertainty associated with the diagnosis of a disease through this process, and as a result of this study, it has been successfully developed to classify each type of pneumonia based upon five important variables: (1) degree of shortness of breath, (2) chest X-ray results, (3) blood analysis results, (4) results of sputum culture, and (5) the immunization record. The decision matrices that were produced by this study have established a systematic means to compare and rank the various pneumonia types with consideration given to symptoms and supporting diagnostic information. The analysis indicates that the decision-making approach is stable when the decision-making process is uncertain and the medical data required is not available. It may be possible to extend and generalize this model to other medical conditions as a practical tool for health care professionals to systematically make multi-criteria decisions to arrive at a more accurately identified diagnosis.

6. FUTURE WORK

By utilizing a broader and more diverse clinical dataset collected from actual hospital environments, this framework may be tested more thoroughly for robustness and generalization. In addition to existing diagnostic criteria, the proposed framework will be further improved by being supplemented with other diagnostic information such as the patient's age and associated diseases, their level of oxygen saturation, and radiological severity scores, to create a more complete clinical picture of patients. Next, the proposed framework could also be coupled with either machine learning or the deep learning approaches to automatically extract relevant features from electronic health records and medical imaging data, thus allowing for semi-automated or real-time decision support. Finally, future research could begin to explore other mathematical fuzzy model numbers, such as interval type-2 fuzzy numbers, Pythagorean fuzzy numbers, and spherical fuzzy numbers, as well as other methods by which to quantify or measure consensus, which would improve how uncertainty is dealt with and the level of agreement between decision-makers in regard to complex medical diagnostic problems.

REFERENCES

Al-Thani, N. A., Al-Ansari, T., & Haouari, M. (2022). Integrated TOPSIS-COV approach for selecting a sustainable PET waste management technology: A case study in Qatar. *Heliyon*, *8*(8), e10274. Advance online publication. DOI: 10.1016/j.heliyon.2022.e10274 PMID: 36061036

Ali, A. M., Abdelhafeez, A., Soliman, T. H., & ELMenshawy, K. (2024). A probabilistic hesitant fuzzy MCDM approach to selecting treatment policy for COVID-19. Decision making: applications in management and engineering, 7(1), 131-144. DOI: 10.31181/dmame712024917

Arslan, A. E., Arslan, O., & Kandemir, S. Y. (2021). AHP–TOPSIS hybrid decision-making analysis: Simav integrated system case study. *Journal of Thermal Analysis and Calorimetry*, *145*(3), 1191–1202. Advance online publication. DOI: 10.1007/s10973-020-10270-4

Ayan, E., & Ünver, H. M. (2019, April). Diagnosis of pneumonia from chest X-ray images using deep learning. In 2019 Scientific meeting on electrical-electronics & biomedical engineering and computer science (EBBT) (pp. 1-5). Ieee. DOI: 10.1109/EBBT.2019.8741582

Azari, A., Nabizadeh, R., Mahvi, A. H., & Nasseri, S. (2022). Integrated Fuzzy AHP-TOPSIS for selecting the best color removal process using carbon-based adsorbent materials: Multi-criteria decision making vs. systematic review approaches and modeling of textile wastewater treatment in real conditions. *International Journal of Environmental Analytical Chemistry*, *102*(18), 7329–7344. DOI: 10.1080/03067319.2020.1828395

Basu, D., Kashid, S., Pawar, S., & Datta, D. (2020, December). An integrated detection and treatment recommendation framework for breast cancer using convolutional neural networks and TOPSIS. In 2020 IEEE 17th India Council International Conference (INDICON) (pp. 1-7). IEEE. DOI: 10.1109/INDICON49873.2020.9342266

Dinesh, & Kumar, S. (2024). Integrated VIKOR-TOPSIS strategy based on picture fuzzy knowledge and accuracy measures with application in waste-water treatment. Evolutionary Intelligence, 17(5), 3891-3920. DOI: 10.1007/s12065-024-00963-2

Ho, L. H., Lin, Y. L., & Chen, T. Y. (2020). A Pearson-like correlation-based TOPSIS method with interval-valued Pythagorean fuzzy uncertainty and its application to multiple criteria decision analysis of stroke rehabilitation treatments. *Neural Computing & Applications*, *32*(12), 8265–8295. DOI: 10.1007/s00521-019-04304-8

Li, H., Yazdi, M., Huang, C. G., & Peng, W. (2022). A reliable probabilistic risk-based decision-making method: Bayesian Technique for Order of Preference by Similarity to Ideal Solution (B-TOPSIS). *Soft Computing, 26*(22), 12137–12153. DOI: 10.1007/s00500-022-07462-5

Liu, X., Peng, Y., Yang, Q., Wang, X., & Cui, N. (2021). Determining optimal deficit irrigation and fertilization to increase mango yield, quality, and WUE in a dry hot environment based on TOPSIS. *Agricultural Water Management, 245*, 106650. DOI: 10.1016/j.agwat.2020.106650

Malekpoor, H., Mishra, N., & Kumar, S. (2022). A novel TOPSIS–CBR goal programming approach to sustainable healthcare treatment. *Annals of Operations Research, 312*(2), 1403–1425. DOI: 10.1007/s10479-018-2992-y

Malekpoor, H., Mishra, N., Sumalya, S., & Kumari, S. (2017). An efficient approach to radiotherapy dose planning problem: A TOPSIS case-based reasoning approach. *International Journal of Systems Science: Operations & Logistics, 4*(1), 4–12. DOI: 10.1080/23302674.2015.1135354

Omrani, H., Alizadeh, A., & Emrouznejad, A. (2018). Finding the optimal combination of power plants alternatives: A multi response Taguchi-neural network using TOPSIS and fuzzy best-worst method. *Journal of Cleaner Production, 203*, 210–223. DOI: 10.1016/j.jclepro.2018.08.238

Pramanik, R., Dey, S., Malakar, S., Mirjalili, S., & Sarkar, R. (2022). TOPSIS aided ensemble of CNN models for screening COVID-19 in chest X-ray images. *Scientific Reports, 12*(1), 15409. DOI: 10.1038/s41598-022-18463-7 PMID: 36104401

Sabaghi, M., Mascle, C., & Baptiste, P. (2015). Application of DOE-TOPSIS technique in decision-making problems. *IFAC-PapersOnLine, 48*(3), 773–777. DOI: 10.1016/j.ifacol.2015.06.176

Štirbanović, Z., Gardić, V., Stanujkić, D., Marković, R., Soković, J., & Stevanović, Z. (2021). Comparative MCDM analysis for AMD treatment method selection. *Water Resources Management, 35*(11), 3737–3753. DOI: 10.1007/s11269-021-02914-3

Sun, X., Douiri, A., & Gulliford, M. (2022). Applying machine learning algorithms to electronic health records to predict pneumonia after respiratory tract infection. *Journal of Clinical Epidemiology, 145*, 154–163. DOI: 10.1016/j.jclinepi.2022.01.009 PMID: 35045315

. Terry, A. F., Etikan, İ., & Sancar, N. (2024). A Different Perspective for Determining the Optimal Treatment Modality in the Treatment of GERD: An Application of the Fuzzy TOPSIS Method Determining the Optimal Treatment Modality in the Treatment of GERD Using Fuzzy TOPSIS Method. DOI: 10.4274/cjms.2024.2024-22

Wang, Y., Liu, Z. L., Yang, H., Li, R., Liao, S. J., Huang, Y., Peng, M.-H., Liu, X., Si, G.-Y., He, Q.-Z., & Zhang, Y. (2024). Prediction of viral pneumonia based on machine learning models analyzing pulmonary inflammation index scores. *Computers in Biology and Medicine*, *169*, 107905. DOI: 10.1016/j.compbiomed.2023.107905 PMID: 38159398

Chapter 5
Healthcare-Based IoB-Driven Continuous Monitoring, Early Prediction, and Better Outcomes

Kathirvel Ayyaswamy
http://orcid.org/0000-0002-5347-9110
Department of Computer Science and Engineering, Saveetha Engineering College, Chennai, India

ABSTRACT

This paper explores how the Internet of Bodies (IoB) can support continuous observation, early prediction of health risks, and improved outcomes for patients, clinicians, and health systems. We first outline the evolution from general Internet of Things (IoT) technologies to IoB in healthcare, and describe the main categories of IoB devices and the types of data they generate. Building on this, we show how continuous streams of physiological, behavioural, and contextual data can be transformed into meaningful insights and risk signals that enable proactive, rather than reactive, care. A conceptual "Monitor–Understand–Act–Learn" framework is proposed to explain how IoB systems collect data, interpret patterns, trigger timely actions, and improve over time through feedback. The paper also examines key benefits, such as better chronic disease management and more personalised support, alongside major challenges related to privacy, security, equity, and usability.

DOI: 10.4018/979-8-3373-8247-0.ch005

1. INTRODUCTION

Building on this foundation, the Internet of Medical Things (IoMT) explicitly connects medical devices, wearables, and clinical information systems, creating integrated digital health ecosystems that can improve access, efficiency, and personalization of care (Matthew et al., 2025; Huang et al., 2023). Healthcare is moving from episodic, hospital-based encounters toward continuous, data-driven care that follows people through their daily lives. Connected sensors, mobile devices, and cloud platforms already underpin the Internet of Things (IoT) in healthcare, enabling remote monitoring, telemedicine, and smart hospital workflows (Singh et al., 2023; Zhu & Zhu, 2023).

The Internet of Bodies (IoB) can be seen as the next step in this evolution. Instead of focusing only on "things," IoB centers the human body and behavior as the interface, connecting networks of devices on, in, and around the body that continuously sense physiological signals, movements, and contexts. Boddington (2021) describes the IoB as the blending of our physical and data selves, where bodies become active nodes in digital networks. Technical work on bioelectronic sensor nodes for the IoB emphasizes ultra-low-power sensing, secure communication, and on-body energy harvesting, so that implants and wearables can operate continuously and safely as part of a dense body-centric network (Chatterjee et al., 2022). Recent reviews further argue that the convergence of micro-electro-mechanical systems (MEMS), bio-MEMS, and networked interfaces enables truly personalized medicine when these devices are integrated into IoB architectures (Marinescu et al., 2025; Mazzeo & dos Santos, 2025)

Several forces are pushing healthcare toward such IoB-driven models. Globally, chronic diseases, aging populations, and workforce shortages are straining health systems, making it difficult to provide timely, high-quality care through traditional, visit-based models alone (Zhu & Zhu, 2023; Singh et al., 2023). IoT and IoMT reviews consistently highlight remote patient monitoring, home-based care, and telehealth as key strategies to reduce hospitalizations, shorten length of stay, and maintain care continuity for people with long-term conditions (Matthew et al., 2025; International Journal of Science and Research Archive [IJSRA], 2024). At the same time, patient expectations have shifted: many now expect care that is more proactive, personalized, and responsive to their everyday lived experience rather than confined to short clinical encounters.

IoB adds two important shifts on top of conventional IoT/IoMT. First, it tightens the coupling between physiological signals, behavior, and digital records. Wearable and implantable sensors can stream high-resolution heart rate, respiratory rate, activity patterns, and sleep metrics; smartphones and ambient sensors contribute contextual cues such as location, environment, and social rhythms (Taherdoost, 2024; Shajari et al., 2023). Second, analytics increasingly move closer to the body. Edge and on-device intelligence mean that basic pattern recognition and anomaly detection can happen in near-real time, enabling feedback, alerts, and micro-interventions without waiting for periodic clinic visits or centralized batch processing (Chatterjee et al., 2022; Matthew et al., 2025).

A recent hospital study using wearable sensors for continuous vital sign tracking showed that such systems can reliably measure heart rate, respiratory rate, and temperature in acutely unwell patients and support earlier recognition of clinical deterioration and virtual ward models (Joshi et al., 2025). Literature reviews of IoT-based vital sign monitoring similarly report that body-worn and home-based sensors can reduce the gaps between measurements, enable trend analysis, and improve clinician situational awareness, though they also caution about data overload and alarm fatigue (Andrade et al., 2024; Taherdoost, 2024). Remote patient monitoring programs that integrate these data streams into telehealth workflows are already being used to support chronic disease management and post-discharge follow-up and are expected to play a central role in value-based care models (Dubey & Tiwari, 2023; Schultz, 2023).

From a technology perspective, IoB-enabled healthcare sits at the intersection of IoMT, wearables, artificial intelligence, and cloud/edge computing. IoMT reviews describe architectures that combine body area networks, secure gateways, and cloud platforms to collect and analyze medical data across home, community, and hospital environments (Matthew et al., 2025; Huang et al., 2023). In parallel, work on AI-based wearable sensors shows how machine learning can turn raw signals into actionable insights, such as detecting arrhythmias, gait changes, or early signs of respiratory compromise in an unobtrusive way (Shajari et al., 2023).

The data involved are deeply intimate: heart rhythms, glucose levels, sleep stages, movement patterns, stress markers, and even implant telemetry can reveal not only health status but daily routines and behaviors. Reviews of IoT in healthcare repeatedly highlight privacy, security, interoperability, and governance as persistent challenges (Singh et al., 2023; IJSRA, 2024). IoMT surveys stress that, without strong security and explainability, large-scale medical device networks could expose patients to cyber-attacks or erode trust in digital health services (Matthew et al., 2025). Boddington's (2021) work on IoB underscores broader ethical questions about data ownership, bodily autonomy, and the risk that continuous body data may feed new forms of surveillance or "prediction economies" if not carefully regulated.

Existing literature tends to fall into two camps. On one side are highly technical treatments focused on hardware, communication protocols, and low-level optimization of IoMT/IoB components (Chatterjee et al., 2022; Marinescu et al., 2025). On the other are broad IoT/IoMT or IoB conceptual and ethical discussions that describe potential opportunities and risks at a high level (Singh et al., 2023; Zhu &

Zhu, 2023; Boddington, 2021). There is comparatively less work aimed at clinicians, health-system leaders, and policy makers that connects the technical capabilities of IoB with concrete care pathways, outcome measures, and practical design choices in a clear, non-technical way (Matthew et al., 2025; Huang et al., 2023; Taherdoost, 2024; Shajari et al., 2023).

Figure 1. IoB-driven healthcare overview

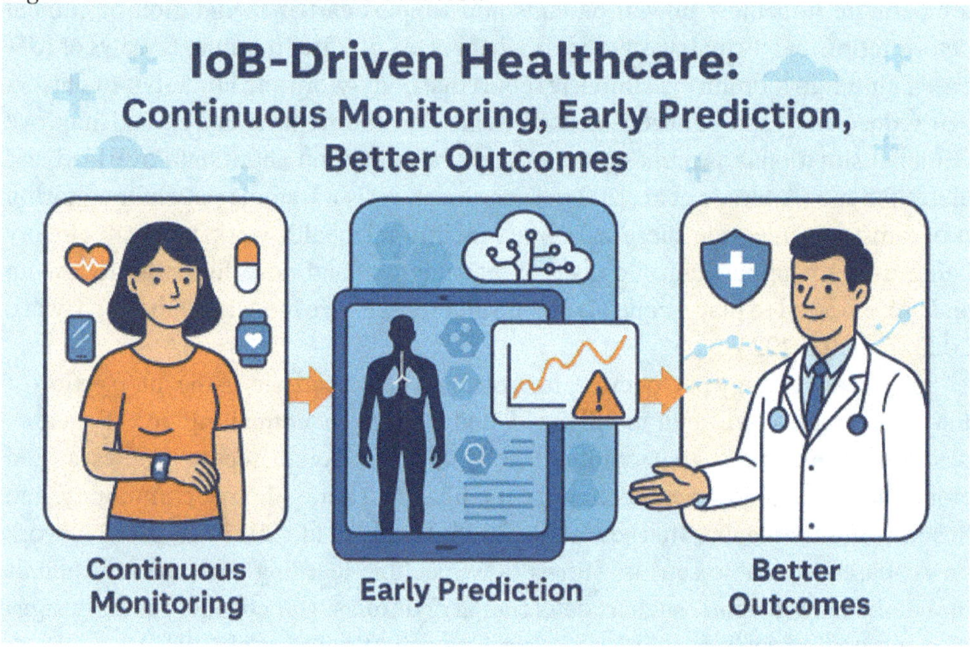

The illustration shows how continuous monitoring with body-worn and ambient Internet of Bodies (IoB) devices feeds data into cloud and edge analytics for early risk prediction, which in turn supports clinicians in making proactive decisions that improve patient outcomes.

2. BACKGROUND: FROM IOT TO IOB IN HEALTHCARE

The journey from IoT to IoMT to IoB is nothing but a gradual procedure through which different technologies in the digital world are getting more and more submerged into a human body-related affair in the area of health care. When the Internet of Things (IoT) was introduced in the healthcare field, the focus was on securing access to bedside monitors, infusion pumps, and hospital equipment externally, in order that one could easily collect data automatically and share it with information systems. Extensive reviews indicate that the IoT in healthcare has matured into a research field encompassing everything from industrial processes to getting smart wards and monitoring vital signs remotely (Rejeb et al., 2023; Singh, 2023). As a result, these systems have already altered healthcare workflows in continuous data acquisition, resource visibility, and replaced manual data entries.

According to recent studies, equipment in hospitals supporting the locations, environment monitoring and location of patients or staff, were now implemented involving numerous communication technologies and sensitive modalities, like RFID, Bluetooth, Wi-Fi, low-power wide-area networks, etc. (Felix & Martins, 2024). Healthcare IoT, which is in its "first generation," is connecting devices around the patient rather than on or in the patient.

A newer concept, that directly addresses the patient-centric needs much more specifically, is known as the Internet of Medical Things. IoMT is a special IoT that includes medical devices, sensors, actuators and clinical systems in a patient-centred architecture (Al Khatib et al., 2024). Reports on IoMT architectures tend to be layered in their approach. This typically entails a perception layer containing medical sensors (ECG, blood pressure, oxygen saturation, etc) and a network layer routing through a gateway. In turn, the data find their way into the application layer which incorporates the information into electronic health records (EHR) and clinical platforms (He et al., 2024; Naghib et al., 2025). In contrast with generic IoT, IoMT must often comply with medical regulations and safety constraints. It has stringent requirements for reliability and latency. Any failure can directly impact a diagnosis or treatment.

The research on IoMT has risen exponentially in the past few years due to the emergence of remote patient monitoring, chronic disease management, telemedicine. Systematic reviews indicate the increasing usage of IoMT for continuous monitoring and management of conditions such as hypertension, diabetes, heart failure, and respiratory disorders (El-deep et al., 2025; Matthew et al., 2025). A lot of these systems use wearable sensors and home monitoring kits linked to the cloud platform. These systems have the ability to automatically measure intelligence. They can analyze for early signs of decompensation. They alert clinicians in advance of impending crises. They also endorse "hospital at home" designs that let stable patients stay home while still under supervision from care teams in parallel. He et al. (2024); Ahmed et al. (2025) state that emerging IoMT applications combine sensor data with AI, as well as machine learning with the aim of providing risk predictions, personalizing treatment plans, or using resources more efficiently.

As IoMT devices get deployed within hospitals, at homes, and even the community settings, their security and privacy requirement become more complex. IoMT environments have less patching and securing of large numbers of heterogeneous mobile ad hoc networks with often resource-constrained devices than classical clinical systems. In a systematic review on intrusion detection in IoMT, a vast range of attacks; device, network and application layer attacks have been discussed. Attacks which include medical devices and data flows comprise eavesdropping, spoofing, denial-of-service and ransomware (Naghib et al., 2025). Due to their sensitive nature and continuous streaming, IoMT data need lighter mechanisms that include cryptography, blockchain-trace audit, AI-based intrusion detection, and other mechanisms to reduce performance impact (El-deep et al., 2025; He et al., 2024). Connecting even more medical devices raises not just technical problems but also governance and trust problems, these issues bring to light.

The Internet of Bodies is the latest advancement of Internet of Things (IoT) and Internet of Medical Things (IoMT). The Internet of Bodies is digital systems applied to and inside the human body. The Internet of Bodies is networks of devices worn on the body, embedded under the skin, or even located inside organs that continuously sense biological signals, and in some cases enable actuation, such as drug delivery or neuromodulation (Datta & Sen, 2023). IoMT refers to medical devices that can physically distance from the patient, such as smart hospital beds and connected imaging equipment. However, IoB pertains to devices that have intimate physical contact with the person, which means being part of the body's extended sensorimotor loop. This covers top-of-the-line wearables including implantable cardiac monitors, neuro stimulators, smart prosthetics, and ingestible sensors that send data after they are swallowed.

According to the expert, microelectronics, MEMS, BioMEMS, and flexible electronics will enable the Internet of Body (IoB). Sensors that can distinguish between very subtle changes are now available as soft, skin-conformable patches or as micro scale implants. They are capable of measuring fine physiological details such as multi-lead ECG, intracranial pressure, local biochemical markers and complex motion. This has been stated by Marinescu and others in 2025 as well as Liu and Liu in 2025. At the same time, body-heat thermoelectric generators and motion-energy harvesting to deliver sustainable power with a view to reducing battery dependency to achieve more practical continuous monitoring (Tabaie & Omidvar, 2023).

In a nutshell, IoB underscores a transition from "around-the-patient" monitoring to "with-the-patient" and "in-the-patient" integration. Previously, external gadgets such as smartwatches and fitness bands were more commonly deployed to get the basic parameters like steps or heartbeat (Khan & Alam, 2021). IoB takes this concept even further by using technology for embedding intelligence into devices that restore or augment bodily functions, including smart prosthetic limbs, biofeedback systems for rehabilitation, and implantable pumps or stimulators that adapt therapy in real time (Marinescu et al., 2025). This can enable highly personalized treatment in healthcare, such as dynamically titrated drug delivery for Parkinson's disease, responsive neuromodulation for epilepsy, or adaptive cardiac pacing guided by real-time physiological feedback.

Researchers discuss how IoB complicates existing frameworks for privacy, data ownership, and responsibility, as the distinction between person and device becomes blurred (El-Khoury & Arikan, 2021; Datta & Sen, 2023). People also worry that the super-detailed biometrics and behavioral data collected by IoB devices could be used for more than just health care targeting marketing, insurance profiling, even surveillance, unless precautions are set to prevent it.

In summary, the path of development from IoT to IoMT and then IoB in healthcare depicts a gradual trend towards deeper interconnection of digital systems with the human body. The first example of IOT in Healthcare connects environments and equipment. IoMT includes clinical-grade devices that directly connect with patients' data and care pathways. IoB takes this idea a step further, creating devices that actually become part of the body's structure. Every phase along this spectrum provides more comprehensive, detailed information and more potent actions. However, it also raises additional risk layers which include safety, cybersecurity, and ethical concerns (Ahmed et al., 2025; El-deep et al., 2025). Because of this, the need for frameworks that utilize IoB to support continuous monitoring, early prediction, and improved outcomes is underscored while respecting human dignity, privacy, and equity. The remainder of the article discusses this evolution and shows how it is possible to design IoB-driven systems that provide clinically meaningful benefits without overwhelming patients, clinicians or health systems.

3. CONTINUOUS MONITORING IN IOB-DRIVEN HEALTHCARE

Continuous monitoring is the practical backbone of IoB-driven healthcare. Instead of checking vital signs or behaviors a few times a day, sensors embedded in wearables, beds, phones, and home devices stream data almost continuously. This shift from episodic to near real-time observation is what allows the system to spot subtle deteriorations, nudge healthy behaviors, and support earlier intervention.

In hospital wards, continuous vital sign monitoring is being used to close the "critical care gap" between the ICU and general wards. Traditional practice still relies on nurses checking vital signs every 4–8 hours and using paper or electronic early warning scores to detect deterioration. This creates long blind spots in which hypoxia, hypotension, or arrhythmias can go undetected. Recent work shows that wearable or contactless systems can dramatically increase the detection of abnormal vital signs and may improve outcomes. A 2025 propensity-matched analysis of surgical patients found that continuous wireless ward monitoring was associated with reduced odds of ICU admission and mortality compared with standard intermittent monitoring (Rowland et al., 2025). A 2024 systematic review and meta-analysis focusing on randomized trials similarly concluded that continuous monitoring on general wards tends to reduce rapid response activations and may shorten length of stay, although the effect on mortality is still uncertain (Bowles et al., 2024). Together, these studies support the idea that continuous data streams can change the trajectory of in-hospital deterioration, even if the exact magnitude of benefit is still being quantified.

New generations of sensors are making this kind of ward-level continuous monitoring far more practical. Portable wireless systems can be worn on the arm, chest, or finger and transmit heart rate, blood pressure surrogates, respiratory rate, and oxygen saturation without tethering the patient to bedside monitors. A 2025 review in BJA Education describes how lightweight wearable patches and portable hubs can maintain near ICU-level surveillance while allowing patients to mobilize, which is critical for recovery (Hicks et al., 2025) (de Waal et al., 2025). From a clinician's perspective, continuous sensors are increasingly seen as a key step in reducing unrecognized deterioration on general wards and even step-down or telemetry units (Michard & Saugel, 2025).

A 2024 study from an Indian tertiary hospital used such a system (Dozee-EWS) to monitor 706 general-ward patients over more than 84,000 hours. Patients who later deteriorated generated substantially more alerts, and the system typically detected concerning trends about 16 hours before clinician-recognized deterioration (Yadav et al., 2024). This kind of contactless continuous monitoring fits very naturally into an IoB architecture: it observes physiology and behavior (lying vs sitting, restlessness) passively, feeds those signals into cloud-based analytics, and returns risk scores and alerts that can guide bedside teams.

The same logic extends beyond hospital walls into chronic disease management at home. IoB-driven remote patient monitoring (RPM) combines home sensors, wearables, and communication platforms so that clinicians can follow patients between visits. A 2025 viewpoint in the Journal of Medical Internet Research highlights RPM as a central tool for chronic disease care in the United States, with rapidly growing deployment in conditions such as heart failure, diabetes, and hypertension (Paul et al., 2025). For chronic obstructive pulmonary disease (COPD), mini-review evidence shows that remote wearables and home oximetry can help detect exacerbations earlier, using changes in respiratory rate, activity patterns, and oxygen saturation to flag high-risk periods (Coutu et al., 2023).

Wearable-based continuous monitoring is not limited to "hard" physiological vital signs. It increasingly tracks functional status and fatigue, which are important for people with chronic disease, shift workers, and older adults. A recent open-access review in Computers in Biology and Medicine synthesizes how multi-modal wearables (measuring ECG, EMG, PPG, motion, and sleep) plus AI can continuously estimate physical and cognitive fatigue, enabling earlier interventions in safety-critical jobs and long-term illness (Kakhi et al., 2025). This kind of monitoring fits neatly into IoB because it links bodily signals with behavior and context: how long someone has been awake, how intensely they have been working, and how their physiological reserves are responding refer Figure 2.

Figure 2. Continuous monitoring workflow in IoB-driven healthcare

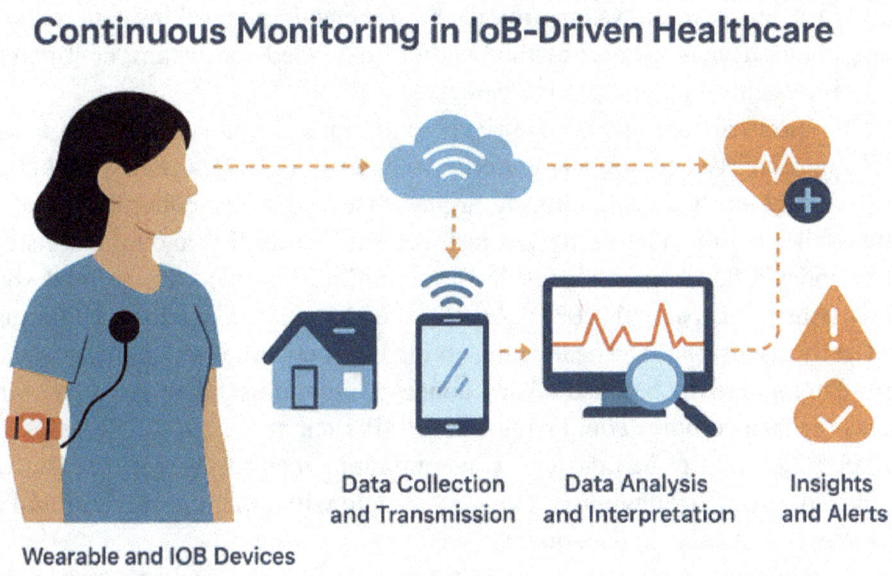

Under the IoB umbrella, all of these streams—vital signs, movement, sleep, social activity—are processed to derive "digital biomarkers" and "digital phenotypes." These are algorithmic features that reflect health states more directly than raw data. A 2025 systematic review in Artificial Intelligence Review shows how passive, non-invasive signals from wearables and smartphones (such as accelerometer data, heart rate variability, and passive activity traces) can be used with machine learning to predict cardiovascular events, neurodegenerative disease progression, stress, and other outcomes in a continuous way (Sameh et al., 2025). The review emphasizes that continuous, passive sensing is particularly well suited to IoB because it does not require active input from patients and can monitor subtle trends over weeks or months rather than single "snapshot" measurements.

Mental and behavioral health are especially strong examples of IoB-style continuous monitoring. Instead of relying only on clinic questionnaires, mental health researchers now use passive sensing from phones and wearables—location variability, call and text patterns, screen time, sleep and activity rhythms—to infer mood and symptom trajectories. A 2025 scoping review in J Med Internet Res summarizes dozens of studies where such data, analyzed with machine learning, were used to monitor depression, anxiety, psychosis, and stress in real-world settings (Shen et al., 2025). A companion commentary in JAMA Network Open discusses how passive smartphone sensing can track broad psychopathology dimensions, but also warns about pitfalls such as data quality, interpretability, and the risk of over-surveillance, and outlines design principles for responsible clinical integration (Webb & Fisher, 2025). In IoB terms, these systems treat everyday behaviors—walking patterns, sleep timing, phone usage—as part of the "body's" extended sensorium, continuously feeding information into predictive models.

At the infrastructure level, IoB-driven continuous monitoring depends heavily on IoT connectivity and human-centred system design. A 2024 review on human-centred IoT-based health monitoring argues that long-term, continuous systems must be tailored to patient needs, not just technical feasibility, and highlights gaps in how today's deployments consider user burden, interface design, and social context (Rashid & Nemati, 2024). Another 2024 article in Intelligent Pharmacy specifically discusses IoT in healthcare, noting how networked devices can simplify day-to-day monitoring but also raising concerns around usability and safety when patients manage complex equipment at home (Parihar et al., 2024). These insights are directly relevant to IoB designs: if a continuous monitoring system is uncomfortable, confusing, or obviously "spying," people will either not use it or will use it in ways that undermine data quality.

As the number of continuous sensors increases, so does the need for robust medical sensing and analytics. Recent reviews on emerging medical sensing technologies describe how smart textiles, implantables, and multi-analyte biosensors are being combined with AI to enable truly continuous, real-time health monitoring for cardiovascular disease, diabetes, and infectious diseases (Kirubakaran, 2025; Soumma et al., 2025)(de Waal et al., 2025; Hicks et al., 2025). Continuous IoB monitoring only adds value if the underlying signals are trustworthy.

The presence of rich, continuous streams poses challenges for interpreting work processes. Meta-analytic work indicates that continuous monitoring detects more variances and may reduce adverse events. However, the effects on hard outcomes depend on the incorporation of alerts into clinical workflow (Bowles et al., 2024). If continuous monitoring does not come with intelligent alerting, it will generate more false alarms leading to alarm fatigue and staff frustration. According to Michard and Saugel (2025), as clinician-oriented commentaries reveal, the current focus is on evolving from historical threshold-based systems to trend-based, multivariate risk score and AI-enabled early warning systems. This, in turn, would focus on combinations of vital signs, with an eye on their trajectories and the relevant baseline pertinent to the patient. There is a similar issue with issues around home RPM. In a 2025 perspective, it is noted that whether or not metrics can be aligned with reimbursement, staffing models, and follow-up pathways, there are not only technical means to stream more and more numbers from people's homes (Paul et al. 2025).

When constant monitoring shifts to the IoB space, privacy, security, and ethics become critical issues. Constant data collection could be able to bring out sensitive information about routine, mental health and social behaviour. According to recent reviews (Parihar et al., 2024; IoT privacy review, 2025).. They also suggest framing clinical deployment as a tool to collaborate but not as surveillance (Webb & Fisher, 2025; Shen et al. 2025). You cannot view these factors as optional. They determine whether continuous IoB systems can be acceptable to patients or clinicians in the first place.

In summary, continuous monitoring transforms IoB-driven healthcare from a static record of past encounters into a living, dynamic representation of each person's physiology and behavior. On hospital wards, it promises earlier detection of deterioration and more efficient allocation of staff time. At home, it enables long-term management of chronic diseases, tracking of fatigue and function, and more responsive mental health care. Wearable and contactless sensors, IoT connectivity, and AI-driven analytics together convert raw data streams into digital biomarkers that can support earlier, more personalized interventions. The evidence base is still evolving and not every deployment improves outcomes by default, but continuous monitoring clearly provides the raw material on which IoB-driven prediction and decision-support systems can be built. The next step, explored in subsequent sections, is how to turn these continuous signals into reliable early warnings and targeted behavioral feedback that truly improve patient outcomes.

4. EARLY PREDICTION AND PROACTIVE CARE

Early prediction is the part of IoB-driven healthcare that really changes the story from "treating sickness" to "protecting health." Once continuous behavioural and physiological data are available, the natural next step is to ask whether subtle changes in these signals can warn clinicians before a crisis appears. Modern digital biomarkers combine heart rate, activity patterns, sleep, mood, medication adherence and environmental context into risk profiles that can be updated hour by hour. Recent work on digital biomarkers for chronic diseases shows how wearable and smartphone-derived signals can be transformed into early warning indicators that support a predictive, preventive and personalised medicine paradigm.

4.1 Digital biomarkers and risk stratification

Reviews of digital biomarker platforms highlight how combinations of heart-rate variability, sleep architecture, gait stability and self-reported symptoms can be used to cluster patients into low-, medium- and high-risk groups that change dynamically over time.

These risk estimates become more powerful when sophisticated analytics are added. Network meta-analyses of machine-learning models for sepsis prediction, for example, show that neural networks and decision-tree–based methods can outperform traditional scoring systems such as SOFA, qSOFA and NEWS in terms of discrimination. However, the same work also underlines that the prediction window matters: algorithms tend to be more accurate in the short term than when they attempt to forecast events many hours in advance. In other words, early prediction is not magic foresight; it is a careful balance between lead time and reliability.

4.2 Predicting deterioration in acute care

In acute settings, early prediction is often framed in terms of early warning scores. Large comparative studies in hospital wards have evaluated several artificial-intelligence-based scores against simpler, transparent tools such as NEWS and NEWS2. The findings are nuanced. Some machine-learning models, such as eCART, achieve higher accuracy and can identify more patients who will deteriorate within the next day, while triggering fewer false alarms.

4.3 Predicting exacerbations in chronic disease

Early prediction is equally important for long-term conditions, where the goal is to avoid slow, cumulative damage and sudden exacerbations. Heart failure is a clear example. Reviews of remote multiparametric monitoring through cardiac implantable electronic devices show that combining several sensor streams—intrathoracic impedance, heart rate, activity level, arrhythmia burden and respiratory patterns—can detect subclinical congestion well before the patient feels short of breath. More recent work on remote monitoring in heart failure reports algorithms that can predict hospitalisation risk weeks in advance, sometimes with average lead times of more than a month, allowing time to adjust medication, reinforce self-care and schedule earlier follow-up.

IoB extends this concept beyond implantable devices. Reviews of chronic-disease monitoring using IoT mobile sensing describe how home blood-pressure monitors, smart scales, spirometers, glucometers and environmental sensors can be linked through cloud platforms and analysed using machine learning to detect early signs of decompensation in cardiovascular disease, chronic lung disease and diabetes. By combining physiological data with behavioural indicators, such as declining step counts, increased phone inactivity or changes in speech, IoB-based predictive models can distinguish a temporary bad day from the beginning of a serious exacerbation.

Recent chronic-disease self-management reviews highlight how artificial intelligence, when wrapped into mobile apps and conversational agents, can give patients personalised recommendations in response to these early warnings.

4.4 From prediction to proactive care pathways

Early prediction only improves outcomes if it is tightly coupled to action. Studies of digital biomarker platforms stress that predictions should trigger structured care pathways that specify what clinicians, nurses, allied health professionals and patients themselves should do at each risk level. In some heart-failure remote-monitoring programmes, for instance, a rising risk score automatically queues a teleconsultation within a fixed time window, prompts medication titration protocols and activates educational messages to the patient.

In IoB-driven systems, proactive care also reaches beyond individual episodes toward long-term behaviour change. When alerts are framed as coaching rather than warnings, patients often perceive them as supportive nudges rather than surveillance. Evidence from mobile-health interventions suggests that persuasive design features, such as goal-setting, timely feedback and social support, can increase adherence and help people sustain lifestyle modifications that reduce long-term risk. Over time, the same behavioural data that feed the prediction models become a record of progress, helping both patients and clinicians to see the effect of small daily choices on future clinical trajectories as shown in Figure 3.

Figure 3. illustrates how IoB-derived predictions can support a collaborative, proactive consultation between patient and clinician

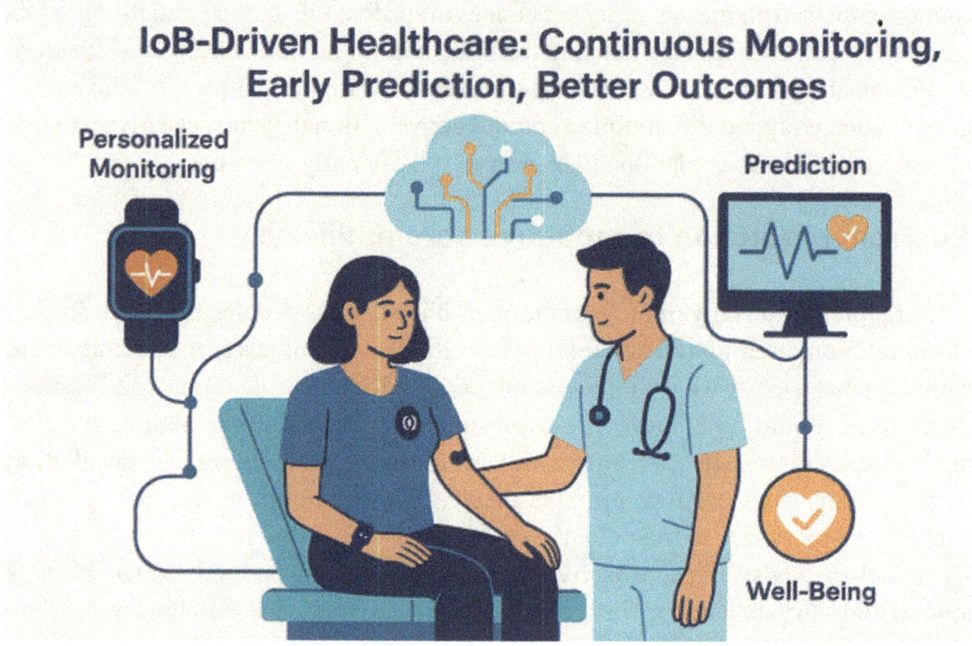

4.5 Challenges, fairness and trust

Despite its potential, IoB-based early prediction raises important challenges. Technical issues include data quality, missingness and drift: a model trained on one set of devices and behaviours may degrade when patients change wearables, routines or environments. Meta-analyses of sepsis and deterioration models emphasise large heterogeneity across studies, limited external validation and a risk that models will appear impressive on retrospective data but perform poorly in new settings. Fairness is another concern. If training data over-represent some populations and under-represent others, prediction errors may be systematically higher for minority groups, potentially widening existing health disparities rather than closing them.

Transparency and clinician oversight are therefore crucial. Comparative work on early warning scores shows that simpler, interpretable tools sometimes perform nearly as well as complex models and may be easier to govern and improve. Position papers on digital biomarkers argue for clear reporting standards, careful calibration, and continuous post-deployment monitoring so that prediction tools remain accurate as clinical practice and patient behaviour evolve.Ultimately, IoB-driven early prediction should be framed as decision support rather than decision replacement:

humans remain responsible for interpreting risk in context, discussing options with patients and making final choices. When that balance is respected, continuous behavioural data, robust prediction models and proactive care pathways can work together to deliver the central promise of IoB-driven healthcare: fewer surprises, fewer crises and better outcomes.

5.FROM TECHNOLOGY TO BETTER OUTCOMES

The real test of any IoB-driven system is simple: does it actually help people live longer, feel better and avoid avoidable crises. Moving from promising technology to better outcomes depends on three things working together: evidence that the tools improve hard clinical endpoints, designs that genuinely support patients in daily life and health systems that can absorb and act on the extra information.

Large-scale studies of remote patient monitoring offer a clear example of how technology can translate into measurable benefit when it is integrated into care pathways. A recent meta-analysis of non-invasive remote patient monitoring in heart failure pooled data from over 16,000 patients across 41 randomised trials and found that such programmes reduced both mortality and first heart failure hospitalisation compared with usual care. Interventions that paired monitoring with structured self-management and education, and used richer communication such as video calls, achieved the biggest reductions in hospital use. (De Lathauwer et al., 2025).That pattern is very much in line with an IoB perspective: data streams by themselves matter less than how they are tied to human contact, coaching and timely decisions.

Randomised trial evidence now shows that carefully designed, IoB-like programmes can change outcomes even in the high-risk "vulnerable phase" just after hospital discharge. The HERMeS trial in Spain tested a mobile-health platform that combined daily telemonitoring of weight, blood pressure and symptoms with scheduled video visits and nurse-led teleintervention for patients with chronic heart failure. Over six months, the intervention significantly lowered the composite of cardiovascular death or worsening heart failure events compared with usual care, with particularly strong effects on cardiovascular mortality and decompensation episodes (Yun et al., 2025). The key design elements mirror the IoB idea: continuous biometric and behavioural data, integrated into a structured remote-care workflow, with clear rules for how clinicians respond to early signs of deterioration.

Beyond single conditions, digital interventions need to show that they work across a wide range of patients and diseases. An umbrella review in The Lancet Digital Health synthesised 34 meta-analyses covering 235 randomised trials of mobile phone interventions for chronic disease management, including diabetes, hypertension, cardiovascular disease and HIV (Sun et al., 2024). Overall, mobile apps and text messaging produced convincing or highly suggestive benefits for several outcomes, such as HbA1c reduction in type 2 diabetes, blood pressure control in hypertension and medication adherence in cardiovascular disease and HIV. At the same time, about 40% of effects were non-significant, and evidence from low- and middle-income countries remained sparse. For IoB-driven healthcare, this is an important message: digital and behavioural data can help, but impact depends heavily on how interventions are targeted, designed and supported.

Telehealth systems that combine monitoring, behavioural support and clinician oversight can also shift softer but important outcomes like self-management and quality of life. A 2023 systematic review and meta-analysis of chronic disease telehealth systems found that programmes offering long-term daily monitoring, feedback and education produced modest but consistent improvements in clinical measures and patient-reported health status across multiple chronic conditions (Xiao & Han, 2023). These systems did more than transmit vital signs: they provided patients with structured feedback, self-care advice and coaching, often based on trends in their own data. This aligns closely with an IoB model where the goal is not just to predict risk for clinicians, but also to nudge and support healthier behaviour for patients in everyday life.

5.1 Patient experience and engagement

Better outcomes are not only about fewer admissions or deaths; they also depend on whether patients can realistically live with these technologies. Studies of remote heart failure programmes, including HERMeS, report high adherence and satisfaction, with many participants valuing the sense of "being watched over" and the convenience of video contacts instead of frequent hospital visits (Yun et al., 2025; De Lathauwer et al., 2025). Similarly, evaluations of telehealth systems for mixed chronic-disease populations highlight improvements in patients' confidence to self-manage and a stronger feeling of partnership with their care team (Xiao & Han, 2023).

From an IoB standpoint, this matters because sustained behavioural data only exist if people keep wearing devices, answering check-ins and engaging with apps. When programmes provide clear feedback, explain why particular prompts are being sent and respect patient preferences, people are more likely to see monitoring as collaborative rather than intrusive. Conversely, if algorithms feel opaque, alerts are frequent but unhelpful or the technology is hard to use, drop-out rates can climb and the quality of data – and predictions – quickly deteriorates.

5.2 Health-system performance and value

At the health-system level, remote monitoring and IoB-style interventions are often promoted as ways to reduce costs and pressure on hospitals. The heart failure meta-analysis by De Lathauwer and colleagues showed reductions in heart-failure hospitalisations and, in some programmes, all-cause admissions, especially where education and self-management modules were built into the service (De Lathauwer et al., 2025). Observational work in accountable-care settings suggests that post-discharge remote monitoring may be associated with lower mortality in selected high-risk patients, even when effects on readmissions are modest, hinting at potential downstream savings from avoided crises and complications.However, systematic reviews of telehealth chronic disease management caution that benefits are not automatic. Some programmes require substantial up-front investment in devices, IT infrastructure and staffing, and the impact on utilisation varies across diseases and designs (Xiao & Han, 2023).

In some settings, telemonitoring has led to more frequent early treatment of exacerbations rather than fewer events overall, which can increase short-term costs even if it possibly prevents later, more severe episodes. For IoB-driven healthcare, this suggests that economic value depends on carefully matching intervention intensity to patient risk and building clear escalation and de-escalation rules into protocols.

5.3 Equity, trust and the risk of a widening gap

Perhaps the most important question for "better outcomes" is: better for whom? A 2024 scoping review in Health Policy examined how digital health technologies intersect with health inequalities in high-income countries (Badr et al., 2024). The authors found that most evaluations focused on differences in access and use across age, socioeconomic status, race and geography, with consistent evidence that those who are older, poorer or digitally excluded are less likely to benefit from digital services. Direct measurement of outcome gaps was much rarer, but the review warned that if health systems move key services and monitoring into digital channels without strong equity safeguards, existing disparities in morbidity and mortality may widen.

For IoB-based systems, this risk is even sharper, because predictive models and behavioural nudges depend on large volumes of high-quality data. If disadvantaged patients are less likely to own compatible devices, have reliable connectivity or feel comfortable with apps, they may be missing from the data that train and refine models. That can lead to biased algorithms whose risk scores are less accurate precisely for the groups who already bear a higher burden of disease. The review by Badr and colleagues argues for embedding an explicit equity lens in digital-health strategy, including targeted support for access and literacy, co-design with underserved communities and routine reporting of outcomes by demographic group, not just overall averages (Badr et al., 2024).

5.4 Putting IoB to work

Overall, the evidence so far suggests that IoB-enabling technologies can improve outcomes when they are embedded in thoughtful care models. Randomised and meta-analytic data show that remote monitoring combined with education, self-management support and live interaction can reduce mortality and hospitalisation in heart failure and improve key risk factors across several chronic diseases (De Lathauwer et al., 2025; Sun et al., 2024; Yun et al., 2025). Telehealth management systems, when sustained over time, can modestly improve both clinical indicators and patient-reported health status across multiple conditions (Xiao & Han, 2023). At the same time, persistent concerns about digital divides and uneven implementation remind us that technology alone does not guarantee fair or universal benefit (Badr et al., 2024).

For IoB-driven healthcare, "better outcomes" will depend on getting the mix right: using rich behavioural and physiological data to trigger timely, human responses; designing tools that patients can and want to use over months and years; aligning incentives so that providers are rewarded for prevention, not just acute care; and building equity and transparency into every stage. When those pieces line up, the promise of IoB is not simply more data, but fewer avoidable crises, more stable chronic disease control and a more proactive, humane model of care.

6. CHALLENGES AND RISKS OF IOB IN HEALTHCARE

The same features that make IoB attractive for healthcare—continuous sensing, intimate coupling with the body and dense data flows—also create a new layer of risk. Unlike traditional health IT, IoB ecosystems blend medical devices, consumer wearables, home sensors and cloud services into a single, highly connected environment. This multiplies the number of points where things can go wrong, technically, ethically and socially.

6.1 Security, privacy and device safety

Security and privacy sit at the centre of IoB risk. Wearable and implantable devices constantly collect physiological, behavioural and sometimes location data, often transmitting them wirelessly to phones or remote servers. A recent survey of security and privacy issues in wearable health monitoring devices shows how these products face attacks at multiple levels: device tampering, eavesdropping on wireless links, spoofing of sensor data, malware in companion apps and misuse of cloud-stored records (Zhang et al., 2025). Because these devices may influence diagnosis, therapy titration or even deliver treatment directly, a successful attack is not just a data breach but a potential patient safety incident.

IoB also inherits the broader cybersecurity fragility of digital health systems. A systematic review of cyberattacks on healthcare organisations highlights how tightly coupled clinical workflows, legacy systems and resource constraints make hospitals and clinics unusually vulnerable (Ewoh & Vartiainen, 2024). The addition of thousands of IoB endpoints—many battery-powered, resource-limited and rarely updated—expands the attack surface further. Compromise of a single gateway or vendor backend could expose highly sensitive, longitudinal body data about large patient populations. For clinicians, even less dramatic failures matter: dropped connections, corrupted data or subtle timing errors can undermine trust in IoB feeds and lead to either inappropriate reassurance or unnecessary alarm.

Traditional security measures are often not a good fit for this environment. Heavy cryptography or complex authentication can drain small batteries or exceed hardware limits in tiny sensors. At the same time, doing too little leaves data streams exposed. Recent work on privacy-preserving healthcare data in IoT argues that new approaches combining techniques like blockchain, deep learning and lightweight cryptography are needed to maintain confidentiality, integrity and availability without overloading devices or networks (Rezaei Bezanjani et al., 2025). For IoB, this means security has to be designed in from the start, rather than bolted on after devices and platforms are deployed.

6.2 Autonomy, consent and surveillance

Because IoB devices sit on or in the body, they touch questions of autonomy and consent more directly than many other digital tools. Continuous sensing can easily blur into continuous surveillance. Once a device is implanted or tightly integrated into rehabilitation or disease management, patients may feel they have little real choice about being monitored. Longitudinal data sets are also attractive for secondary uses such as research, marketing or product development, raising concerns about whether consent is truly informed and ongoing, or whether people are effectively locked into opaque terms-of-use agreements that they cannot meaningfully negotiate.

There is also a risk that predictive models built on IoB data will be used to judge individuals rather than support them. For example, a risk score derived from activity traces, sleep patterns and medication adherence could influence insurance decisions or employment opportunities if safeguards are weak. Even within clinical care, poorly explained predictions can undermine shared decision-making, especially if clinicians are unsure how a risk estimate was produced but feel pressured to follow it. Managing these risks requires not only technical protections, but also clear communication, robust data-governance policies and regulatory oversight that treats body-linked data with particular care (Ewoh & Vartiainen, 2024).

7. A CONCEPTUAL FRAMEWORK FOR IOB-DRIVEN HEALTHCARE

IoB-driven healthcare can easily become a tangle of devices, apps and data streams unless it is organised around a clear, patient-centred logic. A useful way to structure this complexity is to see IoB systems as a continuous cycle with four tightly linked stages: Monitor, Understand, Act and Learn. This cycle runs across settings, from home to hospital and back again, and over time it turns raw signals from bodies and behaviours into better decisions and, ultimately, better outcomes. It also aligns naturally with ideas from learning health systems and data-driven digital health, where continuous feedback between practice and evidence is central to improvement (Cresswell et al., 2025).

The first stage, Monitor, captures the core capability of IoB: continuous sensing on, in and around the body. In practical terms, this includes wearables, implantables, ingestible sensors and ambient devices that collect physiological, behavioural and contextual data during daily life. At this stage the key questions are coverage, comfort and data quality. Systems must be acceptable enough that people will use them for months or years, but robust enough to generate reliable signals. Recent work on sensing and digital biomarkers emphasises that even simple sensors, if used continuously and in combination, can yield rich indicators of health and disease trajectories (Smokovski et al., 2024).

The second stage, Understand, transforms these raw data streams into information that people can actually use. This involves filtering noise, extracting features, building digital biomarkers and estimating risk. For clinicians, this might appear as trend graphs, summary indices or early warning scores; for patients, it may take the form of simple, colour-coded dashboards or personalised feedback messages. The goal is not just statistical accuracy but meaningful interpretation in context. Studies of AI-enabled early warning and chronic-disease management stress that model outputs must be calibrated, explainable and embedded in clinical workflows if they are to support rather than confuse decision making (Edelson et al., 2024; Zhang et al., 2025).

The third stage, Act, is where prediction and insight are linked to concrete changes in care. Actions can range from automated reminders and self-management suggestions through nurse-led teleinterventions to in-person reviews and treatment escalation. In a well-designed IoB pathway, each risk level or pattern has a predefined response plan, so that the system does not simply flag problems but also helps coordinate who does what and when. Evidence from remote heart failure programmes and mobile health interventions shows that benefits on mortality, hospitalisation and risk-factor control are greatest when monitoring is tightly coupled with structured education, coaching and clinician contact, rather than being treated as a standalone technical add-on (Smokovski et al., 2024; Zhang et al., 2025).

The final stage, Learn, closes the loop. Every alert, action and outcome becomes new data for refining both models and workflows. If a particular threshold generates many false alarms, it can be adjusted. If certain patients do not respond well to a standard intervention, the system can be adapted to account for their characteristics or preferences. At scale, this turns IoB deployments into learning health systems in which care delivery and knowledge generation happen together (Cresswell et al., 2025). Importantly, learning should include not only model performance metrics, but also patient experience, equity of access and unintended consequences such as workload or alarm fatigue.

8. FUTURE DIRECTIONS AND RESEARCH OPPORTUNITIES

As IoB matures from isolated pilots to large-scale health ecosystems, the next wave of research needs to focus less on "can we build this device or model?" and more on "how do we make the whole system trustworthy, interoperable and beneficial for diverse patients over years?" This shift points to three broad directions: smarter privacy-preserving data infrastructures, richer representations of the body through digital twins, and more human-centred, explainable intelligence layered on top of IoB data.

8.1 Smarter and more private data ecosystems

A major research frontier is learning from distributed IoB data without centralising sensitive records. Federated learning already shows how hospitals and device vendors can jointly train models while keeping data local, but most studies remain proof-of-concept and only a small fraction are deployed in real-world care (Teo et al., 2024). Future work needs to tackle issues that matter in practice: unstable network conditions, highly heterogeneous devices, unbalanced datasets across sites, and incentives for smaller organisations to participate. There is also a need for standardised evaluation frameworks that measure not just model accuracy, but resilience to attacks, fairness across subgroups and ease of integration into clinical systems.

8.2 From digital biomarkers to digital twins of health

A second direction is to move beyond simple thresholds and risk scores towards richer, personalised models of each person's health state. Digital twin research in healthcare IoT shows how real-time data from sensors can be linked to dynamic virtual replicas that simulate organ function, hospital operations or even whole-population health scenarios (Kabir et al., 2025). For IoB, an obvious extension is the "behavioural and physiological twin" that combines activity patterns, sleep, vital signs, medication use and environmental exposures into a living model that can be probed and updated continuously.

8.3 Human-centred and explainable IoB intelligence

A third set of opportunities lies in making IoB-driven predictions understandable and actionable for both clinicians and patients. Reviews of explainable and interpretable AI in medicine highlight an explosion of techniques, but also note that many explanations are designed in isolation from real users and rarely evaluated in clinical workflows (Frasca et al., 2024). For IoB, research needs to focus on explanations that fit continuous, multi-modal data: showing how a week of disrupted sleep, missed doses and rising resting heart rate combine to trigger a heart-failure alert, for example, rather than just displaying a single risk number.

9. CONCLUSION

IoB-driven healthcare represents a shift from short, isolated clinical encounters to a more continuous, lived relationship between people, their bodies and the health system. By combining devices on, in and around the body with secure connectivity and intelligent analytics, IoB makes it possible to monitor physiology and behaviour in real time, detect risk earlier and support more personalised, proactive care. Across hospital wards, home monitoring programmes and mental and behavioural health applications, emerging evidence suggests that continuous data, when linked to thoughtful care pathways, can reduce deterioration, improve control of chronic conditions and strengthen patients' ability to manage their own health.

REFERENCES

Ahmed, S. F., Sharmin, S., Kuldeep, S. A., & Gandomi, A. H. (2025). Transformative impacts of the Internet of Medical Things on modern healthcare. [CoLab]. *Results in Engineering*, *25*, 103787. DOI: 10.1016/j.rineng.2024.103787

Al Khatib, I., Shamayleh, A., & Ndiaye, M. (2024). Healthcare and the Internet of Medical Things: Applications, trends, key challenges, and proposed resolutions. [MDPI]. *Informatics (MDPI)*, *11*(3), 47. DOI: 10.3390/informatics11030047

Andrade, A. N., Cabral, A. T., Bellini, B., Facco Rodrigues, V., da Rosa Righi, R., André da Costa, C., & Barbosa, J. L. V. (2024). IoT-based vital sign monitoring: A literature review. *Smart Health (Amsterdam, Netherlands)*, *32*, 100462. Advance online publication. DOI: 10.1016/j.smhl.2024.100462

Badr, J., Motulsky, A., & Denis, J. (2024). Digital health technologies and inequalities: A scoping review of potential impacts and policy recommendations. *Health Policy (Amsterdam)*, *146*, 105122. DOI: 10.1016/j.healthpol.2024.105122 PMID: 38986333

Boddington, G. (2021). The Internet of Bodies—alive, connected and collective: The virtual physical future of our bodies and our senses. *AI & Society*, *38*(5), 1897–1913. DOI: 10.1007/s00146-020-01137-1 PMID: 33584018

Bowles, T., Trentino, K. M., Lloyd, A., Trentino, L., Jones, G., Murray, K., Thompson, A., Halpin, S., & Waterer, G. (2024). Outcomes in patients receiving continuous monitoring of vital signs on general wards: A systematic review and meta-analysis of randomised controlled trials. *Digital Health*, *10*, 20552076241288826. DOI: 10.1177/20552076241288826 PMID: 39398891

Chatterjee, B., Mohseni, P., & Sen, S. (2022). Bioelectronic sensor nodes for Internet of Bodies. arXiv. https://arxiv.org/abs/2212.11370

Coutu, F.-A., Iorio, O. C., & Ross, B. A. (2023). Remote patient monitoring strategies and wearable technology in chronic obstructive pulmonary disease. *Frontiers in Medicine*, *10*, 1236598. DOI: 10.3389/fmed.2023.1236598 PMID: 37663662

Cresswell, K., Papoutsi, C., Simon, G. E., Bates, D. W., & Sheikh, A. (2025). Advancing learning health systems: Leveraging routine data for improvement and research. *NPJ Digital Medicine*, *8*, 12. DOI: 10.1038/s41746-024-01045-4

Datta, A., & Sen, S. (2023). Invited: IoB: The vision of the Internet of Bodies. *Proceedings of the IEEE Midwest Symposium on Circuits and Systems (MWSCAS)*, 444–448. DBLPDOI: 10.1109/MWSCAS57524.2023.10405903

De Lathauwer, I. L. J., Nieuwenhuys, W. W., Hafkamp, F., Regis, M., Brouwers, R. W. M., Funk, M., & Kemps, H. M. C. (2025). Remote patient monitoring in heart failure: A comprehensive meta-analysis of effective programme components for hospitalization and mortality reduction. *European Journal of Heart Failure*, *27*(9), 1670–1685. Advance online publication. DOI: 10.1002/ejhf.3568 PMID: 39834044

de Waal, C.. (2025). Accuracy of vital sign monitoring using a photoplethysmography upper arm wearable in hospitalised patients. *Journal of Clinical Monitoring and Computing*. Advance online publication. DOI: 10.1007/s10877-025-01358-z

Dubey, R., & Tiwari, A. (2023). Artificial intelligence and remote patient monitoring in US healthcare market: A literature review. *Journal of Market Access & Health Policy*, *11*(1), 2205618. DOI: 10.1080/20016689.2023.2205618 PMID: 37151736

Edelson, D. P., Churpek, M. M., Carey, K. A., Lin, Z., Huang, C., Siner, J. M., Johnson, J., Krumholz, H. M., & Rhodes, D. J. (2024). Early warning scores with and without artificial intelligence. *JAMA Network Open*, *7*(10), e2438986. DOI: 10.1001/jamanetworkopen.2024.38986 PMID: 39405061

Edelson, D. P., Churpek, M. M., Carey, K. A., Lin, Z., Huang, C., Siner, J. M., Johnson, J., Krumholz, H. M., & Rhodes, D. J. (2024). Early warning scores with and without artificial intelligence. *JAMA Network Open*, *7*(10), e2438986. DOI: 10.1001/jamanetworkopen.2024.38986 PMID: 39405061

El-deep, S. E., Abohany, A. A., Sallam, K. M., & Abd El-Mageed, A. A. (2025). A comprehensive survey on impact of applying various technologies on the Internet of Medical Things. [SpringerLink]. *Artificial Intelligence Review*, *58*(3), 86. DOI: 10.1007/s10462-024-11063-z

El-Khoury, M., & Arikan, C. L. (2021). From the Internet of Things toward the Internet of Bodies: Ethical and legal considerations. Journal of Strategic Contracting and Negotiation, 7(2), 307–314. RSD Journal Ewoh, P., & Vartiainen, T. (2024). Vulnerability to cyberattacks and sociotechnical solutions for health care systems: Systematic review. Journal of Medical Internet Research, 26, e46904. https://doi .org/DOI: 10.1002/jsc.2411

Felix, F. A. S., & Martins, L. E. G. (2024). IoT devices in use in healthcare applications: A systematic literature review. [SpringerLink]. *Research on Biomedical Engineering*, *40*(3-4), 547–561. DOI: 10.1007/s42600-024-00356-5

Frasca, M., La Torre, D., Pravettoni, G., & Cutica, I. (2024). Explainable and interpretable artificial intelligence in medicine: A systematic bibliometric review. *Discover Artificial Intelligence*, *4*(1), 15. DOI: 10.1007/s44163-024-00114-7

He, P., Huang, D., Wu, D., He, H., Wei, Y., Cui, Y., Wang, R., & Peng, L. (2024). A survey of Internet of Medical Things: Technology, application and future directions. Digital Communications and Networks. Advance online publication. sciencedirect. comDOI: 10.1016/j.dcan.2024.11.013

Hicks, M. H., Tore, M., Michard, F., & Khanna, A. K. (2025). Portable wireless monitoring of vital signs in hospital wards. *BJA Education*, *25*(7), 265–272. DOI: 10.1016/j.bjae.2025.04.004 PMID: 40575591

Huang, Y., Wang, J., Wang, S., & Zhang, Y. (2023). Internet of medical things: A systematic review. *Neurocomputing*, *557*, 126719. Advance online publication. DOI: 10.1016/j.neucom.2023.126719

Joshi, M., Iqbal, F. M., Sharabiani, M., Ashrafian, H., Arora, S., McAndrew, K., Khan, S., Cooke, G., & Darzi, A. (2025). Performance of continuous digital monitoring of vital signs with a wearable sensor in acute hospital settings. *Sensors (Basel)*, *25*(9), 2644. DOI: 10.3390/s25092644 PMID: 40363083

Kabir, M. R., Shishir, F. S., Shomaji, S., & Ray, S. (2025). Digital twins in healthcare IoT: A systematic review. *High-Confidence Computing*, *5*(3), 100340. DOI: 10.1016/j.hcc.2025.100340

Kakhi, K., Jagatheesaperumal, S. K., Khosravi, A., Alizadehsani, R., & Acharya, U. R. (2025). Fatigue monitoring using wearables and AI: Trends, challenges, and future opportunities. *Computers in Biology and Medicine*, *195*, 110461. DOI: 10.1016/j.compbiomed.2025.110461 PMID: 40580618

Khan, S., & Alam, M. (2021). Wearable Internet of Things for personalized healthcare: Study of trends and latent research. In Das, H. (Eds.), *Health informatics: A computational perspective in healthcare* (pp. 43–60). Springer., DOI: 10.1007/978-981-15-9735-0_3

Kirubakaran, D. (2025). Review on emerging frontiers in medical sensing: Innovations shaping the future of healthcare. *Biomedical Materials & Devices*, *3*, 385. DOI: 10.1007/s44174-025-00385-3

Liu, J., & Liu, H. (2025). Research on flexible sensors for wearable devices: A review. *Nanomaterials (Basel, Switzerland)*, *15*(7), 520. DOI: 10.3390/nano15070520 PMID: 40214565

Marinescu, M.-R., Ionescu, O. N., Pachiu, C. I., Dinescu, M. A., Muller, R., & uchea, M. P. (2025). Next-gen healthcare devices: Evolution of MEMS and BioMEMS in the era of the Internet of Bodies for personalized medicine. *Micromachines*, *16*(10), 1182. DOI: 10.3390/mi16101182 PMID: 41156428

Marinescu, M.-R., Ionescu, O. N., Pachiu, C. I., Dinescu, M. A., Muller, R., & uchea, M. P. (2025). Next-gen healthcare devices: Evolution of MEMS and BioMEMS in the era of the Internet of Bodies for personalized medicine. *Micromachines*, *16*(10), 1182. DOI: 10.3390/mi16101182 PMID: 41156428

Matthew, A. J., Dhanalakshmi, R., & Vimal, S. (2025). A systematic review of Internet of Medical Things (IoMT) in healthcare. *Sci*, *7*(2), 36. DOI: 10.3390/sci7020036

Matthew, P., Mchale, S., Deng, X., Nakhla, G., Trovati, M., Nnamoko, N., Pereira, E., Zhang, H., & Raza, M. (2025). A review of the state of the art for the Internet of Medical Things. *Sci*, *7*(2), 36. DOI: 10.3390/sci7020036

Mazzeo, A. E. P., & dos Santos, L. W. (2025). Integration of biomedical devices and the internet of bodies revolution. Research. *Social Development*, *14*(5), e48921. DOI: 10.33448/rsd-v14i5.48921

Michard, F., & Saugel, B. (2025). New sensors for the early detection of clinical deterioration on general wards and beyond – A clinician's perspective. *Journal of Clinical Monitoring and Computing*, *39*(2), 435–442. DOI: 10.1007/s10877-024-01235-1 PMID: 39546216

Naghib, M., Chalechale, A., & Gharehchopogh, F. S. (2025). A comprehensive and systematic literature review on intrusion detection systems in the Internet of Medical Things: Current status, challenges, and opportunities. *Artificial Intelligence Review*, *58*(4), 114. Advance online publication. DOI: 10.1007/s10462-024-11101-w

Parihar, A., Prajapati, J. B., Prajapati, B. G., Trambadiya, B., Thakkar, A., & Engineer, P. (2024). Role of IoT in healthcare: Applications, security & privacy concerns. *Intelligent Pharmacy*, *2*(5), 707–714. DOI: 10.1016/j.ipha.2024.01.003

Paul, M. M., Khera, N., Elugunti, P. R., Ruff, K. C., Hommos, M. S., Thomas, L. F., Nagaraja, V., Garrett, A. L., Pantoja-Smith, M., Delafield, N. L., Lizaola-Mayo, B. C., Kresin, M. M., Seetharam, M., Nagarakanti, S. R., & Kaur, M. (2025). The state of remote patient monitoring for chronic disease management in the United States. *Journal of Medical Internet Research*, *27*, e70422. DOI: 10.2196/70422 PMID: 40570326

Rashid, S., & Nemati, A. (2024). Human-centered IoT-based health monitoring in the Healthcare 5.0 era: Literature descriptive analysis and future research guidelines. *Discover Internet of Things*, *4*(1), 26. DOI: 10.1007/s43926-024-00082-5

Rejeb, A., Rejeb, K., Treiblmaier, H., Appolloni, A., Alghamdi, S., Alhasawi, Y., & Iranmanesh, M. (2023). The Internet of Things (IoT) in healthcare: Taking stock and moving forward. *Internet of Things : Engineering Cyber Physical Human Systems, 22*, 100721. DOI: 10.1016/j.iot.2023.100721

Rezaei Bezanjani, B., Ghafouri, S. H., & Gholamrezaei, R. (2025). Privacy-preserving healthcare data in IoT: A synergistic approach with deep learning and blockchain. *The Journal of Supercomputing, 81*(4), 533. DOI: 10.1007/s11227-025-06980-x

Rowland, B., Saha, A., Motamedi, V., Bundy, R., Winsor, S., McNavish, D., Lippert, W., & Khanna, A. K. (2025). Impact on patient outcomes of continuous vital sign monitoring on medical wards: Propensity-matched analysis. *Journal of Medical Internet Research, 27*, e66347. DOI: 10.2196/66347 PMID: 40068153

Sameh, A., Rostami, M., Oussalah, M., Korpelainen, R., & Farrahi, V. (2025). Digital phenotypes and digital biomarkers for health and diseases: A systematic review of machine learning approaches utilizing passive non-invasive signals collected via wearable devices and smartphones. *Artificial Intelligence Review, 58*(2), 66. DOI: 10.1007/s10462-024-11009-5

Schultz, C. (2023). Telehealth and remote patient monitoring innovations in nursing practice: State of the science. Online Journal of Issues in Nursing, 28(2). *Online Journal of Issues in Nursing, 1*(2). Advance online publication. DOI: 10.3912/OJIN.Vol28No02ST01

Shajari, M., Kuruvinashetti, K., Komeili, A., & Sundararaj, U. (2023). The emergence of AI-based wearable sensors for digital health technology: A review. *Sensors (Basel), 23*(23), 9498. DOI: 10.3390/s23239498 PMID: 38067871

Shen, S., Qi, W., Zeng, J., Li, S., Liu, X., Zhu, X., & Lou, X. (2025). Passive sensing for mental health monitoring using machine learning with wearables and smartphones: Scoping review. *Journal of Medical Internet Research, 27*, e77066. DOI: 10.2196/77066 PMID: 40811794

Singh, B., Lopez, D., & Ramadan, R. (2023). Internet of things in healthcare: A conventional literature review. *Health and Technology, 13*(5), 699–719. Advance online publication. DOI: 10.1007/s12553-023-00771-1

Singh, B., Lopez, D., & Ramadan, R. (2023). Internet of things in healthcare: A conventional literature review. *Health and Technology, 13*(5), 699–719. DOI: 10.1007/s12553-023-00771-1

Smokovski, I., Steinle, N., Behnke, A., Bhaskar, S. M. M., Grech, G., Richter, K., Niklewski, G., Birkenbihl, C., Parini, P., Andrews, R. J., Bauchner, H., & Golubnitschaja, O. (2024). Digital biomarkers: 3PM approach revolutionizing chronic disease management—EPMA 2024 position. *The EPMA Journal*, *15*(2), 149–162. DOI: 10.1007/s13167-024-00364-6 PMID: 38841615

Smokovski, I., Steinle, N., Behnke, A., Bhaskar, S. M. M., Grech, G., Richter, K., Niklewski, G., Birkenbihl, C., Parini, P., Andrews, R. J., Bauchner, H., & Golubnitschaja, O. (2024). Digital biomarkers: 3PM approach revolutionizing chronic disease management—EPMA 2024 position. *The EPMA Journal*, *15*(2), 149–162. DOI: 10.1007/s13167-024-00364-6 PMID: 38841615

Sun, S., Simonsson, O., McGarvey, S., Torous, J., & Goldberg, S. B. (2024). Mobile phone interventions to improve health outcomes among patients with chronic diseases: An umbrella review and evidence synthesis from 34 meta-analyses. *The Lancet. Digital Health*, *6*(11), e857–e870. DOI: 10.1016/S2589-7500(24)00119-5 PMID: 39332937

Tabaie, Z., & Omidvar, A. (2023). Human body heat-driven thermoelectric generators as a sustainable power supply for wearable electronic devices: Recent advances, challenges, and future perspectives. *Heliyon*, *9*(4), e14707. DOI: 10.1016/j.heliyon.2023.e14707 PMID: 37025803

Taherdoost, H. (2024). Wearable healthcare and continuous vital sign monitoring with IoT integration. *Computers, Materials & Continua*, *81*(1), 79–104. DOI: 10.32604/cmc.2024.054378

Teo, Z. L., Jin, L., Liu, N., Li, S., Miao, D., Zhang, X., Ng, W. Y., Tan, T. F., Lee, D. M., Chua, K. J., Heng, J., Liu, Y., Goh, R. S. M., & Ting, D. S. W. (2024). Federated machine learning in healthcare: A systematic review on clinical applications and technical architecture. *Cell Reports Medicine*, *5*(2), 101419. DOI: 10.1016/j.xcrm.2024.101419 PMID: 38340728

Webb, C. A., & Fisher, H. (2025). Tracking psychopathology dimensions through passive smartphone sensing—Promises, pitfalls, and pathways to clinical integration. *JAMA Network Open*, *8*(7), e2519054. DOI: 10.1001/jamanetworkopen.2025.19054 PMID: 40608343

Xiao, Z., & Han, X. (2023). Evaluation of the effectiveness of telehealth chronic disease management system: Systematic review and meta-analysis. *Journal of Medical Internet Research*, *25*, e44256. DOI: 10.2196/44256 PMID: 37103993

Yadav, A., Dandu, H., Parchani, G., Chokalingam, K., Kadambi, P., Mishra, R., Jahan, A., Teboul, J.-L., & Latour, J. M. (2024). Early detection of deteriorating patients in general wards through continuous contactless vital signs monitoring. *Frontiers in Medical Technology*, *6*, 1436034. DOI: 10.3389/fmedt.2024.1436034 PMID: 39328308

Yun, S., Comín-Colet, J., Calero-Molina, E., Hidalgo, E., José-Bazán, N., Cobo Marcos, M., Soria, T., Llàcer, P., Fernández, C., García-Pinilla, J. M., Cruzado, C., González-Franco, Á., García-Marina, E. M., Morales-Rull, J. L., Solé, C., García-Romero, E., Núñez, J., Civera, J., Fernández, C., & Fernández, C. (2025). Evaluation of mobile health technology combining telemonitoring and teleintervention versus usual care in vulnerable-phase heart failure management (HERMeS): A multicentre, randomised controlled trial. *The Lancet. Digital Health*, *7*(5), 100866. DOI: 10.1016/j.landig.2025.02.006 PMID: 40374486

Zhang, B., Chen, C., Lee, I., Lee, K., & Ong, K.-L. (2025). A survey on security and privacy issues in wearable health monitoring devices. *Computers & Security*, *155*, 104453. DOI: 10.1016/j.cose.2025.104453

Zhang, K., Jiang, Y., Xi, K., & Sun, N. (2025). Application of persuasive system design in mobile health interventions for chronic disease management: A mini review. *Frontiers in Public Health*, *13*, 1718371. DOI: 10.3389/fpubh.2025.1718371 PMID: 41358248

Zhang, Y., Li, X., Wang, H., & Chen, J. (2025). Advanced applications in chronic disease monitoring using IoT mobile sensing devices. *Frontiers in Public Health*, *13*, 1510456. DOI: 10.3389/fpubh.2025.1510456

Zhao, Y., Du, Y., Liu, Y., Deng, C., & Li, X. (2025). Artificial intelligence in chronic disease self-management: Current applications and future directions. *Frontiers in Public Health*, *13*, 1689911. DOI: 10.3389/fpubh.2025.1689911 PMID: 41358250

Zhu, Z., & Zhu, M. (2023). The usage of Internet of Things in healthcare: A review of mechanisms, platforms, and opportunities from a new perspective. *Journal of Intelligent & Fuzzy Systems*, *45*(1), 1–18. DOI: 10.3233/JIFS-224166

Chapter 6
Breakthroughs in Smart Nursing With Generative AI:
Generative AI Applications in Nursing Practice and Clinical Decision-Making

P. Prakash
http://orcid.org/0000-0003-4879-2222
Velalar College of Engineering and Technology, Erode, India

M. Sobika
http://orcid.org/0009-0005-6827-0116
Velalar College of Engineering and Technology, Erode, India

T. Rajasekaran
Nandha Engineering College, Perundurai, India

M. Sabarish
Velalar College of Engineering and Technology, Erode, India

S. Sasikanth
Vivekanandha College of Engineering for Women, Tiruchengode, India

T. Sivanesh
Velalar College of Engineering and Technology, Erode, India

ABSTRACT

Generative Artificial Intelligence (GenAI) is becoming one of the revolutionary technologies in contemporary healthcare with its significance, to nursing practice and clinical decision making growing more evident as hospitals globally move towards intelligent, automated and data centered care systems. With clinical data expanding at a rate and nurses still encountering heavy documentation demands workforce deficits and increasing patient complexity incorporating GenAI tools has become crucial, for enhancing workflow productivity and elevating patient care quality. This

DOI: 10.4018/979-8-3373-8247-0.ch006

section aims to examine the uses of GenAI, in nursing emphasizing especially its ability to aid clinical decision-making improve risk assessment, automate patient documentation enhance ICU surveillance and produce precise prompt information that assists nurses in making quicker and safer choices at the bedside.

1. INTRODUCTION

Nurses are also involved in some of the complex, cognitively challenging, and physically demanding tasks within the healthcare setting. Some of the tasks include supervising patients, incorporating new advances in the healthcare field, administering medications to the patients, managing different specialties to ensure that the patient receives comprehensive healthcare, communicating with families, as well as documenting all aspects of a patient's health. The modern healthcare environment amplifies these factors such that nurses have to work under more challenging conditions associated with complex patient cases, increased turnover rates, shortages, as well as administrative tasks that distract them from patient interaction (Topol, 2019) (Woo, Ho, Tang, & Tam, 2020).

Generative Artificial Intelligence (GenAI) presents a novel approach for tackling these basic problems (Topol, 2019). Unlike conventional models of Artificial Intelligence that make use of structural data and pre-defined algorithms alone, GenAI utilizes large language models (LLMs) and multimodal artificial intelligence models that enable storytelling in natural language processing, summarization of complex data, document production, trend analyses, and warning alerts for patient deterioration (Garg, Basterrech, Banerjee, & Sharma, 2021).These capabilities are inextricably connected with basic nursing skills in evaluation and judgment, prioritization and decision-making, communication and patient teaching (Gottesman et al., 2020) (Jukanti, 2025).

Recent developments in multimodal fusion enable the GenAI tools to combine various data sources such as vital data, laboratory data, electronic health records, nurse charts, device-telemetry data, and patient self-reported data to present an overarching clinical perspective that cannot be derived from the individual sources of data (Liu et al., 2021) (Pang, Li, Ouyang, Liu, & Tang, 2022). In the Intensive Care Setting, such systems can identify patterns of sepsis, acute respiratory failure or hemodynamic issues long before the same patterns become recognizable to the critical care team (Kline et al., 2022). In the case of nurses simultaneously responsible for the care of multiple patients, such predictive data helps the nurses respond more quickly and think less (Nemati, Ansary, & Nemati, 2020).

Concurrently, the use of GenAI also underscores a range of important moral, legal, and safety considerations. For instance, GenAI systems are capable of providing erroneous information; they can perpetuate any bias in the data used to develop the system or produce outputs that are hard to evaluate (Pruski, 2024). Indeed, their effective utilization in nursing practice can no longer rely on the need to involve the nurse in the design. GenAI must enhance rather than diminish the nursing practice process based upon nursing judgement, empathy, and the therapeutic relationship.

In this chapter, there is a thorough review of the applications of GenAI in nursing and making decisions. It explains how there is benefit in patient assessment, risk prediction, documentation, education, communication, and collaboration of care between specialties. It reviews opportunities in smart ICUs, telecare programs, and AI-assisted programs for nurse training (Chin et al., 2023). It presents a very applicable and ethical way of doing things in healthcare institutions and indicates future areas of investigation in healthcare. It argues with evidence, examples, and theories that GenAI will make a difference in patient care and lighten the load of care providers in making a healthcare system that is safer and highly effective and human-centric (Pawar, O'shea, Rea, & O'reilly, 2020).

2. GENERATIVE AI APPLICATIONS IN NURSING PRACTICE

Generative AI is transforming and revolutionizing nursing practice because it enhances and augments the cognitive and analytical capabilities and communication skills that nurses apply daily. Unlike older generation rule-based computers, current GenAI computers have the ability to document structurally and understand medical language and enable computers to assist nurses in interpreting large data from patients. It is very close to real-life nursing practices in which decisions have to be made quickly and under incomplete data. Table 1 depicts how a comparison review of Generative AI improves key roles in nursing.

Table 1. Impact of generative AI across core nursing functions

Nursing Function	Traditional Approach	GenAI-Enhanced Approach
Patient Assessment	Manual review of vitals, notes, labs	AI-generated summaries, early risk alerts
Clinical Decision-Making	Nurse interprets complex patterns manually	Predictive models highlight subtle trends
Documentation	Time-consuming, typed manually	Auto-drafted notes (SOAP, SBAR) via NLP
ICU Monitoring	Device data reviewed separately	Multimodal fusion detects deterioration early

continued on following page

Table 1. Continued

Nursing Function	Traditional Approach	GenAI-Enhanced Approach
Patient Education	Generic printed materials	Personalized, multilingual instructions
Remote/Home Care	Limited follow-up	Continuous alerts, AI triaging of symptoms

Enhancing Nursing Assessment

Nurses would likely be the first to notice the change in the patient's status, and it is based on those judgments that the course of treatment will be shaped. In that way, GenAI would add value to them as it would consider numerous data sources and use them to develop meaningful summaries to quickly build an insight into the problem (Villanueva-Miranda, Xiao, & Xie, 2025). Once the data is fed into the EHR system by the nurse, the GenAI models would then compare the data with the laboratory results, past data, trends, and the data from the instruments specific to the critical findings about the status of the patient (Topol, 2019).

Subtle clinical deviations, like slight behavioural changes, developing confusion, or elevated breathing efforts, can often occur before physiological changes get measured. How a generative AI picks up on these subtle signs lies in its ability to compare patterns of text from general notes against historical clinical standards. What this does for the nurse, of course, is provide a clearer perspective on potential danger (Nemati et al., 2020).

Supporting Care Planning and Intervention Selection

After analysing the assessment data, the use of generative AI can assist the nurses in intervention development based on guidelines. The advantages in developing the plan include suggestions created by the AI based on clinical guidelines (Jukanti, 2025). For example, based on the signs of the beginning stage of dehydration in the patient's vital signs, the AI can indicate the need for assessments based on increased intake and output or communicating with the healthcare team if the values are abnormal. The process does not eliminate the need for the nurse's decision but instead provides a cognitive aid for safe practices (Chin et al., 2023).

Figure 1. Distribution of GenAI applications in nursing

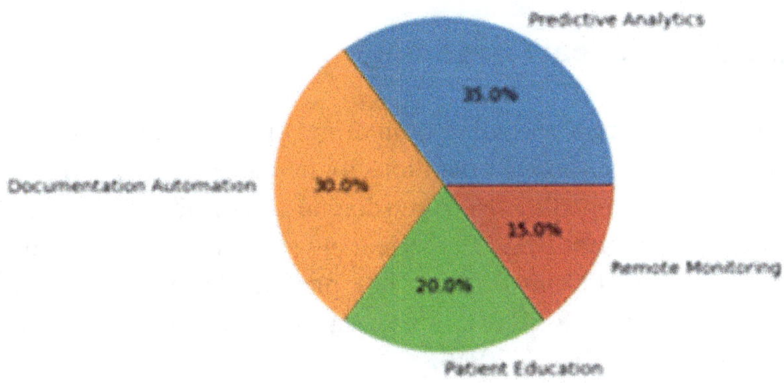

Chart shows a percentage distribution of applications of Generative AI within clinical nursing.

3.GENERATIVE AI IN CLINICAL DECISION-MAKING

Clinical decision-making is an integral component of nursing practice, involving continuous interpretation of dynamic patient data, prioritisation of tasks, and timely escalation of care. Generative AI enhances this decision-making capacity by providing deeper insight into patient trajectories, supporting structured reasoning, and highlighting potential risks before they manifest clinically.

Early Warning and Predictive Surveillance

Early classic models of prediction rely to a great extent on strict criteria. But in numerous cases, there can be a deterioration in a very subtle way with complex patterns. Generation models of AI analysis performed on a massive set of data generated by clinical observations exhibit a much finer level of capability for prediction (Veldhuis, Woittiez, Nanayakkara, & Ludikhuize, 2022). They search for patterns associated with sepsis, ARF, and hemodynamic instability. They identify a number of patterns associated with vitals, labs, nursing aide entries, telemetry (Choudhury & Asan, 2020).

Because generative AI continuously evaluates changes in trajectory rather than isolated values, it can warn nurses of deterioration hours before conventional tools recognise the shift. Research has demonstrated that multimodal AI systems detect sepsis earlier than NEWS or MEWS scores, allowing nurses to initiate early interventions, notify physicians, and activate rapid-response teams in a timelier manner

(Nemati et al., 2020). This enhances patient safety while supporting nurses in high-stakes decision environments.

Strengthening Clinical Reasoning

Nurses often apply rich reasoning to interpret symptoms, anticipate complications, or communicate suspected conditions to the wider clinical team. Generative AI is of great value in generating structured diagnostic considerations from available data. In reviewing a patient who is experiencing shortness of breath, an AI model might generate differential possibilities like pneumonia, pulmonary edema, and COPD exacerbation, with a short rationale anchored in patient recent trends and documented symptoms (Topol, 2019).

Although these suggestions do not list definitive diagnoses, they provide the function of mental tools to guide the nurses in structuring their minds to focus their inquiries in a way that facilitates successful communication among the team present in interdisciplinary rounds.

Delivering Actionable Recommendations

Generative AI systems can be made more effective at aligning "Decision Support With Clinical Protocol." While evaluating the patient data, they can help the clinician make evidence-based decisions regarding the need to reschedule patient reassessments, check fluid volume, or alert the physician when certain parameters are satisfied. (Sutton et al., 2020). These AI-generated prompts reinforce standardised clinical pathways and reduce reliance on memory during demanding shifts (Pawar et al., 2020).

Such recommendations are especially useful in busy units where nurses manage multiple patients with varying acuity levels. The clarity of AI-generated suggestions supports quicker decision cycles and reduces the likelihood of missed interventions. Figure 2 shows a Gen AI assisted clinical decision-making workflow.

Figure 2. Generative AI assisted clinical decision-making workflow

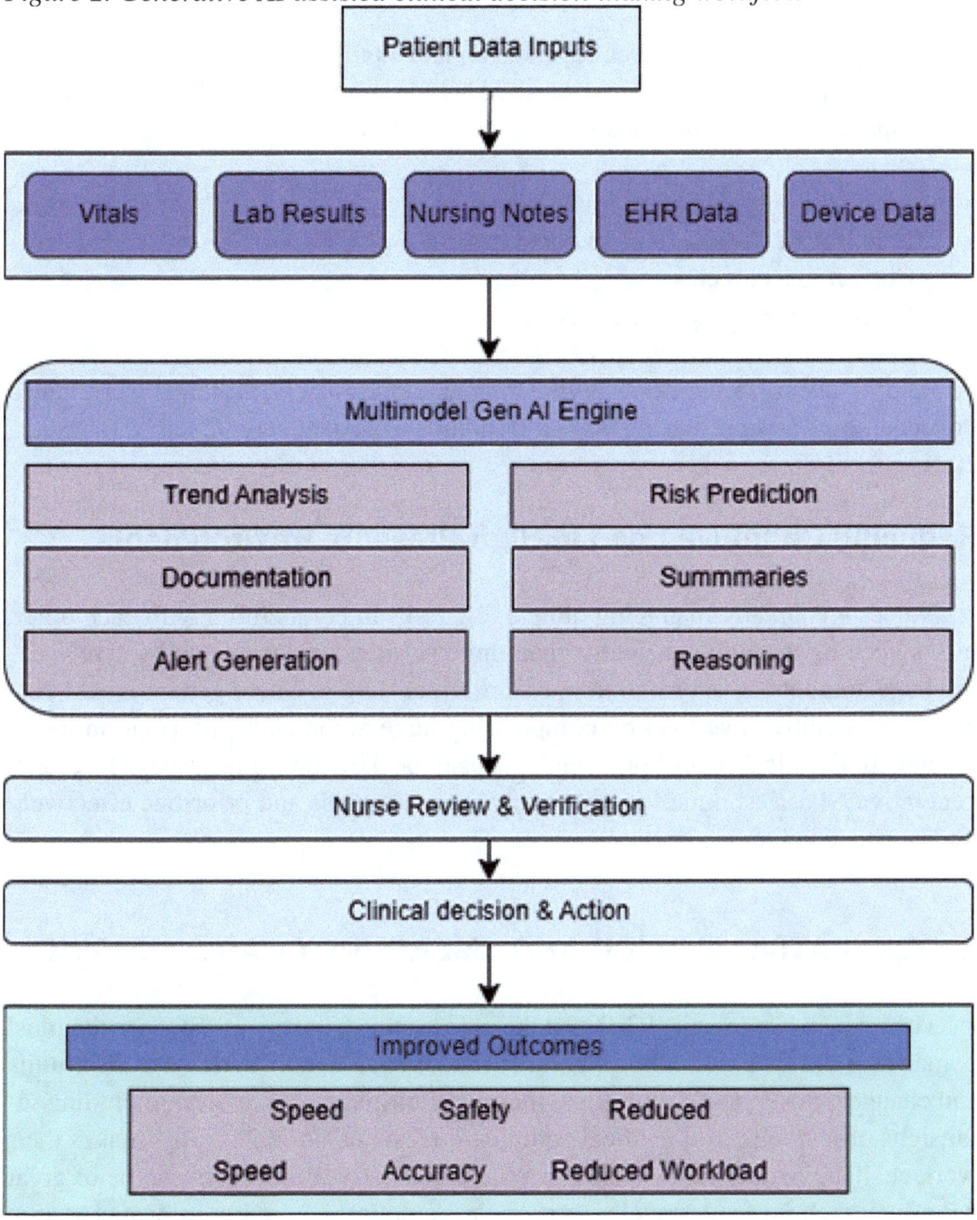

Human Oversight: The Nurse-in-the-Loop Model

High-quality nursing practice depends fundamentally on human judgment. Therefore, generative AI systems must be used within a nurse-in-the-loop framework. This approach ensures that nurses:

- Verify AI outputs before implementation
- Interpret AI explanations in context
- Correct inaccuracies
- Decide when to escalate concerns

Reinforcing nurse autonomy is vital for maintaining safety, avoiding overreliance on technology, and preserving ethical standards in patient care (Chen & Banerjee, 2021).

Reducing Cognitive Load in High-Pressure Environments

Nurses are already managing quite a few tasks in competition with each other, task-switching through constantly changing priorities, and doing so by synthesizing huge amounts of information in record time. Here is where generative AI cuts down on cognitive overload by compressing huge amounts of information into a compressed clinical snapshot, which focuses on key, pressing issues. In effect, generative AI assists nurses to accurately filter out noise and prioritize effectively amidst chaotic clinical situations.

4. GENERATIVE AI IN ICU AND EMERGENCY CARE NURSING

The intensive care unit (ICU) and the emergency department (ED) are the most demanding and data-rich environments in modern healthcare. Patients in these units can change quickly, and nurses must monitor multiple things at once, including vital signs, test results, and medical equipment (Pang et al., 2022). This makes their work challenging and time-sensitive. Where generative AI models can be of great benefit to such professionals by turning vast amounts of patient information into valuable information that can help in making faster and sounder decisions instead of just highlighting numbers that are abnormal in nature.

The multimodal AI system at the ICU level combines wave form analysis, ventilation setting, infusion pump parameter, lab result, nursing documentation, physician orders, and trending vital signs (Kline et al., 2022). By learning patterns on a large-scale dataset such as the MIMIC, the generative model can predict sepsis, acute respiratory failure, hemodynamic instability, and neurological deterioration before conventional methods can. Early identification is crucial because timely interventions within the first hours of deterioration significantly reduce mortality rates. Generative AI thus serves as an additional layer of surveillance that strengthens the nurse's ability to detect abnormal changes rapidly and accurately.

Alarm fatigue in critical care is a major problem because of high volumes of unnecessary alerts that tend to numb experienced staff members, creating a higher chance for missing true emergencies. An important feature of Generative AI, therefore, is its ability to contextualise and correlate multiple signals together, rather than reacting to each signal in isolation based on single parameters, thereby significantly decreasing excessive alarms by replacing numerous false alarms with very few true alarms. For example, a brief drop in oxygen saturation is unlikely to cause any action when viewed in combination with stable respiratory parameters and stable ventilatory settings; however, when accompanied by slight decreases in oxygen saturation combined with subtle increases in respiratory effort and other nursing assessment findings, such as confusion or agitation, the combination of these factors could be identified by generative models as an early warning sign that indicates the potential for impending respiratory failure. The filtering of extraneous alerts and the identification of truly meaningful signals culminates in elimination of excessive notifications and creation of greater focus and quicker response within the critical care environment (Chen & Banerjee, 2021) .

The incorporation of artificial intelligence into smart equipment further improves quality and effectiveness in Intensive Care Units (ICUs). The current equipment in the ICU (ventilators, infusion pumps, smart beds, etc.) produces a large volume of device-level telemetry data. By harmonising these data sources using an Interoperable Framework (HL7/FHIR), the Generative Artificial Intelligence system is able to interpret this data as a whole and provide a complete picture of the patient; rather than just taking a fragmented 'snapshot' of the patient's condition. A complete overview of the patient allows the nurse to be forewarned of any impending intervention(s) for the patient. Using Generative Artificial Intelligence to produce this complete overview of the patient's condition will provide greater accuracy for assessment purposes and greater speed in addressing interventions as they arise.

Patient presentations in the Emergency Department can sometimes be non-specific and time-sensitive, and the hope, of course, is for us to provide care in a time-conscious manner, but the difficulty, of course, is the fact that each person presents for care in multiple different ways, nurse assessments, and vitals at different intervals. The Generative AI model, in this case, helps nurses in the triage process by meshing the following items and presenting this data succinctly in such a manner as to call attention to unique high-risk conditions for immediate attention (Joshi, Pezzotti, & Browne, 2023). Triage accuracy is very important for us as far as providing care in a time-conscious manner, and the Generative AI model helps us provide a more informed perspective of the situation in which patients are presenting for triage assessment.

The reason generative AI deployment makes the biggest difference in the ICU and emergency is because it helps humans achieve better outcomes with their knowledge and skills. Instead of displacing the human experience or intuition, generative AI will democratize large volumes of data so that nurses might create more clear-cut narratives to help them (Moor, Rieck, Horn, Jutzeler, & Borgwardt, 2021). For this reason, generative AI will improve decision-making by decreasing the cognitive overhead on nurses, increasing the safety of the patient, and improving the potential to have better outcomes from the care provided in a critical environment where delay or missed opportunity can lead to drastic consequences.

5. DOCUMENTATION AND WORKFLOW AUTOMATION USING GENERATIVE AI

Documentation plays an essential role within the nursing field when it comes to the continuity and quality of care offered, including the ability to communicate within the health sector and serve as legal evidence of the care offered to patients. In this regard, the documentation of care offered can often be identified as one of the most labor-intensive and time-consuming aspects of the nursing field itself. In this case, the use of generative AI has the ability to radically alter this area by allowing the automation of various documentation aspects while being able to ensure the same standards of clarity, accuracy, and completeness are offered by documentation within the health setting itself (Michalowski, Topaz, & Peltonen, 2025). In the right implementation, the use of AI can ensure reduced documentation work for nurses, which will ultimately optimize the quality of health communication and help solve problems across various members of the health team (Liu et al., 2021). Figure 3 Chart illustrates the way Generative AI improves the efficiency of the nursing profession by lessening the load in the following areas.

Figure 3. Estimated percentage of time saved by GenAI in nursing tasks

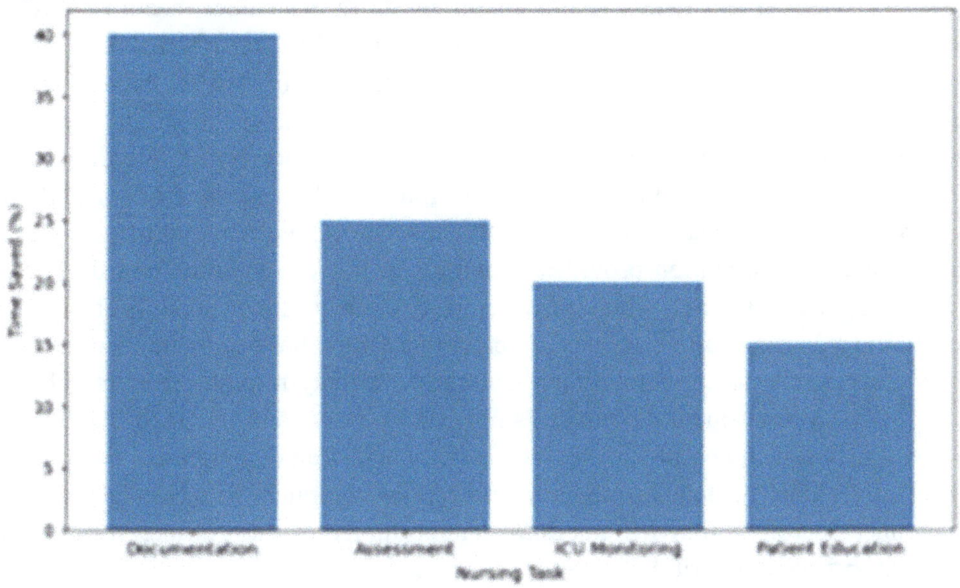

One of the major domains where the use of Generative AI can prove to be beneficial for nurses involves the automated generation of nursing notes. With the use of automated voice recognition systems combined with the ability to perform natural language processing, nurses can voice the results of assessments and happenstance events that may take place when they are at the bedside performing the day-to-day activities related to the patients under their care. The Generative AI can take the results of the nurses' voice input and generate them into a structured form that can include elements such as the SOAP note (Subjective, Objective, Assessment, Plan) and/or system assessments. The generated notes maintained the original clinical integrity of the input provided by the nurses but generated the input in a readable form. (Moore, Garnett, Mason, Onigbinde, & Yurkiv, 2025). While the AI-generated draft is in a structured format, it is still editable, allowing the nurse to take full ownership of their input and to maintain the clinical and legal validity of the documentation.

Another important development is the automatic generation of shift handovers. Quality of handover is known to impact patient safety, and shift transition errors have been identified as contributing factors to adverse events (Pang et al., 2022). Generative AI can create structured handover summaries in the SBAR (Situation, Background, Assessment, Recommendation) from synthesised clinical data captured in the EHR (Electronic Health Record), including historical trends, outstanding issues, pending tests/investigations, and items that require increased priority for monitoring.

By providing all of the information necessary for nurses to have a complete and consistent view of a patient's health, incoming nurse orientation becomes easier and nurse confidence in their ability to make clinical decisions increases. In fast-paced environments, automated nursing documentation using artificial intelligence allows nurses to have full access to patient data and eliminates missed information by creating a shared understanding between nurses and promoting interdisciplinary collaboration among nursing staff from multiple disciplines. Documentation automation has added additional assistance in performing nursing duties. Nursing documentation automation provides reminders to nurses regarding due dates for completing tasks as well as flags any overdue documentation needed. When documentation regarding patient activity indicates that a nurse has documented increased respiratory effort, for Example, then generative AI may remind the nurse of the time frame to re-evaluate the patient's respiratory status and the need for further evaluation based on unit protocols. As a result, nurses can complete nursing duties efficiently, reduce the load on memory storage, stay compliant with clinically-based guidelines; therefore, they will not miss an opportunity to assess or intervene based on their observation period.

The integrity of the documentation must be maintained through documentation automation. The AI-generated content has to state that it is only a draft that will need to be approved by a medical professional before it can be used for final purposes of their record (Gerke, Minssen, & Cohen, 2020). Also, all of the elements of an automated-generated note have to relate to a source of data for patients (e.g., links of audio recordings, lab results, nurse entries to footnotes). Version history and audit trails are also essential to ensure there are records available to verify a professional's documentation for medical malpractice purposes (Pruski, 2024).

For the most part, the use of AI-assisted documentation will result in improvements in both the efficiency and quality of nursing documents while also allowing for the legal protections that must be present in any nursing document to be maintained. However, the effects of generative AI on a nurse's workflow do not stop at documentation; the use of generative AI to simplify administrative processes will allow nurses to focus on more patient-focused activities, therapeutic communication, and the types of clinical reasoning that are done at a higher level. Gradually, this redirection of effort will improve job satisfaction, reduce the chances of nurses experiencing burnout, and enhance the relational aspects of nursing that technology can never replace. Therefore, automating documentation should not be considered as a simple time-saving device, but rather, it is a means to free nurses to perform those types of care items that will benefit from the nurse's emotional intelligence, clinical judgment, and holistic involvement with the patient.

6. GENERATIVE AI FOR PATIENT ENGAGEMENT AND COMMUNICATION

Effective communication is at the heart of nursing practice. In addition to ensuring the accuracy of their clinical work, nurses must establish trust, alleviate fears and uncertainties, and empower patients to make decisions about their care (Chin et al., 2023). Through generative artificial intelligence (GenAI), nurses have access to all three functions: personalised education for individuals, multi-lingual environments for cultural inclusion, and detailed, logical guides tailored to the individual's level of understanding/Involvement.

Historically, patient education materials have been written for generalised populations and are often too text-heavy and do not meet the needs of diverse populations who may not have the ability to read. GenAI can change this by providing real-time responses for patients, answering questions about their health, clarifying complex medical jargon, and generating instructions that are accessible and culturally aware (Nutbeam, 2023).

One of GenAI's most powerful tools is its capacity to restate or reformat complex medical information into an easy-to-understand format for patients. For example, GenAI can translate the medical term "acute exacerbation of chronic obstructive pulmonary disease" into language that is much easier to understand, such as "Your lungs are having more trouble than they should be." Following the easier definition, GenAI will provide an uncomplicated list of what to watch out for as warning signs. The ability to create and convey this simplified information improves the patient's understanding, and thus their compliance to their treatment regimen. Nurses may further edit these translations to add to patient-specific preferences, cultures, and/or hospital protocols.

The use of GenAI has the potential to allow communication between people who speak different languages in a way that it has never been historically possible. In several geographic locations, patients and health care providers often experience miscommunication, medication errors, and a negative patient experience due to a language barrier. By providing the ability to translate nursing instructions into many different languages using generative AI tools, nurses have the ability to build a better relationship with their patients and families who do not speak the same language as them. Many times, nurses utilize visual aids when educating their patients. The creation of visual aids through Generative AI enables the generation of visual diagrams and illustrated step-by-step instructions using text-based input and converting them into images. These visual aids improve the process of educating patients regarding procedures, self-care techniques, medication management, and chronic disease management.

Generative AI also enables the use of intelligent clinical conversational agents in patient facing virtual environments that provide initial general information, respond to frequently asked questions and perform low risk symptom checks prior to escalating any identified concerns to the nurse. In addition to simplifying patient access to information, these agents assist in managing chronic medical conditions by providing timely reminders to monitor blood pressure, glucose levels, and adherence to prescribed medications through a built-in reminder system. The agent will also alert the nurse should any potentially problematic patterns emerge through giving a summary of what has been reported to be occurring with the patient as well as giving information about their last device results. This type of system will support greater continuity of care by enabling a nurse to provide oversight for many patients when using home based and/or remote monitoring programs.

Although AI will never completely replace human oversight, there is concern that AI may oversimplify or misinterpret clinical decisions. Accordingly, systems should be designed such that if there is any uncertainty or high risk associated with output, such output will always require a referral to the human clinician. This will help maintain therapeutic integrity in nurse-patient communication and trust in the caregiver relationship. Ultimately, generative AI improves efficiency in communication, and enables nurses to spend greater amounts of time on empathetic support, counseling, and being a supportive presence—all aspects of care that cannot be replicated by any technology.

7. GENERATIVE AI FOR NURSING EDUCATION AND WELLBEING

The nursing profession is changing at an unprecedented pace as a result of advancements in healthcare technology. Future nursing professionals will need a thorough understanding of clinical informatics, AI systems, digital health technologies, and data-informed decision-making in order to remain relevant. Generative AI will support the new generation of nurses in their ability to engage in simulation-based learning, establish personalised study pathways, automate assessments, and provide ongoing support for continued professional growth. As such, generative AI will assist in breaking down barriers within more traditional methods of teaching nursing by providing more flexible and adaptive educational opportunities that reflect the complexities of real-world practice.

AI-simulation scenarios generated through generative AI are uniquely beneficial for Learning experience (Chen & Banerjee, 2021). Unlike traditional static case studies, generative AI technology creates Clinical scenarios that are Dynamic and Branching based on a learner's actions in the simulation experience. As an example, a New Student Nurse doing an Assessment on a patient with Chest Pain, Depending on how quickly the Student Nurse reacts to the assessment (a delay for example would result in a worsening Hypothetical condition), the New Student Nurse would receive different results. If the Student Nurse acted appropriately by conducting the assessment quickly, the scenario would return to prior state or become stabilised. The Dynamic nature of Generative AI learning experiences enables students to explore multiple ways to practice Clinical Reasoning, Communication Skills, Teamwork and Prioritisation skills, provided they have a safe environment to practice their skills. A significant benefit of generative AI in Education is the capacity for generative AI technologies to create Personalised Learning Pathways. The Technology uses the learner's performance record to identify skills the learner has difficulty mastering and recommends courses, Quizzes, and Case Studies based upon the area(s) of difficulty. A learner having difficulty completing a Respiratory Assessment may only need targeted tutorials on respiratory topics to successfully master that skill set. By providing more effective approaches to Personalise Skill Development based upon a learner's unique needs the efficiency and effectiveness of the Learning experience are improved.

Generative artificial intelligence (AI) can also be used to provide automated feedback during formative assessments. AI applications can evaluate students' documentation, identify vague language or recommend terminology based on scientific evidence, and identify missing elements in students' documentation for example: lack of details regarding an assessment, lack of clinical reasoning or supporting evidence. By using generative AI this way, instructors can attend to more complex forms of instruction than simply correcting students' work. Generative AI is not intended to replace the role of faculty members in overseeing their students' education, but rather to lessen the administrative burden on faculty while increasing the effectiveness of their communication and education.

Furthermore, generative AI has positive impacts on nurses' health and is helping nurses remain in the profession during challenging times such as burnout, compassion fatigue, or stress at work potentially hindering nurses' ability to provide high-quality care. Generative AI systems use natural language processing technologies to evaluate reflective writing, monitor communications, review notes of wellness checks, and identify linguistic indicators of stress, frustration, or emotional exhaustion (Rani, Vishnoi, & Mishra, 2023). If generative AI is utilized ethically (e.g., with the informed consent of nurses to allow analysis of personal data and with stringent security measures), generative AI can facilitate earlier interventions such as peer-support recommendations, schedule changes, or mental health resources.

Nurses may use AI-based wellness tools, in the form of reflective journaling assistants, to aid in overcoming emotionally challenging situations. The assistants may offer supportive prompts, help in the summary and analysis of the emotional components of a situation, as well as offer possible strategies for overcoming. Thus, these AI colleagues will enhance healthy reflection as well as assist in the ability of the AI to boost the psychological resilience of an individual. However, these wellness tools will need to incorporate adequate privacy measures to secure the misuse of employee emotional information by an employer and/or manager. Thus, in the training of nursing students as well as the protection of nursing practitioners, the use of generative artificial intelligence (AI) allows for the development of a means by which overall well-being will be enhanced in the development of the resilience and skills of nurses, as well as retaining humanistic ideals associated with the practice of nursing.

8. ETHICAL, LEGAL, AND GOVERNANCE CONSIDERATIONS IN GENERATIVE AI FOR NURSING

Although the integration of generative AI into nursing has the promise of opening up new vistas for further improvements in the way healthcare is delivered, there are some crucial challenges that pertain to ethics, governance, as well as legality that need to be addressed proactively before implementing these tools. The nursing profession has some foundational values that include ethical obligations, advocacy, as well as caring relationships. The development as well as performance of AI tools within nursing needs proper structures that are allied with human dignity, autonomy, as well as justice (Nasir, Khan, & Bai, 2024). Table 2 illustrates the primary risks associated with generative AI within nursing practices, as well as the complimenting measures that can ensure its safe application within the healthcare domain.

Table 2. Major risks of generative AI in nursing and mitigation strategies

Risk	Description	Mitigation Strategy
AI Hallucinations	Incorrect summaries or sugesstions.	Human verification; clear XAI explanations
Privacy & Data Leakage	Misuse/exposure of sensitive health data	Encryption; consent; strong access controls
Algorithm Bias	Unequal predictions across groups	Diverse datasets; bias audits; fairness tools Nurse-in-the-loop protocols
Overdependence on AI	Reduced nurse critical thinking	Nurse-in-the-loop protocols
Workflow Disruption	Alerts overload; poor integration	Workflow redesign; alert optimization

Ethical Foundations for AI in Nursing

Nursing ethics prioritise beneficence, non-maleficence, autonomy and justice. The design and use of generative AI must comply with these ethical principles. The principle of beneficence means that AI should improve patient outcomes and provide enhanced methods for delivering care. The principle of non-maleficence requires that AI not introduce new types of harm to patients by providing inaccurate clinical recommendations, disseminating false information and/or violating patient privacy. Autonomy refers to maintaining patients' preferences, their consent and respect for their values (Nasir et al., 2024). To comply with the principle of justice, AI developers and healthcare organisations must use their AI tools to treat all populations fairly and without propagating structural biases. Thus, nursing generative AI systems must be developed transparently, they should not manipulate patient data nor create deceptive information about patients. In addition, it is just as critical to maintain the human connection between the nurse and their patient; algorithms cannot replace the nurse-patient therapeutic relationship (Gerke et al., 2020).

Data Privacy, Consent, and Security

Healthcare practitioners deal with a wide variety of sensitive personal health information regarding their patients. Generative artificial intelligence (AI) solutions utilize enormauls amounts of sensitive personal health information to operate optimally, as well as to facilitate applications such as Electronic Health Records (EHRs) and Continuous Health Monitoring (CHM), Safeguarding the privacy of a individual's health data is critical to maintaining data integrity and supporting trust between the healthcare provider and the individual. Ethical use of generative Artificial Intelligence (AI) requires compliance with applicable data protection laws, and also includes written policies governing how healthcare providers may use, collect, store, access, and retain individual health data. Patients should be aware that AI tools are being used to help provide care for them, particularly when the AI is being used to support decision making (Nasir et al., 2024) . By providing transparent communication between the patient and the healthcare provider, the patient can better understand the role that AI plays in their health and provide informed consent where appropriate. As advocates for patients, nurses have a crucial responsibility to communicate this to patients and to support patient autonomy (Gerke et al., 2020).

Explainability, Transparency, and Nurse Trust

One of the main difficulties with generative AI is that it is opaque. Most AI technologies function as "black boxes" which yield results without offering a clear rationale. It is essential for nurses to understand the rationale behind an Alert, Summary, or Suggestion that a generative AI produces (Kline et al., 2022) (Chin et al., 2023). A lack of clear rationale greatly increases the likelihood of clinical errors happening with generative AI, and decreases nurse confidence in using generative AI. It is important for AI to be concise, clinically understandable, and all the supporting evidence that supports why a warning or recommendation is being issued. For instance, if the system produces an early sepsis warning, the system should identify what clinical values or observations were involved in coming up with that warning (for example, rising lactate levels, falling blood pressure trends, nurse-documented confusion, etc.). When AI generates a transparent explanation of its output, and nurses have a better chance of verifying the AI output, correcting any errors that are associated with the AI output, and safely incorporating AI recommendations into a nurse's clinical judgment.

Bias, Fairness, and Equity in Clinical AI

The potential for bias in artificial intelligence (AI) systems can occur when the training data used to build those ai systems exhibit an imbalance in the distribution of population, access to health care, or clinical documentation practices. Without mitigating measures, Generative AI has the potential to recommend courses of action systematically that are not accurate for certain demographic populations, which may, over time, negatively affect the health care equity. Mitigating measures that have been identified include the use of diverse and representative training data, continuous monitoring of model outputs by demographic variable, and the embedding of techniques that promote algorithmic fairness into the model development process. When caring for vulnerable populations, nurses occupy a unique vantage point to detect inequities in AI behaviour. Observations and input from nurses should inform cycles of improvement for algorithms to ensure that AI contributes positively to equitable care.

Legal Accountability and Professional Liability

The legal implications of AI use in nursing practice is still evolving. As AI recommendations play a role in influencing the decisions that nurses make regarding their practice, there are questions about who is ultimately responsible for the recommendations made by the AI and what happens if those recommendations do not produce the desired results. Nurses are legally responsible for their practice decisions, including those that may have been influenced by AI. Therefore, AI tools must be clearly defined as decision-support rather than autonomous decision-makers. Each Health Care Organization will have to establish policies that define the roles, responsibilities, and escalation pathways for when the outputs from AI are in question. It will be important for health care organizations to work with their legal department, clinical governance board, and nursing leadership to define the boundaries of use for AI, create documentation trails to maintain accountability, and ensure that clinical authority is not improperly delegated to AI systems.

Regulatory Frameworks and Standards

Globally, government authorities are setting up the right framework to ensure that artificial intelligence is adopted in a safe way within the health care sector. The European Union has published the AI Act, the FDA has proposed guidelines for adaptive learning systems, and WHO has also established guidelines for ethics of artificial intelligence usage in health care. The essential requirements of these guidelines include: Transparency, Safety, Fairness, and Accountability (TSA). All of these requirements: Outline specific requirements to be followed during clinical evaluation (clinical evaluation), as well as additional requirements which depend on risk categorization, as well as requirements related to post-market surveillance (risk categorisation). For health care providers to be within compliance of requirements set by the foregoing framework, emphasis has to be placed on ensuring the completion of assessment requirements mentioned above, which assess potential risks of health care providers' generative artificial intelligence systems. In making health care providers attempt to be in compliance regarding foregoing standards of practice, patient safety regarding AI-based enhanced nursing will improve, as will the credibility of artificial intelligence within health care services.

9. IMPLEMENTATION FRAMEWORK FOR HOSPITALS USING GENERATIVE AI

In order to create conducive conditions for the application of generative AI in nursing, organizations need to evaluate their capabilities from their current knowledge base. The first level of implementing generative AI at a hospital will include assessment of what is available within their infrastructure for generative AI, its potential for adaptation, and what might be limiting its adoption. In this case, hospitals would need to focus on five key dimensions: quality of data, data exchange capabilities, patient participation, internet accessibility, and compliance with regulations. Data will also need to be interoperable, which will include development of good network infrastructure at hospitals to enable sharing of health information by medical practitioners.

Phase One: Readiness Assessment

As a measure of the success of the implementation of generative AI for hospitals, there will possibly be a need for investment in terms of technology development under the following: provision of access to the internet for healthcare providers; provision of adequate digital literacy skills for all healthcare providers in relation to the benefits of generative AI technology. In addition to developing the necessary technology, hospitals will also need to ensure that the organization has enough leadership support to allocate adequate resources for the development of technologies for the use of generative AI. Without funding to promote the growth of the necessary technologies, hospitals are unlikely to be able to implement successful use of generative AI.

Phase Two: Pilot Implementation

To validate usability of AI, initial deployment of systems should occur within controlled pilot projects - such as a specific unit or a small group of clinicians working together; this allows pilot organisations to check/assess the usability of the AI, identify changes that have to be made to existing workflows, collect feedback from users and assess outcomes. For example, the areas of the organisation where AI pilot studies typically take place are: documentation automation, early warning systems or AI-assisted handover; while conducting a pilot, organisations should track metrics related to time savings, alert accuracy, speed of response and nurse satisfaction. Nurses must be engaged and involved with the design, development and evaluation processes from the very beginning of the project, this involvement ensures that AI tools will be more clinically relevant and will consequently be incorporated easily into the nurses' daily workflow.

Phase Three: Workforce Training and Capacity Building

To successfully implement and adopt AI in a clinical setting, hospitals need to provide nurses with in-depth training on how best to use, interpret and verify the output from AI, find and fix problems with AI models and understand the limitations of AI; training should also teach nurses how to work safely with human beings and AI by using simulation-based learning methods to effectively gain a greater understanding of AI; organisations should also continuously provide an environment where nurses can improve their skills in working with the growing technology (Joshi et al., 2023).

Phase Four: Full Integration and Workflow Optimisation

Once hospitals have successfully completed their pilot initiatives, they may incorporate Artificial Intelligence (AI) technologies into all hospital departments. To achieve maximum effect from these new tools, workflow redesign and modification must also accompany implementations. For instance, predictive early warning systems should be tied to existing standardised escalation protocols. Draft documentation produced by AI systems would need to be tied directly into Electronic Health Record (EHR) workflows. AI should complement, not interfere with, Nursing workflows. When systems generate too many alerts or notify at inappropriate times, these alerts become counterproductive. Continuous evaluation serves as a mechanism to match AI-supported workflows to reality.

Phase Five: Continuous Monitoring, Governance, and Quality Management

Generative AI also needs continuous monitoring for appropriate safety and fairness outcomes along with reliable performance. When the patient population or clinical practice is modified, there is potential for a model drift to occur. The establishment of performance metrics or dashboards by hospitals can allow hospital personnel to identify types and patterns in alert frequency, false positive indicators and overrides made by clinicians, disparities within predictive analytics and final clinical outcome Results. Governance committees review incidents with the use of AI technologies, approve updates to these technologies, monitor nurses' experience in order to gain a voice in improving AI technologies and oversee adherence to ethical and regulatory requirements. Members of these committees must include nursing leadership, ethicists, clinical informatics professionals, data scientists, legal counsel and patient representatives.

Importance of a Human-Centered Implementation Philosophy

During deployment, every hospital should adopt a human-centered approach to care delivery. While Generative AI can play an assisting role in the provision of clinical expertise, it cannot replace the nurse's responsibility for making the final decision based on their knowledge and experience. The nurse will continue to be the main decision-maker responsible for merging AI insight with their complete understanding of the whole patient. Therefore, in order for an implementation framework to be effective, it must be able to provide the nurse with the ability to be an empowered, autonomous and ethical provider. By doing this, AI can increase the nurse's ability to provide compassionate and safe care while providing equitable access to that care.

10. CASE STUDIES OF GENERATIVE AI IN NURSING PRACTICE

As healthcare providers start to look to Generative AI to support their nursing practice, there are numerous documented case studies in the literature that show that Generative AI has the potential to improve efficiencies around workflow, protect the clinical decision-making process and enhance early detection of patient deterioration, facilitate remote management of patients, and decrease documentation workloads. Many deployments of Generative AI are still in the very early stages; however, there is considerable evidence in documented case studies from hospitals, research institutions and community-based programs that demonstrate the ability for Generative AI to create significant gains in all of these areas, but more importantly, in the area of enhancing patient safety and transforming how nurses do their work.

Case Study: Documentation Automation in a Medical-Surgical Unit

Nursing documentation has received the greatest immediate and quantifiable returns from generative AI. A large academic hospital completed a pilot study with an AI documentation tool that converted audio recordings of nurses talking at the bedside into structured nursing notes. This encouraged nurses to record assessments, interventions and patient responses verbally while the AI tool produced drafts for the nurse in standardised formats such as SOAP and system-based templates. The nurses were required to review and edit the draft for clinical and legal issues before submission. When the pilot study was completed, nurses indicated they saved between 20 and 30 minutes of time each shift; consequently, nurses had more interactions at the bedside with patients, were able to communicate more effectively with family members and felt less time pressure at the end of each shift to complete charting activities. Nurse satisfaction ratings also increased, with participants stating documentation felt less burdensome and more aligned with real-time patient care. Furthermore, the improved clarity and consistency of documentation improved communication between disciplines, making for an easier transfer at hand-off times. As a result, the hospital has introduced the use of the AI tool to other nursing units and has demonstrated that meaningful efficiencies can be achieved through the responsible use of generative AI.

Case Study: Early Sepsis Detection in Critical Care

An ICU at a tertiary hospital developed an intuitive, inter-operative multi-modal artificial Intelligence (AI) system that utilized sensor data collected through nurse observations, via telemetry, from laboratory reports, and across telemdiacle systems. The System's core capability was to generate a risk scoring and alert warning to indicate the likelihood or risk of developing sepsis. Included within the alerts were explanatory details regarding the reasoning behind the prediction, including actual data trends and patterns from individual patient records and assessments by nurses (e.g., a downward trend in blood pressure, increased lactate, behavioural changes reported in nursing assessments) (Villanueva-Miranda et al., 2025) (Gottesman et al., 2020). Through the use of a multi-modal AI system, the ICU identified patients with a high probability of deteriorating 3 to 6 hours before the traditional scoring process flagged abnormalities. The initial alert enabled nurses to conduct a formal evaluation sooner and, if necessary, notify the physician in a timely manner so that sepsis bundles (standardised management protocols for treating sepsis) could be initiated immediately. The retrospective analysis of ICU transfers from the ward was also associated with a substantial but clinically meaningful reduction in the mortality rate of patients who received prompt intervention. It determines the use of generative AI and the potential for GenAI to enhance timely, accurate clinical decisions made by critical care teams.

Case Study: Virtual Nurse Support for Chronic Disease Management

In order to help patients who were allocated a community health program for Diabetes, Chronic Obstructive Pulmonary Disease (COPD), and Hypertension, to check and control their respective conditions using Tele-Health, the virtual assistant using the concept of generative Artificial Intelligence (AI) was introduced. With the help of the virtual assistant, patients were able to communicate and update the respective symptoms, home device readings, and reminders for taking medications and following lifestyle changes every day of the week. Depending on the input from the patients, the AI performed an evaluation and made prioritized report summaries for the respective nurses who are handling patients' cases (Moor et al., 2021). In the case of patients' data, when there are critical and unusual data identified, alert notifications were sent to the respective nurse through the AI, and the reasoning behind the data visualization for alert notification was explained, and the nurse could call the patients as follow-ups or adjust the current handling procedure by actively engaging Medical Doctors with the respective patients when necessary. Nurses and patients alike expressed appreciation for the additional support provided to them when using the technology and felt it provided them an opportunity to reduce gaps between clinic visits. It is evident from this case study that generative AI has the potential to extend nursing services into the home and assist in managing chronic diseases by improving care processes through better continuity of care (Liu et al., 2021).

11. FUTURE RESEARCH DIRECTIONS IN GENERATIVE AI FOR NURSING

The rapid development of generative AI shows great potential for transformation; however, much work still must be done to better understand the best method for designing, using safely, and applying generative AI to nursing practice. Learning routes for future research, technology development, and nursing leadership exist within the current body of knowledge regarding generative AI's use in nursing.

Development of Nursing-Specific Language Models

Most of the current generative AI tools that have been developed and utilised by all types of healthcare professionals have been trained on datasets that are not refined enough or specific enough for nursing. Most of them have been based on general medical datasets or general language datasets. Future research should focus on developing nursing-specific LLMs that are trained using high-quality, anonymised nursing documentation, care plans, assessments, and decision pathways (Topol, 2019). These will provide more accurate documentation support, improved generation of handovers, and more relevant decision-support outputs (Jukanti, 2025).

Advancements in Multimodal Clinical Reasoning

Future AI models will include not only text-based reasoning, but will also integrate modalities such as audio, image, sensor data, waveforms, and environmental cues. Research on how multimodal AI systems imitate bedside observational reasoning, such as detecting laboured breathing, changes in tone of voice, or subtle shifts in neurological function that experienced nurses are able to intuitively identify is necessary (Nasir et al., 2024). These advances have the potential to change how clinical monitoring is conducted, especially in Intensive Care Units (ICU) and Emergency Departments (Moor et al., 2021).

Human–AI Teaming and Decision-Making Dynamics

Further research will also be necessary to understand how the use of AI in the context of the immediate clinical decision-making process by nurses would affect their cognitive load, the accuracy of their prioritising of cases and trust patterns regarding AI; their escalation behaviours regarding patient care and their communications with other disciplines (Shortliffe, Sepùlveda, & Patel, 2022). Identifying the most appropriate models for the interaction between AI and the human clinician will be a key factor in the design of AI systems that will enhance, rather than disrupt, the clinical workflow.

Ethical Governance and Policy Frameworks

As the generative AI technology matures and becomes more integrated into the daily clinical activities, new challenges related to regulation and ethics will arise regarding the need to develop governance structures that allow for the growth of innovation but also protect the public's health and safety; the legal obligations associated with decisions made by AI-assisted clinicians and; equity and fairness in the treatment of patients. Such studies will assist in developing policy frameworks to allow for the responsible application of these technologies across a wide variety of healthcare settings.

Long-Term Workforce Impacts

Ultimately, it is crucial to establish how generative and non-generative AI technologies will impact upon nurse retention rates (and factors contributing to burn-out), sense of professional identity (including, but not limited to), and how satisfied they feel in their work. In addition to potentially decreasing administrative workloads; however, using AI could also place greater emphasis on physician/nurse oversight, monitoring or digital accountability and thus create new pressures that may exist among nurses. Longitudinal studies are needed to assess if AI will improve the resilience of the nurse workforce or whether it will create new challenges requiring an organisationally based intervention approach.

12. CONCLUSION

Throughout the 21st century, one of the most influential technological advancements on the profession of nursing has been generative AI, which has advanced to include an extensive range of capabilities beyond automation. The generative

AI capability supports advanced reasoning when applying clinical judgement to complex data/information sets; generates patient-specific clinical narratives; and supports clinical assessments, documentation, communication, and decision-making with relevant clinical circumstances. Implementation of generative AI in real-world settings has resulted in measurable outcomes, i.e. decreased documentation compliance; earlier identification of decline/deterioration; improved management of chronic diseases; improved communication across nursing care teams; etc. While the ethical, legal, and governance requirements for successfully deploying generative AI must be in place to ensure patient safety, transparency, equitable application, and accountability; hospitals should utilise structured implementation models that include comprehensive assessments of the organisational readiness to implement generative AI, pilot studies, ongoing evaluation and monitoring, engagement of multiple professional disciplines to develop training, and using a human-centred design approach.. Every stage of the adoption and development of Artificial Intelligence (AI) must place Nurses at the centre of this process, as they are the key evaluators, users, and advocates for patient safety. Generative AI will redefine Nursing Practice and generate new possibilities as the technology continues to grow and develop. Newer technologies and developments include generating nurse-specific language and building a multimodal decision support engine for Nursing practice. There will be new AI technology tools that will provide nurses with an increased number of opportunities to engage in compassionate patient care and to share their work with other healthcare professionals, allowing them to be part of a more intelligent Healthcare Ecosystem and allowing them to further support the value of human connection within Nursing. Ultimately, the integration of Generative AI technology should support and re-establish the importance of our connection to one another in Nursing and will provide opportunities for the development of healthcare systems that allow for enhanced patient care at all levels.

REFERENCES

Chen, K. K., & Banerjee, A. (2021). *The digital transformation of medical education* (Vol. 14). SAGE Publications Sage UK.

Chin, M. H., Afsar-Manesh, N., Bierman, A. S., Chang, C., Colón-Rodríguez, C. J., Dullabh, P., & Hightower, M. (2023). Guiding principles to address the impact of algorithm bias on racial and ethnic disparities in health and health care. *JAMA Network Open, 6*(12), e2345050–e2345050. DOI: 10.1001/jamanetworkopen.2023.45050 PMID: 38100101

Choudhury, A., & Asan, O. (2020). Role of artificial intelligence in patient safety outcomes: Systematic literature review. *JMIR Medical Informatics, 8*(7), e18599. DOI: 10.2196/18599 PMID: 32706688

Garg, L., Basterrech, S., Banerjee, C., & Sharma, T. K. (2021). *Artificial intelligence in healthcare*. Springer.

Gerke, S., Minssen, T., & Cohen, G. (2020). Ethical and legal challenges of artificial intelligence-driven healthcare. In *Artificial intelligence in healthcare* (pp. 295–336). Elsevier. DOI: 10.1016/B978-0-12-818438-7.00012-5

Gottesman, O., Futoma, J., Liu, Y., Parbhoo, S., Celi, L., Brunskill, E., & Doshi-Velez, F. (2020). *Interpretable off-policy evaluation in reinforcement learning by highlighting influential transitions*. Paper presented at the International Conference on Machine Learning.

Joshi, M., Pezzotti, N., & Browne, J. T. (2023). Human–AI relationship in health-care. In *Explainable AI in Healthcare* (pp. 1–22). Chapman and Hall/CRC. DOI: 10.1201/9781003333425-1

Jukanti, M. (2025). Ai in healthcare: Revolutionizing medical diagnosis. *Journal Of Engineering And Computer Sciences, 4*(7), 1087–1093.

Kline, A., Wang, H., Li, Y., Dennis, S., Hutch, M., Xu, Z., Wang, F., Cheng, F., & Luo, Y. (2022). Multimodal machine learning in precision health: A scoping review. *NPJ Digital Medicine, 5*(1), 171. DOI: 10.1038/s41746-022-00712-8 PMID: 36344814

Liu, X., Gao, K., Liu, B., Pan, C., Liang, K., Yan, L., & Pan, S. (2021). Advances in deep learning-based medical image analysis. *Health Data Science, 2021*, 8786793. DOI: 10.34133/2021/8786793 PMID: 38487506

Michalowski, M., Topaz, M., & Peltonen, L. M. (2025). An AI-Enabled Nursing Future With No Documentation Burden: A Vision for a New Reality. *Journal of Advanced Nursing*. PMID: 40129115

Moor, M., Rieck, B., Horn, M., Jutzeler, C. R., & Borgwardt, K. (2021). Early prediction of sepsis in the ICU using machine learning: A systematic review. *Frontiers in Medicine*, *8*, 607952. DOI: 10.3389/fmed.2021.607952 PMID: 34124082

Moore, S. J., Garnett, A., Mason, K., Onigbinde, E., & Yurkiv, H. (2025). Nurses' Perceptions on the Usability of Electronic Health Records: A Scoping Review. *Science of Nursing and Health Practices = Science Infirmière et Pratiques en Santé*, *8*(1), 57–86. DOI: 10.62212/snahp.130

Nasir, S., Khan, R. A., & Bai, S. (2024). Ethical framework for harnessing the power of AI in healthcare and beyond. *IEEE Access : Practical Innovations, Open Solutions*, *12*, 31014–31035. DOI: 10.1109/ACCESS.2024.3369912

Nemati, M., Ansary, J., & Nemati, N. (2020). Machine-learning approaches in COVID-19 survival analysis and discharge-time likelihood prediction using clinical data. *Patterns (New York, N.Y.)*, *1*(5), 100074. DOI: 10.1016/j.patter.2020.100074 PMID: 32835314

Nutbeam, D. (2023). Artificial intelligence and health literacy—Proceed with caution. *Health Literacy and Communication Open*, *1*(1), 2263355. DOI: 10.1080/28355245.2023.2263355

Pang, K., Li, L., Ouyang, W., Liu, X., & Tang, Y. (2022). Establishment of ICU mortality risk prediction models with machine learning algorithm using MIMIC-IV database. *Diagnostics (Basel)*, *12*(5), 1068. DOI: 10.3390/diagnostics12051068 PMID: 35626224

Pawar, U., O'shea, D., Rea, S., & O'reilly, R. (2020). *Explainable AI in healthcare*. Paper presented at the 2020 international conference on cyber situational awareness, data analytics and assessment (CyberSA). DOI: 10.1109/CyberSA49311.2020.9139655

Pruski, M. (2024). Ethical challenges to the adoption of AI in healthcare: A review. *The New Bioethics : a Multidisciplinary Journal of Biotechnology and the Body*, *30*(4), 251–267. DOI: 10.1080/20502877.2025.2541438 PMID: 40779305

Rani, K., Vishnoi, H., & Mishra, M. (2023). *A mental health chatbot delivering cognitive behavior therapy and remote health monitoring using NLP and AI*. Paper presented at the 2023 International Conference on Disruptive Technologies (ICDT). DOI: 10.1109/ICDT57929.2023.10150665

Shortliffe, E. H., Sepùlveda, M.-J., & Patel, V. L. (2022). Framework for the evaluation of clinical AI systems. In *Intelligent systems in medicine and health: the role of AI* (pp. 479–503). Springer. DOI: 10.1007/978-3-031-09108-7_17

Sutton, R. T., Pincock, D., Baumgart, D. C., Sadowski, D. C., Fedorak, R. N., & Kroeker, K. I. (2020). An overview of clinical decision support systems: Benefits, risks, and strategies for success. *NPJ Digital Medicine*, *3*(1), 17. DOI: 10.1038/s41746-020-0221-y PMID: 32047862

Topol, E. J. (2019). High-performance medicine: The convergence of human and artificial intelligence. *Nature Medicine*, *25*(1), 44–56. DOI: 10.1038/s41591-018-0300-7 PMID: 30617339

Veldhuis, L. I., Woittiez, N. J., Nanayakkara, P. W., & Ludikhuize, J. (2022). Artificial intelligence for the prediction of in-hospital clinical deterioration: A systematic review. *Critical Care Explorations*, *4*(9), e0744. DOI: 10.1097/CCE.0000000000000744 PMID: 36046062

Villanueva-Miranda, I., Xiao, G., & Xie, Y. (2025). Artificial Intelligence in Early Warning Systems for Infectious Disease Surveillance: A Systematic Review. *Frontiers in Public Health*, *13*, 1609615. DOI: 10.3389/fpubh.2025.1609615 PMID: 40626156

Woo, T., Ho, R., Tang, A., & Tam, W. (2020). Global prevalence of burnout symptoms among nurses: A systematic review and meta-analysis. *Journal of Psychiatric Research*, *123*, 9–20. DOI: 10.1016/j.jpsychires.2019.12.015 PMID: 32007680

Chapter 7

Generative AI-Powered Automation of Nursing Documentation and Patient Reporting:

Enhancing Accuracy, Efficiency, and Clinical Decision Support

Rocky Kumar
http://orcid.org/0009-0002-6995-2037
Poornima University, Jaipur, India

Neeraj Kushwaha
https://orcid.org/0009-0006-3201-2833
Poornima University, Jaipur, India

Himanshi Sharma
http://orcid.org/0009-0007-8458-6836
Poornima University, Jaipur, India

ABSTRACT

Nursing documentation is an important part of the delivery of healthcare services and supports the following: clinical communication, continuity of care, patient safety and regulatory compliance. However, the growing demands for documentation within electronic health record (EHR) systems have played a significant role in the creation of administrative burden, inefficient use of workflow, and professional burnout among nurses. In high acuity clinical environments, delays or inconsistencies in documentation may have an adverse impact on care coordination and patient

DOI: 10.4018/979-8-3373-8247-0.ch007

outcomes. Recent progress in generative artificial intelligence (AI), especially large language models and natural language processing techniques, creates new possibilities to automate and augment the documentation of nursing and reporting from patients. This chapter looks at the role of generative AI-powered automation plays in the improvement of the accuracy, efficiency, and clinical utility of nursing documentation. Key applications discussed include automatic clinical document generation, voice enabled documentation, shift to shift handoff reporting, real-time integration of patient monitoring data and structured patient status summarization in an EHR system. The chapter goes on to discuss some of the methodological considerations of how to implement AI-assisted documentation such as fine-tuning AI models on de-identified clinical data, metrics for evaluation, and human in the loop validation to ensure clinical safety and accountability. Ethical, legal and regulatory issues, including data privacy, algorithmic bias, transparency and nurse responsibility are critically examined. Through the use of illustrative case scenarios based on empirical data, this chapter discusses the use of generative AI as a clinical co-pilot to support nurses without adding to the documentation burden while maintaining professional judgment. Overall, the chapter offers a mix of practical and scholarly insights for clinicians, healthcare administrations, and policymakers attempting to responsibly integrate generative AI into nursing documentation and clinical decision support.

1. INTRODUCTION

Nursing documentation is one of the pillars of contemporary healthcare systems and is crucial for clinical communication and patient care. Accurate and timely nursing records not only provide continuity of care for the most part of multidisciplinary teams but also participate importantly in providing care for patient safety, quality assurance, regulatory compliance and medico legal accountability. With the complexity of healthcare delivery growing and the growing use of electronic health record (EHR) systems, the scope and volume of nursing documentation have grown significantly, with big demands on nursing professionals (Topaz & Pruinelli, 2017).

Despite the advancement in digital health technologies, nursing documentation is labour-intensive, time-consuming, and a challenging task. Nurses are frequently expected to juggle direct patient care with a large amount of documentation, which can cause inefficiencies in the workflow and a general increase in cognitive load.

Studies have shown that activities required for documentation are able to take up a significant percentage of working hours of nurses and as a result, oftentimes reduce the amount of time they have available to devote to patient centred care (Sinsky et al., 2016). These challenges have been compounded in high acuity clinical environments where timely and accurate documentation is so important to patient outcome.

Recent advances in artificial intelligence (AI), in particular generative AI and large language models (LLMs) hold out exciting prospects in transformative effects on the process of nursing documentation but likewise patient reporting behaviours. By facilitating the automated, context-aware and consistent generation of clinical text, generative AI can play an important role in improving the accuracy of documentation, mitigating administrative burden and facilitating real-time clinical decision-making. This chapter explores in-depth the role of generative artificial intelligence (AI) empowered automation in documentation and reporting of patient care, in this instance, in the example of improved efficiency, enhancing accuracy, and clinical decision support of patient records.

Figure 1. Evolution of Nursing Documentation Systems from Manual Records to AI-Driven Automation

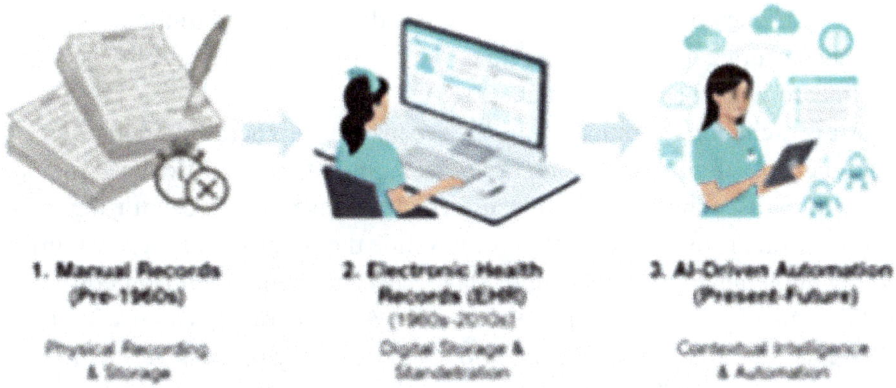
1. Manual Records
Physical Recording
& Storage
2. Electronic Health
Records (EHR)
Digital Storage &
3. AI-Driven Automation
(Present-Future)
Contextual Intelligence
& Automation

This chapter has been organized to give an orderly and application discussion of generative AI in nursing documentation. Section 2 introduces the basics of nursing documentation and reporting of patients and emphasizes their clinical, legal, and operational importance. Section 3 presents fundamental ideas about generative artificial intelligence which apply in healthcare settings. Sections 4 to 8 are focused on a nursing-specific application such as AI-based documentation automation, intelligent reporting of patient information, accuracy improvement, efficiency of nursing, and clinical decision support. Section 9 covers ethical, legal, and regulatory considerations, and then goes on to present some illustrative case scenarios drawn from real world scenarios in Section 10. The chapter concludes by synthesizing some of the key insights and provides implications for nursing practice and healthcare policy.

1.1 Background Of Nursing Documentation In Modern Healthcare

Nursing documentation has transitioned from handwritten notes and charts to paper-based Nursing documentation has gone from handwritten notes and charts to paper-based systems to sophisticated electronic systems that fit into hospital information systems. Traditionally, nursing notes were used to document vital signs, medication administration, patient assessments, care plans and progress notes. In the contemporary health care settings, these records are implemented in EHR platforms that support sharing of data, data interoperability and regulatory reporting (Kutney-Lee & Kelly, 2011).

Modern-day documentation of nursing is not limited only to record keeping. It is a tool for communication between healthcare providers, evidence-based practice, quality improvement programs, clinical research and population health analytics. Regulatory frameworks and accreditation standards only add to the importance of strong and accurate documentation, and link it directly to patient safety and quality of healthcare impact (Ratwani et al., 2018).

However, challenges inherent in this recent development in technology of the development of a digital documentation system, such as difficulty of use, fragmented working processes and overloading information have emerged with the growing dependence on the use of this technology. While the purpose of EHRs was efficiency, EHR implementation and design flaws have frequently contributed to macros added documentation burden on nursing staff. As such, there is a growing need for intelligent systems that would be able to standardize the process of documentation while preserving the clinical accuracy and relevance.

1.2 Challenges In Manual And Semi-Automated Nursing Records

Manual and semi-automated nursing documentation systems are associated with numerous ongoing problems which adversely affect clinical workflows and care delivery. The manual documentation is prone to error like illegibility, incomplete entries, delayed recording and discrepancy in the terminologies. These issues could have a negative impact on the safety of patients and the co-ordination of their care, as well as increasing the risk of adverse clinical events (Carayon et al., 2020). Semi-automated systems such as the use of templates for EHR documentation have been one way of overcoming some of the limitations of manual records but these tend to be rigid and interrupt the workflow. Nurses may be forced to use complex interfaces, be given limited choices they are not able to use to adequately cover the context of the patient situation, or be asked to copy information from one place to another, within the record.

Such practice is not only taking much more time to document but is also a contributing factor to cognitive fatigue and professional burnout (Dall'Ora et al., 2020). In addition, traditional methods of documentation are not intelligent nor do they have predictive capabilities in the here and now. They are dominated as passives, as parties in which information is collected rather than being active in clinical information intelligence. Sociotechnical and cultural differences - The distinction in sociotechnical and cultural factors in human behaviour also restricts the success of implementing them in the dynamic clinical environment. These challenges reveal the need of advanced solutions for automation that are compatible with nursing flow of work and clinical reasoning processes.

1.3 Emergence Of Generative AI In Clinical Workflows

Generative AI is a breakthrough technology that emerged in the healthcare industry thanks to the advance in natural language processing, deep learning and transformers. Large language models may be able to understand the context of the clinical scenario, produce a coherent narrative of the medical situation and synthesise information from a wide variety of sources of data (Brown et al., 2020; Singhal et al., 2023). These capacities have a lot of potential in the nursing profession, however, in terms of documentation and patient reporting automation. Generative AI systems can be used in assisting with the generation of clinical notes in real time either from structured data and/or voice inputs but, more importantly, medical devices. Simulating the spoken assessments or the sensor data into uniform cases of nursing notes, AI powered tools are prone to cut down on the number of manual data inputs and make them more data-driven. In addition, these systems can detect inconsistencies and missing information and can ensure that clinical documentation standards are followed. Beyond documentation, generative AI helps to contribute to clinical workflow to generate intelligent summaries and patient summaries, generate predictive alerts for patient care, and patient decision support recommendations. When combined with EHR systems, the automation driven by AI can help to increase the situational awareness of nurses and clinicians to help in proactive care intervention, and better patient outcomes. However, the use of generative AI in the clinic also has to be done with due considerations for trust, explainability and human oversight.

1.4 Motivation And Objectives Of The Chapter

The major source of inspiration for this chapter also is the ever-increasing burden of documentation in the nursing profession as well as the need for innovative methods of solution that would also increase the efficiency without compromising the quality of care. As healthcare systems become more integrated with digital technologies, there is an important opportunity to leverage the generative capabilities of artificial intelligence to revolutionize the nursing documentation process to become a smarter, more supportive and value-driven process.

This chapter seeks to offer a detailed analysis of generative AI automation of full-fledged AI in nursing documentation and patient reporting. The objectives of this chapter are as follows:

(i) To Study the Limitations of Traditional and Semi Automated Nursing Documentation Systems.
(ii) To assess the usefulness of generative artificial intelligence in promoting the accuracy, efficiency, and standardization of nursing documentation.
(iii) To introduce the methodology of the implementation of AI-assisted nursing documentation systems in the clinical environment.
(iv) To assess the use of generative AI in clinical decision-making as well as in workflow for patient reporting.
(v) To evaluate the ethical, legal, and accountability issues related to the adoption of AI in nursing practice.

2. FUNDAMENTALS OF NURSING DOCUMENTATION AND PATIENT REPORTING

Nursing documentation and patient reporting is the backbone to the clinical communication and healthcare delivery. These are systematic records of patient condition, nursing assessment, intervention, and outcomes creating systems of coordinated actions of inter-professional teams. In the modern worlds healthcare systems, Nursing documentation has a dual purpose of a clinical record as well as legal record, a quality assurance record and as a source of research and policy development data. As the acuity of patients and the complexity of healthcare rise, the accuracy, completeness and timeliness of the nursing documentation has become important factors in the determination of quality of care and patient safety (McGonigle & Mastrian, 2021).

Patient reporting, which has much to do with nursing documentation, but also the structured presentation and communication of patient-related information in the transition of care, handovers, and clinical reviews. Effective patient reporting supports the continuity of care; helps reduce information loss and facilitates informed clinical decision making. Together, the nursing documentation and patient's report help to provide a common clinical narrative that is used to guide care delivery to the patient.

Figure 2. Categories and Structure of Nursing Documentation and Patient Reporting

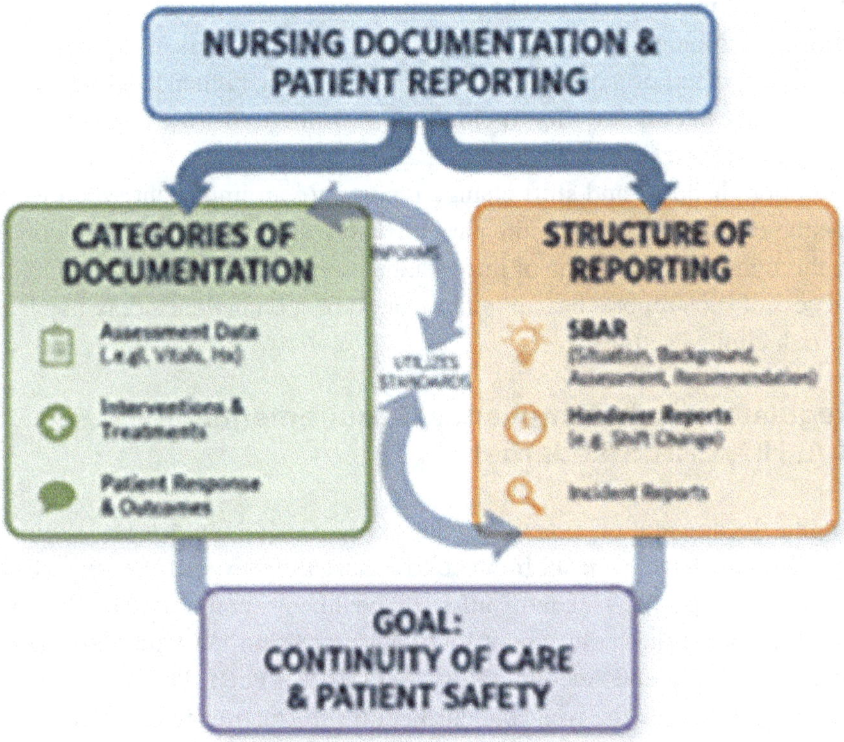

2.1 Types Of Nursing Documentation

Nursing documentation is a collection of a variety of nursing records and each has a unique clinical and administrative function. One of the more common forms is narrative nursing notes Descriptive account of patient conditions Observed Symptoms and Interventions using nursing knowledge and skills. These notes allow nurses to record information that is in a context and in a qualitative design is impossible to record via a structured field.

Another necessary category is flowing sheets and charts which represent methods and ways for recording vital signs, intake and output, administering of medication and other routine assessment. Flow sheets help in analysing trends and help clinicians in easily detecting the changes in the state of the patients. Care plan is more structured form of documentation, which includes patient problems, nursing diagnoses, goals, nursing actions, and anticipated outcomes which facilitate evidence-based care and goal-oriented care.

With the use of electronic health records, structured and quasi-structured documents have come to the fore. These include checklists, dropdown menus, standardized terminologies and coded data elements based on clinical standards. While structured documentation offers facilities for supporting higher-level issues of data consistency and interoperability, it can impose limitations for expressivity if they are poorly conceived (Topaz & Pruinelli, 2017).

In addition, handoff and shift change reports are an important type of nursing documentation and reporting to the patient. These summaries facilitate continuity of care through communication of important patients' information with transitions. The success of such reports has an immediate impact on patient safety in particular in high-risk clinical settings.

2.2 Regulatory And Compliance Requirements (HIPAA, Hl7, EHR Standards)

Nursing documentation practices adhere to strict regulatory and compliance requirements that have been set in place to ensure the privacy, integrity of patient data, and encourage the standardisation of healthcare communications. In most healthcare systems, the requirement that data protection laws such as the Health Insurance Portability and Accountability Act (HIPAA) be followed is mandatory. HIPAA sets guidelines for what patient health information is to be confidential, secure and used and holds healthcare professional, including nurses, to the legal and ethical standards.

Interoperability standards such as Health Level Seven (HL7) is important in making it possible to easily communicate medical information between heterogeneous healthcare information systems. HL7 standards are used to facilitate the organization of a representation and transmission of clinical data so that the documentation of nursing can be accurately shared throughout the department and across organizations. Similarly, Fast Healthcare Interoperability Resources (FHIR) also came around and is a modern juice of realizing the actual access and integration of the data in a digital health ecosystem. Electronic health record standards also provide the documentation requirements for data completeness, audit trails, time stamping, and role-based access requirements. Compliance with these standards ensure that nursing records are reliable, traceable and legally defendable (Ratwani et al. 2018). However, dealing with regulatory requirements often creates an additional layer of complexity in documents, which overshadows on requiring intelligent automation solutions that can ensure compliance without placing an additional administrative burden on the same.

2.3 Role Of Nursing Notes In Patient Safety And Care Continuity

Nursing notes play a pivotal role in safeguarding the safety of patients and ensuring the continuity of care Nursing notes are an essential part of patient safety and need to ensure continuity of care across healthcare settings. Accurate documentation enables risk of patients to be promptly recognised, e.g. clinical deterioration and medication error, or the unmet needs of care When assessment and intervention of nursing are recorded properly, a nurse is able to make an informed decision with thorough knowledge of the patient's condition (Carayon et al., 2020).

Care continuity is dependent on effective information transfer during change of shift, Inter department referrals and discharge planning. Nursing notes are a major source of information about the patient during these transitions, losing the communication and information is less. Studies have proved that poor or insufficient documentation is one of the major causes of adverse events and avoidable medical errors (Shortliffe & Sepulveda, 2018).

Furthermore, nursing documentation fosters the emergence of collaboration between disciplines by utilization of the common clinical reference point for physicians, pharmacists, therapists and allied health professionals. In complicated care pathways e.g. critical care or chronic disease management well-kept notes are better to enhance co-ordination and contribute to better patient outcomes. As healthcare systems focus on value-based care to a higher degree, the role of nursing documentation in quality assessment and evaluation of outcomes has also been more prominent.

2.4 Limitations Of Traditional Documentation Practices

Despite the fact that it is so important, there are a number of limitations in the way nursing documentation is carried out traditionally, by way of the practice of quality of care. Manual documentation is essentially time consuming and prone to errors such omission, inaccurate and delayed entries. Handwritten records can have legibility issues which can lead to errors in interpretation and clinical mistakes. Semi-automated digital systems, although bringing improvements to the paper-based ones, often entail new problems.

Template-based documentation may be limiting to clinical expression and a secondary factor to redundant data entry. Poorly designed EHR interfaces can interrupt nursing work processes, causing frustration, cognitive overload, and diminished job satisfaction (Dall'Ora et al., 2020).

Another major drawback is that the traditional documentation systems are passive. These systems are mostly information storage systems, except that they do not deliver real-time intelligence, predictive intelligence, or decision support. As a result, nurses have to manually synthesise data from different sources to detect patient risks or trends. This lack of automation and lack of contextual awareness highlights the need for advanced, AI-enabled documentation systems which are able to provide for proactive and efficient nursing practice.

Table 1. Comparison of Manual vs Digital Nursing Documentation

Aspect	Manual Nursing Documentation	Digital Nursing Documentation
Data Entry	Handwritten, time-consuming	Electronic, faster data entry
Accuracy	Prone to errors and omissions	Improved accuracy with validation
Legibility	May be unclear or illegible	Clear and standardized
Accessibility	Limited physical access	Real-time, multi-user access
Interoperability	Poor information sharing	Supports data exchange (HL7/FHIR)
Compliance Support	Difficult to audit	Built-in compliance and audit trails
Decision Support	Not available	Enables integration with CDS tools

3. OVERVIEW OF GENERATIVE ARTIFICIAL INTELLIGENCE IN HEALTHCARE

Generative Artificial Intelligence (AI) has become a world-changing paradigm in the healthcare industry, which has provided the capacity to machines to produce human-like text, speech, images & clinical content in a structured format. Unlike traditional rule-based or discriminative examples of artificial intelligence that are mainly concerned with classification or prediction, generative artificial intelligence models possess the capabilities to synthesize (i.e. create new information) through the learning of different and complex patterns from big data sets. In a healthcare setting, these capabilities are increasingly being used to automate documentation, clinical decision-making and the delivery of patient-centered care (Rajkomar et al., 2019).

The transformation of generative artificial intelligence into the workflow of healthcare is motivated by the exponential increase in clinical data such as electronic health records, medical images, physiological signals, and unstructured text, i.e., narrative text.

Nursing documentation, which includes extensive use of free text notes or hand-off reports, and patient narratives, are just some of the areas where generative AI applications are a particularly good fit. By allowing for contextually relevant and semantically rich content creation, there is tremendous potential for generative AI to make documentation more accurate, efficient and clinical ready.

Figure 3. Generative AI Pipeline in Healthcare Applications

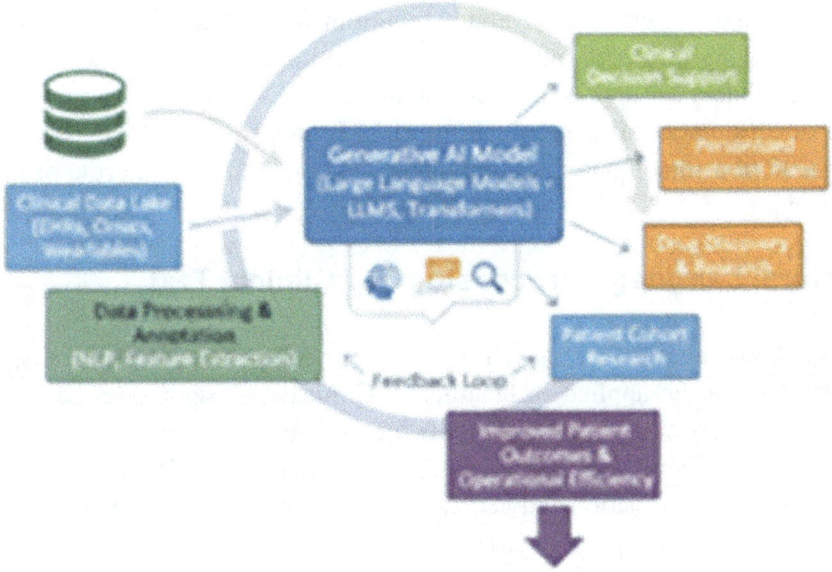

3.1 Generative AI Concepts And Models (LLMs, Transformers)

Building on the issues of documentation outlined above, this section is a focus on generative AI techniques that are relevant to the nursing workflows. At the heart of the Generative AI systems of today is the transformer architecture systems that has transformed the study of Natural Language Processing by its abilities to strengthen long-range dependencies and contextual relationship in the text. The transformer architecture was introduced in the year 2017 by Vaswani et al. The transformer architecture uses self-attention mechanisms that allow the modeling of models that are sensitive to the importance of different tokens in a sequence, providing them a tendency to capture the semantic meaning than the previous recurrent models and convolutional models.

Large Language Models (LLMs), for example those that depend on the GPT architecture, are models that have been trained on massive amounts of corpses of texts and fine-tuned for domain-specific purposes, including CLU. These models can be used to create coherent, contextually relevant and grammatically correct clinical narratives that are very well-suited for automating the nursing documentation and patient reporting tasks (Brown et al., 2020).

In healthcare applications, LLMs are often adapted with the use of healthcare datasets to assure its coaching to medical terminology, medical documentation requirements and also ethical conversion requirements. The generative capabilities of this technology allow for automated note drafting and clinical summarisation and structured data extraction from unstructured clinical data. However, given the life-and-death situation of clinical settings, LLMs are usually applied as a helping hand instead of a standalone decision maker, since it reaffirms the role of human supervision.

3.2 Natural Language Processing For Clinical Text

Natural Language Processing (NLP) is a major component allowing generative AI applications to be applied in healthcare. Clinical text such as nursing notes, discharge summaries and progress report etc. is naturally complex and includes domain-specific terminology, abbreviations and context. NLP techniques make interpretation, transformation and generation of such text easy, in Favor of an enormous array of clinical applications (Kreimeyer et al., 2017).

In case of the documentation of the nursing documentation, NLP allows to extract automatically the key clinical entities in order to extract symptoms, interventions, medications, and patient responses. Advanced NLP models can also conduct semantic analysis to extract relationships between clinical concepts in order to aid in understanding context. Generative NLP systems go further by having the effect of creating narrative summaries that relate to clinical intent but still adhere to documentation standards.

Recent research shows how generative models based on NLP are capable of similar performance to clinical text written by a human, created on the basis of a good quality healthcare dataset (Thirunavukarasu et al., 2023) in coherence and relevance. These advancements place NLP as a base technology to automate the documentation of nursing processes and improve the accuracy of reporting for patients.

3.3 Speech-To-Text And Multimodal AI In Nursing

Speech-to-text technologies are a profoundly important enabler for the generative AI-powered nursing documentation. Nurses commonly use verbal communication as part of the patient assessment process, the delivery of care, and in interdisciplinary work with other health professionals. By transcribing spoken inputs into structured or narrative text, speech recognition systems decrease the need for manual data input, and enable nurses to save notes of care as they occur.

Modern speech-to-text systems, with the roof over their head, driven by deep learning and transformer, have shown to be highly accurate even in a clinical, noisy setting.

When incorporated with generative AI systems, these could be used to turn sombre speech in the form of standardized nurse notes, which are able to incorporate clinical context and words autonomously. This capability puts an additional lot in the documentation efficiency, but without affecting the clinical documentation (Topol, 2019). Beyond speech, multimodal AI systems are mixtures that kind of data of multiple sources (such as physiological sensors, medical units, imaging systems, textual records, etc.). In the nursing practice, the use of multimodal AI for offering full reporting off patient is synthetic in crucial essential in laying down the vital signs, observational and narratives the provided for f clinical reporting. Such systems allow for the ability to cause proactive monitoring and provide for the ability to impacted clinical intervention particularly in high acuity areas such as intensive care unit settings.

3.4 Trust, Explainability, And Human-In-The-Loop AI

Despite the potential of generative AI, there needs to be a careful evaluation of trust, transparency, and accountability, especially when being used in healthcare. Clinical environments require explainable and reliable AI systems which clinicians want to understand and validate. The "black box" nature of deep learning models makes them hard to comprehend, clinically accept and regulatory compliant (Floridi et al., 2018).

Explainable AI (XAI) approaches attempt to boost the transparency into the model behaviour, the path to decision and level of confidence. In the case of nursing documentation systems, explainability can mean making the source data used to produce text explicit, or find areas of uncertainty. Such features allow nurses to check and correct content produced by AI for the purpose of enhancing levels of trust and clinical accuracy (Ghassemi et al.,2021). The human in the loop (HITL) paradigm is considered by many to be one of the best practices for generative AI deployment in healthcare. Under the above approach, AI systems can assist with documentation tasks and reporting tasks with nurses lending the final word in content validation and clinical decision making. HITL frameworks point towards the fact that generative AI should not replace professional judgment but should help to scaffold generative AI in line with ethical principles and patient safety requirements (Shortliffe & Sepulveda, 2018).

In principle, the ethic law comprises the incorporating of trust-aware designing, explanations and human supervision is necessary for the responsible integration of generative AI in the nursing workflow. These considerations not only help in ensuring safe and ethical deployment, but also increase the acceptance and sustainability of the use of AI for healthcare applications over a long period of time Amann et al. (2020).

3.5 Methodological Readiness Of Generative AI For Clinical Documentation

The use of generative artificial intelligence in clinical documentation must be prepared methodologically to ensure the safety of generative techniques, their reliability and clinical relevance. Major language models used in medical fields require fine-tuning on domain-wide and de-identified medical corpora, in order to correctly capture the medical terminology or the steps of the nursing workflow and nuances. De-identification strategies can be a critical part of preserving patient privacy and allowing for real world clinical text to be used in model training/validation.

In addition, methodological readiness is the establishment of validation protocols prior to the deployment. This includes testing the outputs of models considered against standards in the clinical documentation, checking semantic correctness and ensuring alignment with nursing practice guidelines. Without this kind of methodological underpinning, generative AI systems may not only generate incomplete, biased or clinically inappropriate documentation. Therefore, methodological preparedness can be seen as a basic prerequisite for incorporating generative AI in nursing documentation work flows. (Singhal et al.,2023).

4. AI-DRIVEN AUTOMATION OF NURSING DOCUMENTATION

The increasing complexity of healthcare delivery and the amount of clinical data have put a greater responsibility of documentation on disciplinary practitioners of the Medicine profession in Nursing. Traditional documentation practices, even with electronic health record (EHR) systems backing them up, are often labour intensive, fragmented and subject to inefficiencies. Artificial intelligence-powered automation has been found to be a possible solution to overcome these challenges by converting the nursing documentation into a more intelligent, adaptive & flow-aligned process. Generative AI technologies in particular can support the automated generation, validation and standardization of clinical documentation while capturing clinical intent and professional judgement of nurses (Rajkomar et al., 2019).

AI-driven automation in nursing documentation is not meant to be a substitute for nurses but to supplement their ability to deliver care, by reducing time spent on repetition of administrative work, minimize mistakes and enable real time clinical insights generation. By combining generative models with EHR systems, medical devices and voice interfaces, healthcare organizations have the chance to boost accuracy, efficiency and clinical usability when recording this information. The subsequent subsections look at the key dimensions of automation via facial recognition in nursing documentation.

Figure 4. AI-Enabled Nursing Documentation Workflow Integrated with EHR Systems

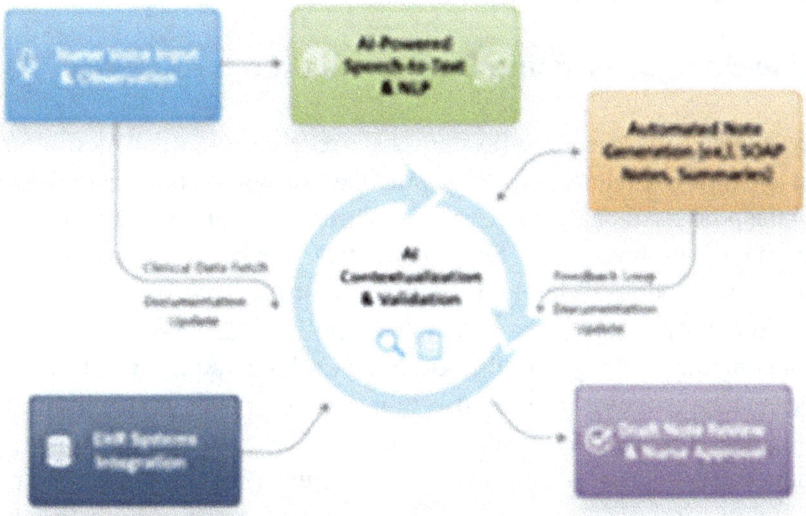

4.1 Automated Clinical Note Generation

Generative start-up: Automated clinical note creation is one of the most significant generative AI uses in nursing documentation. Nursing notes are traditionally held together as narrative descriptions of patient assessments, interventions, responses and outcomes. Associated with the clinical context, these free-text entries are key components of recording the clinical context but are also time-consuming to complete manually. Generative AI models, especially large language models that are trained on clinical corpora, can help write nursing notes out of structured inputs, past patient data and other contextual cues (Singhal et al., 2023).

In practice, automated note generation systems use various sources of data such as vital signs, medication, laboratory results, and prior nursing notes to generate coherent and context-aware notes. These draft notes can then be reviewed, edited and approved by nurses for clinical accuracy and accountability. Such systems decrease redundancy, increase consistency and enable nurses to focus more on direct patient care.

Empirical studies show that AI-assisted documentation may be a decisive reduction in charting time with the same or better quality of documentation (Sinsky et al., 2016). In addition, standardized generation of notes helps to promote interoperability and secondary use of the data, such as quality measurement and clinical research. However, for effective implementation, where the model is trained carefully, domain adaptation is employed, and continuous validation is performed to avoid any inaccuracy or contextual misinterpretation.

4.2 Voice-Enabled Nursing Documentation

Voice-enabled documentation systems have received more and more attention as a natural and intuitive interface to nurse practice. Nurses often use verbal communication in the process of patient assessments, care coordination, and communication within the interdisciplinary team. Speech to text: Driven by advances in deep learning and transformer models, technologies like speech-to-text can transcribe a real-time clinical observation that doctors make to a digital record.

When combined with generative AI, voice-enabled systems reach well beyond text-to-speech type transcription, converting the raw form of speech into structured and standardised forms of nursing documentation. For example, the results of spoken assessment can be converted automatically to written progress notes, care plans, or handoff reports to appear formatted. This way one has less typing to do, the workflow is less interrupted, and supports documentation at the point of care (Topol, 2019).

Voice-enabled documentation is especially helpful for use in high acuity areas like emergency departments and intensive care units that impose time constraints and cognitive load. Nevertheless, there are challenges such as noise in the background, different accents, and the strict privacy level required. Ensuring data security and complying with healthcare rules is the key to widespread adoption at voice-based AI systems.

4.3 Real-Time Data Capture From Medical Devices

Modern healthcare environments are growing predominantly interconnected medical devices and sensor networks that have a continuous generation of patient data. Vital sign monitors, infusion pumps, wearable and bedside devices produce huge amounts of real-time data of use in nursing care. AI-powered documentation systems can automatically capture, interpret and integrate this data into the nursing records, reducing the need for manual data entry and increasing the accuracy of the data (Bibri, 2021).

Real-time data capture can then be used to document dynamic and reflective of the current clinical status of the particular patient. For instance, vital signs changes can be automatically entered and put into context within nursing notes and abnormal readings can be an alert or prompt for further assessment. By combining the information synthesized by the device with a narrative documentation, generative AI systems help to facilitate complete and timely reporting of the patient. This automated integration is also having the effect of clinical decision support by giving nurses actionable insights, which are drawn out of a continuous monitoring. However, issues in interoperability, data quality issues are to be overcome ensuring reliable performance of the systems. Having the standardized forms of the data and powerful integration frameworks are both critical for implementation at scale.

4.4 Error Detection, Correction, And Standardization

Documentation errors such as omissions, discrepancies and inaccurate entries pose significant risks to the safety of patients and continuity of care. AI driven automation incorporates high-end features in the identification and correction of errors by analysing patterns in documentation, cross-referencing data sources and identifying anomalies. Generative AI systems can be applied to identify missing data, provide recommendations for data correction, and remind nurses to follow up on ambiguous data entries (Carayon et al., 2020).

Standardization is also another key benefit of AI-enabled documentation. By translating content created using content to clinical terminologies, coding systems and standards documentation, AI systems ensure consistency and interoperability. Standardized documentation facilitates data sharing between care settings and also assists in secondary use of data such as for analytics and reporting.

Despite such advantages in the plasticity of Over-standardization can be a danger of oversimplifying complicated clinical narratives. Therefore, a balance between structure and flexibility in AI systems is needed for the AI systems to allow nurses to express nuanced clinical judgement. Human supervision is still required to ensure that automated standardisation is enhancing rather than constraining professional practice.

4.5 Workflow Integration With EHR Systems

Seamless Integration with EHR systems is a key to the success with AI-supported Nursing Documentation. Dispersed and not well integrated solutions may disrupt work processes and fail to focus adoption on users. Good integration entails that the documentation produced by artificial intelligence is compatible with existing clinical processes, data standards, and user interfaces (Ratwani et al., 2018).

AI-enabled documentation software is also increasingly becoming part of EHR platforms themselves, allowing nurses to be able to access automation features without switching systems. Such integration helps us in real time documentation, to reduce the duplication and to improve the usability of the application. Furthermore, there are such interoperability standards as HL7, FHIR, etc. that help in data exchange between AI and EHR to ensure that systems are scalable and compliant.

From the organizational point of view, the process of workflow integration includes stakeholder engagement, training and ongoing evaluation. Clinically, nurses should be actively involved in system design and system implementation in a way that is based in clinical need. When implemented properly, AI-driven automation within EHR systems can make a big impact in improving documentation efficiency, data quality and clinical decision support.

4.6 Methodological Framework For Generative AI In Nursing Documentation

The effective integration of generative AI into nursing documentation must be provide generative AI as a valuable tool to ensure clinical accuracy, accountability and safety. This framework will commonly start with training and tailoring of the models, whereby large language models are re-trained on de-identified data from nursing records, electronic health records and standardized clinical terminologies. Domain-specific fine-tuning enables nurse language, documentation standards and clinical reasoning in the appropriately appropriate setting to all be considered in the model.

The second section of the framework is the data governance. Secure data pipelines, access controls, and data anonymization mechanisms to ensure healthcare regulations and patient privacy are met Generative AI systems need to run in controlled environments that allow for auditability and traceability of the content that's been generated (Translation Path 2020). Evaluation and validation form the third part. AI generated documentation should be measured by both quantitative and qualitative measures including documentation completeness, semantic accuracy, performance of entity extraction and nurse validation checklists. Human-in-the-loop mechanisms are at the core of this structure and ensure that medical history images are revealed, corrected, and approved by nurses before being finalized and documented.

This collaboration, which not only keeps things professionally accountable but also utilizes the power of automation to avoid the administrative load, is a viable option to keep in mind (Thrall, 2024).

5. INTELLIGENT PATIENT REPORTING AND MONITORING SYSTEMS

Intelligent patient reporting and monitoring systems are one specific area of utilizing AI-driven automation in healthcare that is especially important in the field of nursing practice. While traditional patient reporting is highly manual - document-based and periodic assessments, intelligent systems use artificial intelligence in order to produce dynamic, real-time, context-aware insights about patients. These systems combine the data from electronic health records, medical devices and interactions with patients to facilitate continuous situational awareness and auto Clinical decision making (Rajkomar et al., 2019).

For nurses, however, patient reporting is not only a documentation task, but a cognitive process where tasks are synthesised such as making sense of the observations made and interpreting the trends and information to tell the stories to the care team needed to work together to produce actionable information. The use of AI-enabled patient reporting systems complements this process by automating the collection and analysis of patient-related data, as well as its summary and interpretation, which improves the process efficiency and mitigates the risk of information flooding. The following subsections investigate important constituents of intelligent patient reporting and monitoring architectures in today's healthcare contexts.

Figure 5. Intelligent Patient Reporting and Continuous Monitoring Architecture

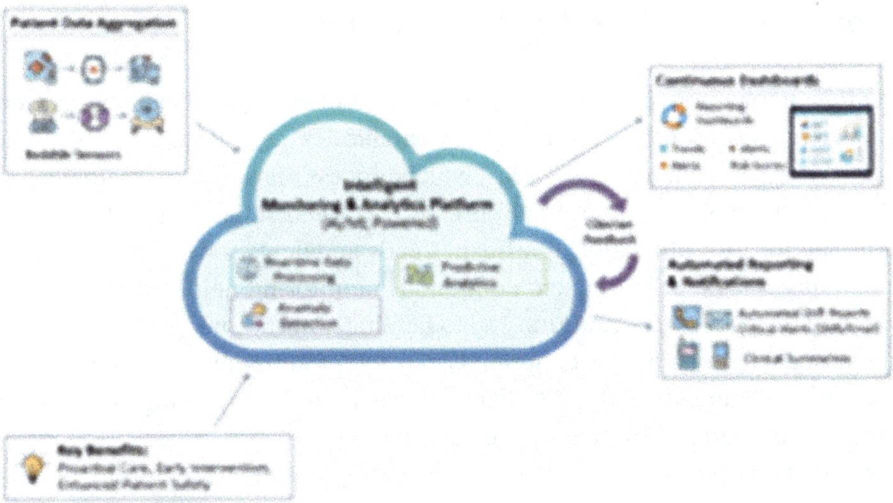

5.1 Automated Patient Status Summarization

Automated patient status summarization is a fundamental function for intelligent reporting systems made possible through generative artificial intelligence and natural language processing technologies.

In clinical settings with a high volume of data and high turnover of patients, review of volumes of files is needed by nurses to familiarize with the current status of a patient. Automated summarization systems solve this problem by summarizing complex clinical data in clinically relevant summaries. Generative AI models which look at structured data such as vital signs, laboratory values, medication and text from nursing and physician notes to create a holistic summary of the patient. These summaries might be focused on current clinical status, recent changes, interventions in progress and issues pending. By providing synthesized information, AI-driven summaries aid in efficient handovers, interdisciplinary communication and informed decision-making (Kreimeyer et al., 2017).

For practising nurses, automated summaries are an effective way to reduce cognitive burden and enhance situational awareness especially over shift changes and care transitions. However, the quality of such summaries relies on the quality of the data that is used, as well as the training of the model and how well it can be validated by humans. Consequently, automated patient summaries are most effective when they are used as decision supporting tools with nurse oversight instead of as autonomous reporting mechanisms.

5.2 Continuous Patient Monitoring Using AI

Continuous monitoring of patients is the hallmark of intelligent healthcare systems, with development of sensors technologies, wearable devices, and networked medical devices. AI-driven monitoring systems, which process real-time physiological data such as the patient's heart rate, blood pressure, oxygen saturation and respiration patterns and look for clinically significant trends and deviations.

In nursing-related environment, continuous monitoring helps to improve early detection of the patient deterioration and to facilitate timely interventions. Machine learning models are an approach to analysing longitudinal data streams in which normal variability and pathological changes are distinguished, giving nurses actionable insights instead of raw data (Liu et al., 2019).

This capability is especially useful in pillowcase of high acuity environments (i.e., intensive care units, post-op wards, as well as remote patient monitoring programs). By overlaying the output of continuous monitoring with patient reports, AI systems create dynamic documentation of the changing clinical state of patients. However, to ensure they are implemented effectively, there needs to be good interoperability, alert management approaches and training so alarm fatigue and clinical relevance are ensured.

5.3 Predictive Alerts And Early Warning Systems

Predictive alerts and early warning systems are an important step in the intelligent reporting of patients and are a radical shift from the reactive approach to healthcare to a more active approach. Traditional methods of early warning are based upon fixed thresholds and scoring instruments and are not necessarily sensitive to subtle or complex patterns of deterioration that are present in a patient. AI-driven systems, on the contrary, are systems that use predictive analytics and deep learning to detect risk trajectories using multivariate data (Topol, 2019).

For nurses, early warning signs of possible adverse events like sepsis, respiratory failure, or falls can be provided through the use of predictive alerts. These alerts are generated by analysing the historical and real-time data to estimate the risk probabilities, and nurses can prioritize the assessments and interventions based on it. Incorporating predictive warnings into reports for patient care increases clinical decision support and encourages the early escalation of care (Shortliffe & Sepulveda, 2018).

Despite the benefits, predictive systems are difficult to calibrate so that sensitivity and specificity are properly balanced. Excessive or inappropriate context of alerts may cause an alarm fatigue and a lack of clinical trust. Therefore, human-in-the-loop validation and continuous evaluation of the system is necessary for safe and effective usage.

5.4 Patient-Centered Reporting And Personalization

Patient-centered care focuses on individual treatment with shared decision-making process and respect for patient choice. Intelligent Patient Reporting Systems help to support this paradigm by enabling personalized reporting based on the clinical profile of the individual patient, the care goals and communication needs. Generative AI models can adjust the content of report according to patient demographics, diagnoses and care plan to ensure that the content is relevant and provide clear information. In the world of nursing instruction, personalized patient reports have the advantage of enhancing the communication with the patient and family as well as assisting in patient education, engagement and adherence to care plans. AI-generated summaries may be customized for different audiences (including, e.g., clinicians, patients and caregivers) with distinct required level of detail and technical complexity (Floridi et al., 2018).

However, there is a growing ethical issue with personalization involving data privacy, bias and equity. Ensuring that personalization driven by AI is a critical task for healthcare organizations to make sure that they don't reinforce any disparities or exclude any vulnerable population. Transparent design and inclusive data practices are relevant in order to maintain the ethical standards in patient-centered reporting.

Table 2. AI Techniques Used in Patient Reporting Systems

AI Technique	Application in Patient Reporting	Nursing Impact
Natural Language Processing (NLP)	Automated patient summaries and note synthesis	Reduces cognitive load
Machine Learning	Trend analysis and risk prediction	Supports early intervention
Deep Learning	Pattern recognition in continuous monitoring	Improves accuracy
Generative AI (LLMs)	Narrative report generation and personalization	Enhances documentation quality
Predictive Analytics	Early warning and alert systems	Improves patient safety
Multimodal AI	Integration of sensor, text, and device data	Comprehensive reporting

5.5 Risk Management And Failure Scenarios In AI-Based Patient Reporting

Despite its benefits, patient reporting systems using artificial intelligence entail some risks which need to be managed proactively. Failure scenarios could be mis- documentation due to lack of complete data, incorrect context of AI model and poor or too many notifications leading to alert fatigue. Algorithmic bias and excessive reliance on systems could also put the safety of patients at more risk if not properly addressed.

Some of the risk mitigation strategies are human-in-the-loop validation, continuous model monitoring and threshold calibration for alerts. Auditing of AI's outputs on a regular basis, as well as structured feedback from nursing personnel, are important to identify limitations in the system and to improve performance. By taking into account the risk management in the design of the systems and the way they are governed, healthcare organizations can ensure that safe and responsible instances of AI-driven patient reporting tools can be implemented.

6. ENHANCING ACCURACY AND DATA QUALITY THROUGH GENERATIVE AI

Accuracy and data quality are needed as a prerequisite to provide safe and effective and evidence-based healthcare. In the context of nursing practice, errors in documentation and inconsistency of data may have an impact on patient safety as well as disturb continuity of care and its impact on clinical decision making. As healthcare systems are increasingly relying on digital records and insights that can be derived from analytics, the quality of nursing documentation acts as a critical factor in determining whether or not healthcare systems are trustworthy. Generative artificial intelligence provides sophisticated functionality to improve the accuracy and semantic clarity as well as data consistency of documents through the automation of detecting any errors, maintaining standardization, and providing contextual interpretations (Topaz & Pruinelli, 2017).

One key difference between generative AI systems and conventional documentation tools is that generative AI systems are active in terms of analyzing and synthesizing clinical information. Through the application of large language models, natural language processing, and knowledge-based constraints, these systems can assist with nurses producing quality documentation enclave of clinical intent and in compliance with set standards. The following subsections discuss some of the mechanisms by which generative AI improves the accuracy and quality of data in nursing documentation.

Figure 6. Accuracy Improvement Cycle Using Generative AI in Nursing Documentation

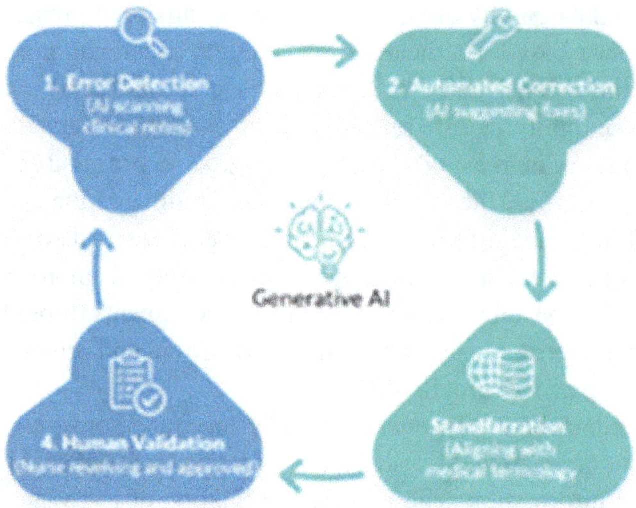

6.1 Reduction Of Documentation Errors

Documentation errors are an ongoing problem in the practice of nursing, and include omissions, inaccuracies, inconsistencies and delayed documentation. Manual documentation is especially prone to human error especially given time constraints, the burden of cognitive load, and interruptions in the process.

Even electronic documentation systems, if poorly designed or poor integration might add to data entry errors and redundancy (Carayon et al., 2020). Generative AI systems try to overcome such problems by becoming automatic mechanisms of detecting errors and validating information.

By using a cross-referencing of different data sources such as vital signs, medication administration golf log, and lab results, using AI models, it could be detected when there are discrepancies in the data and remind nurses to check or change an entry. For example, when there is a discrepancy between a recorded intervention and a recorded medication data or an entry time stamp on the medical records system, the medical records system can produce a flag for verification.

Furthermore, generative AI assists with real-time documentation assistance to eliminate the need for reliance on retrospective documentation, which is a known cause of documentation errors. Studies suggest that, with the help of AI, documentation can be made more complete and timelier, which subsequently can enhance the overall quality of data and patient safety (Sinsky et al., 2016). However, the efficacy of the error reduction mechanisms relies on steady training of the model, clinical validation, and human supervision.

6.2 Standardized Clinical Terminology And Coding

Standardization of clinical terminology and clinical coding is a key to interoperability, data exchange, and oversight of healthcare data for secondary use. Nursing documentation is often composed of a wide range of terminologies, abbreviations and writing styles, which may make comparison and consistency between settings of care difficult. Synonymy Standardization Healthcare Artificial intelligence (AI) based systems such as those in NLP can ensure standardization by the meeting documentation with recognized clinical vocabulary/ coding.

Through natural language processing and knowledge representation techniques, AI models are able to map free-text notes in nursing and categories such as nursing diagnoses, intervention and outcome terminology. This is a capable feature that enhances semantic consistency, supports integration with electronic health records, clinical decision support systems (McGonigle & Mastrian, 2021).

Standardized documentation also increases data usability with quality measurement, research and policy development. However, strong standardization may have one disadvantage in an attempt to oversimplify complex clinical narratives. Generative AI is addressing this concern where people say there is a balance between the structured coding and expressive narrative and nurse will document some nuance clinical observation and will write it in terms terminologies are as consistent as.

6.3 Context-Aware And Semantic Understanding

Context-awareness and semantic understanding of the context is what makes generative AI different from traditional documentation tools. Nursing documentation is often tradable and encodes implicit clinical reasoning, situational context and patient specific detail that is difficult to summarise using predetermined templates. Generative models of AI, on the other hand, when trained on large scale of clinical text, can understand the context and generate documentations that represent underlying clinical meaning.

For example, this is how the precision of understanding certain terms in diseases could be made possible through context-aware systems where variables such as patient history, ongoing condition, and treatment history can be used to distinguish between otherwise similar terms. They are also able to derive relationships between symptoms, intervention and outcome, leading to more coherent and clinically relevant documentation (Kreimeyer et al., 2017). Such semantic understanding makes the nursing notes more fascinating and more useful for the users - other users such as clinicians and analysts, etc.

In addition, context-aware documentation for personalized patient reporting and decision support, such as meeting the patient's unique clinical profile to ensure that the generated content is appropriate for the resulting content. Nevertheless, keeping the semantic accuracy is an issue that must be resolved through effective training datasets availability, domain-specific fine-tuning and mechanisms to control the bias and misinterpretation.

6.4 Data Consistency Across Care Transitions

Care transitions and shifts of care such as unit transfers and discharges are among the major points of vulnerability for loss of information and inconsistency in data. Poor documentation or inconsistent documentation during transitions can result in a breakdown of communication and adverse patient outcomes. Generative AI systems are used in helping to better data consistency by automating handoff summaries and making sure documentation components are aligned.

AI-powered handoff tools can be used to synthesize essential information about a patient into a standardized summary that is routinely updated on a real-time basis, reducing the need for manual transcription and from being memory-based reporting. Through the use of data from multiple different sources, these systems encourage continuity of care across clinical settings and teams of providers (Shortliffe & Sepulveda, 2018). Moreover, the consistency of the longitudinal data is simplified using generative AI since the patient narratives between episodes of care are kept. This capability is particularly useful for chronic disease management as well as complex care pathways where it is important to have a proper historical context which can be useful for an effective decision-making process. Making sure data is consistent between transitions is ultimately going to improve patient safety, care quality and clinical efficiency.

7. IMPROVING NURSING EFFICIENCY AND REDUCING BURNOUT

Nursing efficiency and workforce well-being have become highly important issues within healthcare systems of this modern world, especially in consideration of the issues of increasing patient complexity and staffing shortage and increased administration duties. Documentation requirements (although a key component in maintaining patient safety and compliance with regulations, documentation requirements are a huge contributor to the workload and cognitive load of nurses).

Numerous studies have found that documentation burden has been an important cause of occupational stress, burnout and reduced job satisfaction among nursing professionals (Dall'Ora et al., 2020). Artificial intelligence fuelled automation, through the use of generative AI in particular, is a possible strategic plan in order to improve the efficiency of the nursing profession while reducing the effects of burnout. By streamlining documentation processes, cutting down the number of unnecessary tasks and easing clinical reasoning AI-enabled systems can assist nurses with gaining back time and mental capacities to use up on direct patient care. This section pertains to the contribution of generative AI in the optimization of time, cognitive load, and job satisfaction and of AI as co-pilot of nursing in the making (Booth et al.,2023).

Figure 7. Impact of AI Automation on Nursing Efficiency and Burnout Reduction

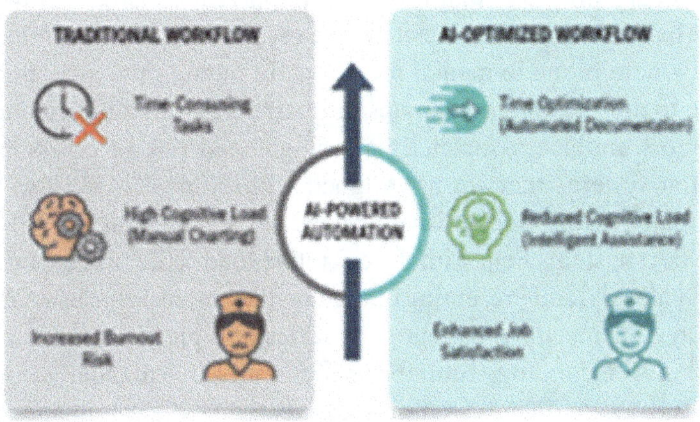

7.1 Time Optimization In Nursing Tasks

Time management is a basic decision maker for the efficiency of nursing. Nurses are constantly managing several tasks such as patient assessments, administering medications, coordinating care, and documentation. Studies have revealed that a large percentage of time spent in nursing is spent on activities involving documentation, and most of the time this negatively affects contact with the patient (Sinsky et al., 2016).

AI driven documentation automation addresses this imbalance head-on by lowering the amount of manual data entry and the work that occurs and can be done at the point-of-care instead of later. Automated clinical notes generation, voice-enabled charting, and interfacing with medical devices permit nurses to record information quicker and in a more precise manner. By reducing repetitive procedures and removing the need for retrospective charting, AI systems are involved in substantial time saving Pavuluri et al. (2024).

Time optimization is also helpful in increasing the predictability of workflow and reducing the fragmentation of jobs. When documentation processes are respectfully incorporated into the nursing routines, nurses are less likely to be interrupted and have a more run of events between the care activities. These improvements in efficiency are not only good for the individual, but can lead to team-based care coordination and operational improvement in the healthcare organization.

7.2 Cognitive Load Reduction

Cognitive load is the mental effort in processing information making observations; this theory proposes that this is an important construct in that cognitive overload can have a significant effect on the efficiency with which learners work hence making them prone to mental problems. In nursing practice, high cognitive load is linked to multitasking, high rates of interruptions and information overload and these factors are also associated with heightened risk of errors and burnout. Documentation systems that are not aligned with clinical workflows add to this difficulty by placing further cognitive demands (Carayon et al., 2020).

Generative AI systems help with the cognitive load reduction by automating the information synthesis, and presenting clinically relevant insights in a condensed and structured way. For instance, patient summaries and predictive alerts that can be generated using AI technology limit the need for nurses to manually review lengthy records. Context-aware documentation supports the next stage in supporting clinical reasoning is context-aware documentation, whether in the form of highlighting important data points and potential concerns.

By taking on some of the more routine cognitive aspects of nursing and delegating them to AI systems, nurses are able to become more focused on higher-order clinical judgment and patient-focused work. This redistribution of cognitive work helps to enhance safe delivery of care and professional satisfaction. However, it's crucial to get it right, in order to really, really achieve the benefit of a substantial reduction cognitive load that is needed to avoid being too reliant on the automation or too alerting.

7.3 Impact On Job Satisfaction And Care Quality

There is a strong relationship between job satisfaction and workload balance, autonomy of nurses, and perceived influence for patient outcomes. High documentation burden and administrative overloading have been linked repeatedly to lower job satisfaction and greater intentions to leave the organisation (Dall'Ora et al., 2020). AI-driven automation has the potential to help in reversing these trends, through helping nurses spend more time on meaningful clinical activities.

When documentation tasks are made streamlined though, nurses will record that they have seen their engagement with patients increase and that they are more aligned with their professional values. Improved documentation accuracy and timeliness also contributes to improved quality of care as clinical decisions are based on reliable and up-to-date information. In case of value-based care models, such improvements translate into an improvement in patient outcomes and organizational performance (Topol, 2019).

Importantly, the positive impact of AI on job satisfaction depends on the acceptance and trust of users. Systems that are felt to be invasive, unreliable or out of alignment with clinical need may worsen, instead of ameliorate, frustration. Therefore, the participatory design and the continuity of training is essential to make sure that AI tools help rather than hinder the practice of nursing.

7.4 AI As A Nursing Co-Pilot

The concept of AI being the nursing co-pilot is a concept that drives the idea of collaboration rather than replacement. In this paradigm, AI systems are used as partner systems that assist nurses' documentation, decision-making and care coordination. Generative AI tools generate recommendations, draft documentation and identify potential risks and nurses have the ultimate authority and responsibility for clinical decisions (Shortliffe & Sepulveda, 2018).

Perceiving AI as a co-pilot is in line with both ethical and professional values by maintaining human judgment and accountability. It also promotes trust and acceptance of AI by setting the context of AI as a supportive force instead of a competitive one. In practice, the co-pilot model makes it possible to offer adaptive assistance in the form of support, depending on individual nurse's preference, experience and the clinical situation.

As AI technologies continue to evolve, the nursing co-pilot concept brings home the importance of human-centered design, transparency and explainability. By instilling these principles into the AI-enabled systems, healthcare organizations are able to obtain as much efficiency gain as possible, without having to compromise the well-being of their nurses and the safety of their patients.

Table 3. Impact of AI Automation on Nursing Performance Metrics

Performance Metric	Traditional Documentation	AI-Enabled Documentation	Observed Impact
Documentation Time	High	Reduced	Improved efficiency
Error Rate	Moderate to high	Lower	Enhanced patient safety
Cognitive Load	High	Moderate	Reduced burnout risk
Job Satisfaction	Variable	Improved	Higher retention
Patient Interaction Time	Limited	Increased	Better care quality
Workflow Interruptions	Frequent	Fewer	Smoother care delivery

8. CLINICAL DECISION SUPPORT ENABLED BY GENERATIVE AI

Clinical decision support systems (CDSS) are an integral part of modern healthcare and they help clinicians make informed, timely, and evidence-based decisions. In the practice of nursing there is a continual, dynamic interaction of decision making in the areas of assessment of the patient, prioritization for patient care, choice of intervention and evaluation of the patient outcome. Traditional CDSS have mostly been based on rule-based logic and static alerts-which while useful are both mostly limited and context-aware and adaptable. Generative artificial intelligence is bringing forth a paradigm shift in the sense of supporting context sensitive, adaptive and explainable decision support that is more in tune with the complexities of real-world nursing care (Shortliffe & Sepulveda, 2018).

By levering capabilities such as large language models and predictive analytics, in addition to real-time data streams, generative AI-enabled CDSS can be levered to synthesize large amounts of clinical information on top of the existing data and present information in real time which is actionable at point of care. These systems provide an adjunct beyond nursing judgment by providing recommendations, risk assessments, and summary of evidence and improve clinical accuracy, efficiency, and patient safety. The following subsections discuss the dimensions of generative AI-enabled clinical decision support in nursing (Rodman & Topol 2025).

Figure 8. Generative AI–Based Clinical Decision Support Architecture

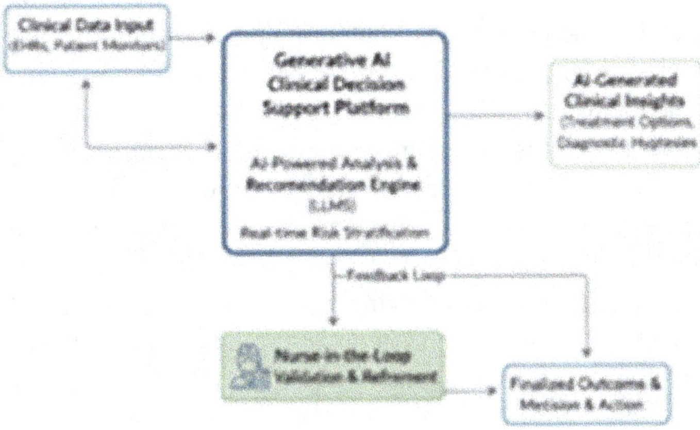

8.1 AI-Assisted Clinical Recommendations

AI-assisted clinical recommendations involve the use of generative models that offer context-aware recommendations based on the condition of individual patients. Unlike classic alert systems that have fixed thresholds for triggering alerts, with generative AI technology the doctor can analyse longitudinal data on the patient, nursing notes, laboratory results, and vital signs and respond with nuanced recommendations. For nurses, this ability becomes a tool in informed decision-making, for example, in the prioritization of care, selection of intervention and escalating concern.

Generative AI systems could help write suggested actions of care or develop highlights of the best practice intervention based on the current patient's status and historical patterns. For instance, an AI system can advise that a patient needs to be monitored more frequently due to subtle indications that they are worsening or advise an evidence-based intervention for managing their symptoms. Pre-eminently, these recommendations are expounded as supportive rather than prescriptive in any way, thereby respecting the autonomy of the profession (Rajkomar et al., 2019).

The utility of recommendations made with the help of AI relies on transparency and explainability. In order to evaluate the relevance and safety of suggestions to their practice, nurses need to be able to understand the rationale behind these suggestions. Consequently, well-designed systems incorporate some type of contextual explanations, confidence indicators or links to supporting evidence, resulting in trust and clinical acceptance Singhal et al. (2023).

8.2 Risk Stratification And Outcome Prediction

Risk stratification and prediction of outcomes are examples of some of the most powerful ways to use generative AI for clinical decision support. Nursing practice often requires the identification of patients at risk of adverse events such as clinical deterioration, infection, falls or readmission. In the classroom mainly taught risk assessment tools, since they often rely on static scoring systems which cannot produce complex interactions amongst variables in the patient population.

Generative AI models improve risk stratification because they use multivariate and longitudinal data, and detect evolving patterns of risk. Machine learning and deep learning methods allow these systems to forecast outcomes on subtle trends and correlations that cannot necessarily be visualized through manual review (Liu et al., 2019).

For nurses, predictive insights are used to support proactive planning to care and timely intervention. When incorporated into the workflow of a nurse's job, predictive alerts can prioritize patient assessments as well as direct resource allocation. But, the nature of predictive system design really needs to have a balance between sensitivity and specificity to avoid alarm fatigue. Human supervision is critical to contextualize the predictions and draw appropriate measures so that the recommendations come from AI to complement but not replace the clinical judgment.

8.3 Integration With Evidence-Based Practice

Evidence-based practice (EBP) is one of the pillars of quality nursing care and focuses on integration of the best available evidence, clinical expertise, and patient preferences. Generative AI facilitates the use of EBP as it allows for quick access to the relevant research findings, clinical guidelines and recommendations for practice. With natural language processing technologies, AI programs are able to summarise the evidence and match this with patient-specific contexts.

In the field of clinical decision support, generative AI can be used to dynamically incorporate updated evidence into a recommendation during practice where integrins are designed to ensure that practice in the field of nursing aligns as it reflects the current standard of care. For example, based on their input, AI-produced summaries may include indications to guideline-aligned interventions, or point to recent evidence of relevance to a patient's condition. This capability is less demanding on the cognitive effort of searching and appraising literature, to make timely and informed decisions (Topol, 2019).

Nevertheless, combining the AI and EBP need to be properly validated and governed to avoid the spread of outdated or biased information. Transparent sourcing, regular updates, and clinician review is key to the integrity of integration of AI-supported evidence.

8.4 Human-AI Collaboration In Decision Making

Human-AI collaboration is a distinctive standard among responsible clinical decision support. In training such as nursing, where care decisions most of the time have to do with ethics, patient's comfort, and situational judgement, AI systems should become their collaborative partners and not autonomous agents. The human-in-the-loop model guarantees that the control over decision-making process lies with nurses while also making use of insights from AI (Floridi et al., 2018).

Collaborative decision support systems are adapted according to the feedback of the user which learns based on their interactions with nurses so that it will become more relevant and applicable with time. This back-and-forth feedback loop helps to build trust and helps in the improved performance of the system. In addition, collaborative models are consistent with professional development, including provision of educational feedback and reinforcement of evidence-based reasoning. In terms of ethics, human-AI collaboration is consistent with accountability and patient safety requirements. Nurses are in charge of the final decisions and the AI systems are used for additional information and analysis support. As generative AI continues to evolve, it is key to promote effective collaboration as part of the puzzle of maximizing benefits whilst minimizing risks.

8.5 Limitations Of AI-Based Clinical Decision Support Systems

While the generative AI contribution to improved clinical decision support makes good sense, it is sown with limitations. AI models may not display uncertainty for complicated and/or novel clinical scenarios, and this can result in incomplete or inappropriate recommendations. Contextual issues such as patient preferences, ethical considerations and situational judgement may not be fully represented in automated systems.

Furthermore, relying too much on the recommendations from AI can compromise important clinical thinking when human oversight is reduced. Therefore, the AI-based decision support systems must design them as assistive tools rather than autonomous decision-makers. Clear delineation of responsibility, transparency of model outputs and continuous involvement of nurse staff are important so that it is ensured that AI is working in support of rather than substituting professional medical judgement.

9. ETHICAL, LEGAL, AND PRIVACY CONSIDERATIONS

The embedding of generative artificial intelligence in nursing documentation and patient reporting presents major ethical, legal and privacy issues in association with its clinical benefits. Healthcare is a high-stake field where data sensitivity and trust with patients and accountability of professionals is of paramount importance. While the efficiency and the decision support provided by AI-driven automation is good, there had been concerns of data protection, algorithmic bias, transparency and AI-assisted responsibility for outcomes. The consideration of these issues is important in the safe, ethical and sustainable adoption of generative AI in the nursing practice (Floridi et al., 2018).

Ethical frameworks of governance have been centered on the concept that AI systems that are incorporated into healthcare must be respectful of patient autonomy, it must be fair, and maintain accountability. As front-line users of AI-enabled systems, nurses have a vital role in ensuring these principles are upheld because they can support rather than compromise patient-centered care if they do not percent correct in their use of the technology (Morley et al., 2019).

9.1 Patient Data Privacy And Security

Patient data privacy and security are important ethical and legal concerns in healthcare systems that involve artificial intelligence. Nursing documentation includes highly sensitive information including clinical assessments as well as personal identification and social context, which makes it a prime target for data breach and misuse. Generative AI systems may need access to massive data amount related to patient data for them to train and process information and data in real-time, which is a greater potential attack surface for potential security threats. Regulatory frameworks such as Health Insurance Portability and Accountability Act (HIPAA) require stringent regulatory control of data access, storage and data sharing.

Compliance requires use of encryption, role-based access control, audit trails, secure data transmission mechanisms, etc. AI systems embedded in electronic health records should comply with these safeguards to avoid unauthorized disclosure and maintain patient confidentiality (Ratwani et al., 2018).

Beyond any technical measures to safeguard against patients, ethical stewardship of data involves openness about how patient data are done within AI systems. Patients and healthcare professionals should be informed of data collection practices, secondary use of data, and of the potential risks. In order to trust that nursing documentation is being done by AI, strong security practices and accountability structures should be in place.

9.2 Bias, Fairness, And Transparency In AI Models

Algorithmic bias is an important ethical issue for generative AI applications. AI models that are trained on historical healthcare data may inadvertently learn about and reinforce existing disparities on the basis of race, gender, socioeconomic status or health conditions. In terms of nursing documentation and decision support, biased output may affect the quality-of-care prioritization, risk assessment, and communication quality and may cause health inequities to be exacerbated (Mittelstadt et al., 2016).

To ensure that fairness is taken into account, it is necessary to pay attention to the dataset they want to use, bias is caught, and periodically their model is evaluated. The transparency into AI systems is also paramount, especially in a clinical setting where people expect explainable and justifiable decisions to be made. Explainable AI approaches, one approach to this challenge, are an attempt to provide insight into the reasoning of the AI, putting the power into the hands of nurses to understand and critically consider AI generated recommendations or documentation. From a nursing perspective, the principles of transparency are tied to the concept of professional judgment as well as ethical responsibility. Nurses need to be able to question, validate, and override the output of AI when necessary, in order to ensure that the soothing decisions continue to be set in the needs of sufferers and the ethical norms.

9.3 Regulatory Compliance And Accountability

Regulatory compliance extends beyond data protection and to include system validation and clinical safety while also providing accountability of AI-assisted outcomes. Increasing healthcare regulators require evidence-based evaluation of AI systems before and after implementation. Generative AI tools that are used to nursing documentation and decision support must exhibit reliability, accuracy, and compliance with clinical standards.

Accountability in AI-enabled systems is a complex issue because decision making involves interaction between humans and machines. While AI will produce recommendations or drafts of documents, nurses and healthcare organizations remain legally liable for any clinical decision and its subsequent outcome to the patient. There is a need for clear governance frameworks establishing roles, responsibilities and liability within AI assisted workflows. (Shortliffe & Sepulveda, 2018). Institutional policies should address system monitoring, incident reporting and continuous improvement to ensure compliance of the regulations and ensuring patient safety. Such measures score the belief of trust and legitimacy in AI Artificial intelligence-driven Nursing systems.

9.4 Ethical Role Of Nurses In AI-Driven Systems

Through their multiple roles as workers in and advocates of the patient's interests, nurses find themselves at a special position in relation to ethics in AI-powered healthcare systems. Professional nursing ethics promote the values of compassion, autonomy and beneficence values which are required to act as an alert for professional adoption and usage of AI technologies. Nursing personnel are responsible for ensuring that AI tools improve and not undermine the human aspects of care.

In practice, this ethical role of Nurses comprises validating the AI-generated documentation, being mindful of any errors or biases and advocating for the patient preferences in support with the Artificial Intelligence decision-making. The nurses are part of the ethical governance as well, because they engage in the design, evaluation and policy development of the system. Their clinical expertise and understanding of the context are a critical part of fitting AI systems into the real-world care needs (Mastrian, 2021).

Education and training are important in empowering nurses in this position. Ethical AI literacy enables nurses to deliver confidently with AI system, know when a system is limited and maintain professional responsibility. As the adoption of AI increases, it will be the role of nurses in their role as ethical leaders that will help create responsible and patient healthcare innovation.

Table 4. Ethical Challenges and Mitigation Strategies

Ethical Challenge	Description	Mitigation Strategy
Data Privacy	Risk of unauthorized access to patient data	Encryption, access control, audit trails
Algorithmic Bias	Disparities in AI outputs	Diverse training data, bias audits
Lack of Transparency	Black-box decision-making	Explainable AI techniques
Accountability	Unclear responsibility for AI outcomes	Human-in-the-loop governance
Patient Trust	Reduced confidence in AI systems	Transparency and informed consent
Professional Autonomy	Overreliance on automation	Nurse oversight and validation

9.5 Regulatory And Legal Accountability In AI-Assisted Nursing Documentation

The use of generative AI to help nursing documentation falls under complex regulatory and legal frameworks. Compliance with healthcare regulations such as HIPAA as well as AI governance guidelines under development means that AI systems must be shown to be secure, transparent, and reliable in terms of data. From a legal viewpoint, nurses are the ultimate accountable authors of clinical documentation, even if AI tools have been used to create drafts to assist them in doing so.

Healthcare institutions need to create government policies that outline roles, responsibilities, and liability in AI-supported workflows. Documentation audit trails, version control and validation logs are necessary for supporting medico-legal accountability. By defining structures of accountability organizations can foster trust and ensure lawful and ethical uses by AI in nursing documentation (El Arab & Al Moosa, 2025).

10. CASE STUDIES AND REAL-WORLD IMPLEMENTATIONS

The following case scenarios are used as examples and are synthesized from peer-reviewed empirical studies, as well as deployment in hospitals and implementations of AI-enabled nursing documentation systems. These scenarios are not single-site experimental trials and are based on evidence from the real world and publicly published evaluations of generative AI applications in clinical practice.

The journey of generative artificial intelligence from experimental prototypes to real-world clinical use in nursing documentation and patient reporting. Healthcare organizations across the world are increasingly adopting artificial intelligence (AI) powered solutions into the day-to-day nursing process to make sense of the documentation burden, improve the quality of care, and even assist in making decisions by the nurse. Case studies of smart hospitals and digitally sophisticated healthcare systems share some valuable information on operational feasibility, benefits and issues around AI enabled nursing documentation. This section discusses representative operational real-world applications, with consequences and real-world experiences gained noted

10.1 AI-Based Nursing Documentation In Smart Hospitals

Smart hospitals make use of the strength of interconnected digital technologies, such as electronic health records, Internet of Medical Things (IoMT) and artificial intelligence to enable data-driven and patient centered care in hospitals. In this sort of setting, the documentation systems based on AI have been rolled out for automating the normal charting activities and assisting in the better-quality data. In one representative implementation of smart hospital, generative AI tools were combined with an EHR system of the hospital, to help nurses document patient assessments and interventions. The system utilized structured inputs from vital sign monitors, medication administration records and its laboratory systems, and unstructured nursing notes to generate a draft clinical documentation. Nurses reviewed and validated the notes produced by the AI system and ensured that there is both accuracy and accountability at a clinical level. Post implementation evaluation demonstrated significant improvement in the time spent in documentation and completeness of nursing records. Nurses reported greater efficiency of the work flow and alleviation of cognitive burden, particularly during the time of high acuity shifts. Further that, the use of standardized documentation facilitated the communication across disciplines and enabled subsequent analytics for quality improvement purposes (Rajkomar et al, 2019).

However, some challenges were also noticed, including initial resistance to adoption, the need for continued system training and data privacy and trust issues. These results should give importance to the user-centered design, feedback mechanism, and governance mechanisms regarding the smart hospital deployments.

10.2 Voice-Assisted Clinical Reporting Case Study

Voice-assisted clinical reporting - generative AI intended to decrease fatigue and enhance real-time documentation. In a given case study carried out at a tertiary care hospital, voice enabled artificial intelligence AI systems were implemented in order to accommodate nursing documentation in the patient assessment and handoffs.

The solution made use of state-of-the-art speech-to-text models linked to natural language processing and generative artificial intelligence with the ability to translate verbal observations to structured nursing notes. Nurse utilized secure voice interfaces to record the assessment at the bedside and AI system automatically structured the information into standardized EHR fields.

Evaluation results showed that there were significant improvements on documentation timeliness and accuracy. Nurses commented to voice assisted reporting enabled nurses to keep the patient experience as they were recording care, therefore enhancing the patient experience. Additionally, the system minimized the use of retrospective charting that is famously known to be associated with documentation errors (Topol 2019).

Despite all these advantages, the implementation process confirmed practical difficulties in terms of noise in the background, variability in speech patterns, and the need for a strict authentication mechanism to guarantee the security of the data Fixing these problems required working on the systems in iterative fashion as well as user training. Overall, the case study proved that voice-assisted artificial intelligence systems can play a fruitful role in nursing documentation when carefully embedded in the course of clinical work.

CONCLUSION

Generative artificial intelligence-enabled automation represents an individual and prominent progress in the medical documentation and patient reporting in current healthcare systems. As has been covered throughout this chapter, generative AI is delivering useful solutions for age-old problems such as unnecessary documentation burden, inconsistencies in data quality, inefficiency of workflow and limited clinical decision support. By allowing for the automated creation of clinical notes, intelligent patient status summary and real-time patient monitoring, as well as predictive decision support, generative AI contributes to the accuracy of patient care documentation in nursing and contributing to providing patient Centre clinical care delivery as well. Importantly, the process of incorporating generative AI into the workflow of the nursing profession should be done with due consideration of ethical, legal, and regulatory considerations.

Tracking the trust between healthcare professionals and patients, ensuring data privacy, minimizing algorithmic bias, and holding healthcare professionals accountable and transparent are some of the major considerations to ensuring the sustainability of trust. The idea of human-in-the-loop paradigm is the main criterion of responsible adoption paradigm that, in turn, promotes the role of nurses as an ultimate decision makers and ethical custodians of care.

This chapter contributes to the knowledge base of nursing informatics through the integration of the methodological, managerial perspectives, and ethical viewpoints of generative AI-enabled documentation. It provides practical insights for healthcare professionals who are healthcare administrators, clinicians, and decision-makers that are seeking to implement AI in ways that are responsible and maintain the roles of nursing autonomy and patient safety. The way the chapter itself supports the core position of nurses in the future of intelligent healthcare systems is through posing AI as a co-pilot, not as the plane's replacement. From an organizational point of view, the number of nurses at risk of nurse burnout and the lack of job satisfaction and the poor continuity of care between clinical settings can be minimized with the help of AI-driven documentation systems. When implemented as a collaborative co-pilot less than a replacement of professional judgement there will be a strengthening nursing practice and support on evidence-based decision making. In conclusion, proper use of generative AI in the documentation of patient care and patient reporting is well-placed to bring about more resilient, efficient and human-centred healthcare systems and places the invaluable technology in harmony with the primary values and responsibilities of the nursing profession.

REFERENCES

Amann, J., Blasimme, A., Vayena, E., Frey, D., & Madai, V. I. (2020). Explainability for artificial intelligence in healthcare: A multidisciplinary perspective. *BMC Medical Informatics and Decision Making*, *20*(1), 310. Advance online publication. DOI: 10.1186/s12911-020-01332-6 PMID: 33256715

Bibri, S. E. (2021). Artificial intelligence-driven smart sustainable healthcare. *Sustainable Cities and Society*, *72*, 103098. DOI: 10.1016/j.scs.2021.103098

Booth, R. G., Strudwick, G., McBride, S., O'Connor, S., & López, A. L. (2023). How artificial intelligence can improve nursing practice. *Nursing Outlook*, *71*(2), 101912. DOI: 10.1016/j.outlook.2022.101912 PMID: 36690529

Brown, T. B., Mann, B., Ryder, N., ... (2020). Language models are few-shot learners. *NeurIPS*. https://doi.org//arXiv.2005.14165DOI: 10.48550

Carayon, P., Hoonakker, P., Hundt, A. S., & Salwei, M. E. (2020). Work system design for patient safety. *Applied Ergonomics*, *82*, 102914. DOI: 10.1016/j.apergo.2019.102914

Dall'Ora, C., Ball, J., Reinius, M., & Griffiths, P. (2020). Burnout in nursing. *Journal of Advanced Nursing*, *76*(12), 3364–3376. DOI: 10.1111/jan.14539 PMID: 32503559

El Arab, R. A., & Al Moosa, O. A. (2025). Systematic review of cost effectiveness and budget impact of artificial intelligence in healthcare. *NPJ Digital Medicine*, *8*(1), 172. Advance online publication. DOI: 10.1038/s41746-025-01722-y PMID: 40858882

Floridi, L., Cowls, J., Beltrametti, M., Chatila, R., Chazerand, P., Dignum, V., Luetge, C., Madelin, R., Pagallo, U., Rossi, F., Schafer, B., Valcke, P., & Vayena, E. (2018). AI4People—An ethical framework. *Minds and Machines*, *28*(4), 689–707. DOI: 10.1007/s11023-018-9482-5 PMID: 30930541

Ghassemi, M., Oakden-Rayner, L., & Beam, A. L. (2021). The false hope of current AI in healthcare. *The Lancet. Digital Health*, *3*(11), e745–e750. DOI: 10.1016/S2589-7500(21)00208-9 PMID: 34711379

Ghassemi, M., Oakden-Rayner, L., & Beam, A. L. (2021). The false hope of current approaches to explainable artificial intelligence in health care. *The Lancet. Digital Health*, *3*(11), e745–e750. DOI: 10.1016/S2589-7500(21)00208-9 PMID: 34711379

Kreimeyer, K., Foster, M., & Pandey, A.. (2017). Natural language processing systems for clinical text. *Journal of Biomedical Informatics*, *65*, 14–29. DOI: 10.1016/j.jbi.2017.07.012 PMID: 28729030

Kutney-Lee, A., & Kelly, D. (2011). The effect of hospital EHR adoption. *Health Services Research*, *46*(3), 884–905. DOI: 10.1111/j.1475-6773.2010.01231.x

Liu, X., Faes, L., & Kale, A. U.. (2019). Deep learning in healthcare. *The Lancet. Digital Health*, *1*(6), e271–e297. DOI: 10.1016/S2589-7500(19)30123-2 PMID: 33323251

McGonigle, D., & Mastrian, K. (2021). *Nursing informatics and the foundation of knowledge* (5th ed.). Jones & Bartlett., DOI: 10.21019/9781284231542

Mittelstadt, B. D., Allo, P., Taddeo, M., Wachter, S., & Floridi, L. (2016). Ethics of algorithms. *Big Data & Society*, *3*(2), 2053951716679679. Advance online publication. DOI: 10.1177/2053951716679679

Morley, J., Floridi, L., Kinsey, L., & Elhalal, A. (2019). From what to how: An initial review of publicly available AI ethics tools, methods and research to translate principles into practices. SSRN *Electronic Journal*. DOI: 10.2139/ssrn.3830348

Pavuluri, S., Sangal, R., Sather, J., & Taylor, R. A. (2024). Balancing act: The complex role of artificial intelligence in addressing burnout and healthcare workforce dynamics. *BMJ Health & Care Informatics*, *31*(1), e101120. DOI: 10.1136/bmjhci-2024-101120 PMID: 39181545

Rajkomar, A., Dean, J., & Kohane, I. (2019). Machine learning in medicine. *The New England Journal of Medicine*, *380*(14), 1347–1358. DOI: 10.1056/NEJMra1814259 PMID: 30943338

Ratwani, R. M., Savage, E., & Will, A.. (2018). Identifying EHR usability problems. *Journal of the American Medical Informatics Association : JAMIA*, *25*(7), 834–844. DOI: 10.1093/jamia/ocy024

Rodman, A., & Topol, E. J. (2025). Is generative artificial intelligence capable of clinical reasoning? *Lancet*, *405*(10480), 689. DOI: 10.1016/S0140-6736(25)00348-4 PMID: 40023638

Shortliffe, E. H., & Sepúlveda, M. J. (2018). Clinical decision support in the era of AI. *Journal of the American Medical Association*, *320*(21), 2199–2200. DOI: 10.1001/jama.2018.17163 PMID: 30398550

Singhal, K., Azizi, S., Tu, T., Mahdavi, S. S., Wei, J., Chung, H. W., Scales, N., Tanwani, A., Cole-Lewis, H., Pfohl, S., Payne, P., Seneviratne, M., Gamble, P., Kelly, C., Babiker, A., Schärli, N., Chowdhery, A., Mansfield, P., Demner-Fushman, D., & Natarajan, V. (2023). Large language models encode clinical knowledge. *Nature*, *620*(7972), 172–180. Advance online publication. DOI: 10.1038/s41586-023-06291-2 PMID: 37438534

Singhal, K., Azizi, S., Tu, T., Mahdavi, S. S., Wei, J., Chung, H. W., Scales, N., Tanwani, A., Cole-Lewis, H., Pfohl, S., Payne, P., Seneviratne, M., Gamble, P., Kelly, C., Babiker, A., Schärli, N., Chowdhery, A., Mansfield, P., Demner-Fushman, D., & Natarajan, V. (2023). Large language models encode clinical knowledge. *Nature*, *620*(7972), 172–180. DOI: 10.1038/s41586-023-06291-2 PMID: 37438534

Sinsky, C., Colligan, L., & Li, L.. (2016). Allocation of clinician time. *Annals of Internal Medicine*, *165*(11), 753–760. DOI: 10.7326/M16-0961 PMID: 27595430

Thirunavukarasu, A. J., Ting, D. S. J., Elangovan, K., Gutierrez, L., Tan, T. F., & Ting, D. S. W. (2023). Large language models in medicine. *Nature Medicine*, *29*(8), 1930–1940. DOI: 10.1038/s41591-023-02448-8 PMID: 37460753

Thrall, J. H. (2024). Challenges of implementing artificial intelligence–enabled programs in the clinical practice of radiology. *Radiology. Artificial Intelligence*, *6*(5), e240411. DOI: 10.1148/ryai.240411 PMID: 39259022

Topaz, M., & Pruinelli, L. (2017). Big data and nursing. *Nursing Outlook*, *65*(1), 104–112. DOI: 10.1016/j.outlook.2016.10.003 PMID: 28106594

Topol, E. (2019). High-performance medicine. *Nature Medicine*, *25*(1), 44–56. DOI: 10.1038/s41591-018-0300-7 PMID: 30617339

Vaswani, A., Shazeer, N., Parmar, N., ... (2017). Attention is all you need. *NeurIPS*. https://doi.org//arXiv.1706.03762DOI: 10.48550

Chapter 8
AI-Enabled Virtual Nursing Assistants:
Seq2Seq LSTM Neural Networks for Digital Healthcare

Suha Khalil Assayed
http://orcid.org/0000-0002-9924-0324
National Kaohsiung University of Science and Technology, Taiwan & The British University in Dubai, UAE

Chin-Shiuh Shieh
http://orcid.org/0000-0003-3187-458X
National Kaohsiung University of Science and Technology, Taiwan

Shashi Kant Gupta
http://orcid.org/0000-0001-6587-5607
National Kaohsiung University of Science and Technology, Taiwan & Centre for Research Impact & Outcome, Chitkara University Institute of Engineering and Technology, Chitkara University, India

ABSTRACT

Background: The rapid growth of artificial intelligence (AI) is reshaping the quality of delivering the healthcare services, creating new opportunities to support patients beyond traditional clinical environments. Unfortunately, not all individuals can access medical services equally and efficiently. This research aims to develop a virtual nursing assistant by utilizing a neural network model to provide patients with immediate and effective answers to medical inquiries. Methods: In this study we adopted a generative artificial intelligence (AI) powered by neural network layers. The architecture starts with encoding the input of health enquiry into the embedding layer. We utilized the MedQud dataset from Kaggle website, it includes

DOI: 10.4018/979-8-3373-8247-0.ch008

47,457 medical question-answer pairs covering questions about treatment, diagnosis and side effects. Results: The proposed model performs well during the training phase. However, during the execution phase, the performance metric shows a higher precision score (40%) compared to the recall and F1-score. Conclusions: The healthcare industry can implement an affordable conversational assistant to help patients with medical inquiries by adopting a virtual nursing assistant that utilizes a sequence model with encoder-decoder architecture. In the future, the model will be enhanced to expand the dataset and incorporate a speech mechanism, enabling users to interact with the system through voice commands.

1 INTRODUCTION

In today's era, the artificial intelligence (AI) is being utilized across a wide variety of domains. For example, it's being used in education and learning (Baidoo-Anu & Ansah, 2023; (Assayed, Alkhatib, & Shaalan, 2024)) in banking systems (Umamaheswari & Valarmathi, 2023) and in healthcare and medical applications (Lee & Yoon, 2021; Assayed, Shieh, & Gupta, 2025) While the 4th Industrial Revolution emphasized on improving the technology through the state-of-art networking and artificial intelligent systems as well as improving speed up the customers' satisfactions and maximizing the company profits, the 5th Industrial Revolution, continued working on this goal but by focusing on human-centric values in enhancing human lives by contributing positively to human wellbeing, equity and sustainability (Noble et al., 2022). As a result, researchers and developers are currently paying more attention to novel technologies such as artificial intelligence (AI) and Internet of Things (IoT) applications, that can effectively collaborate with humans in order to maximize both human and technological strengths toward Society 5.0 (Ziatdinov et al., 2024) Notably, Industry 5.0 includes several digital technologies that can significantly contribute to the health sector by enhancing digital health solutions through the integration of intelligent systems with human intelligence (Nahavandi, 2019). However, this contribution aligns with the vision of the World Health Organization (WHO) on the regional digital health in improving the health outcomes by developing and promoting digital health infrastructures and solutions (World Health Organization, 2022).

Within Healthcare 5.0, various smart sensors and agents have been integrated into medical services, enabling applications such as remote patient monitoring and smart health solutions (Mbunge, Muchemwa, & Batani, 2021; Assayed & Maheshwari, 2023). This has led to a substantial increase in the volume of available health data. To analyze data behavior and predict diseases, researchers have applied a range of machine learning and deep learning models within different health agents (Khanna et al., 2023; Al Sadi & Balachandran, 2023)

The Healthcare 5.0 framework closely aligns with the objectives of the World Health Organization (WHO), offering benefits to a wide range of individuals, such as patients, students, and parents. Both emphasize improving well-being and advancing health equity for all people.

According to the World Health Organization (World Health Organization, n.d), the health equity is achieved successfully when all can attain their full potential for both health and well-being. However, not all people can afford the nursing assistance immediately and equally. For instance, some people might need answers to medical enquiries immediately and urgently, while unprivileged students might may lack access to some of educational medical resources (Alfakhry et al., 2023). Henceforth, this research aims to have a virtual nursing assistant by developing a neural network model to provide people with immediate and effective answer to their medical inquiries, utilizing an affordable sequence-to-sequence (Seq2Seq) model integrated with multiple neural network layers.

2 TECHNICAL BACKGROUND

2.1 Sequence Models

A sequence model is a type of neural network particularly designed to handle sequential or time series data like stock price, text and audio data. In these sequences, predicting what comes next, depends on the data that precedes it. Therefore, the order of the data as well as the time are essential for making accurate predictions. Remarkably, the sequence neural network models consist of models that takes sequential data as input and produce a sequential output, or they are least applied in one side of the input or output as sequential data. In fact, the sequence models play an important role in enhancing applications and tasks within the field of natural language processing (NLP).

2.1.1 Sequence-to-one Model

This model receives a sequence input from time series or sequential data and generates one output. For example, detecting the blood pressure for the patient over specific timeframe; the input is time series data, and this data can be learned to identify the patterns in order to predict whether the blood pressure is normal or not (1 or 0) as illustrated in Figure 1.

Figure 1. An example of sequence-to-one model (blood pressure reading).

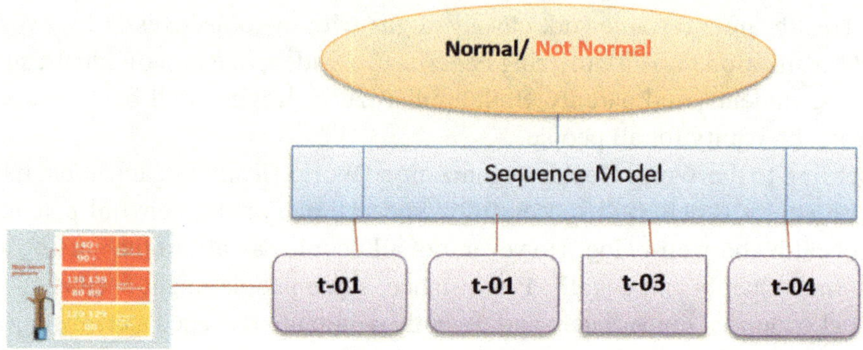

2.1.2 One-to-Sequence Model

This This model produces a sequential output from non-sequential input. For example, predicting the medical X-ray image, as the input is one X-ray image with only one-time step as it's analyzed the image all at once, so in this example the time is not important as no historical data is used, as the predicted output is produces sequentially for describing and analyzing the image. Figure 2 explains this model by generating a sequential text description from a given image (broken bone).

Figure 2. An example of one-to- sequence model for predicting the medical image description.

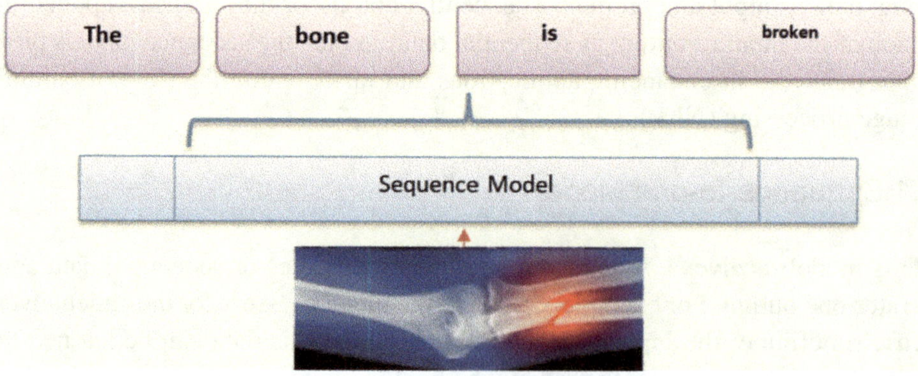

2.1.3 Sequence-to-Sequence Model

This model processes the sequential input to generate a sequential output. The input and output sequences differ in length, as seen in applications like machine translation, text summarization and chatbots. Its architecture includes two main components: the encoder and the decoder. Figure 3 depicts an example of translating a sequence from English to Portuguese. The input sequence includes 6 words “When can I take my medicine” and the output to Portuguese translation is only five words “Quando posso tomar meu remédio”.

Figure 3. Seq2Seq model in Machine Translation (From English to Portuguese)

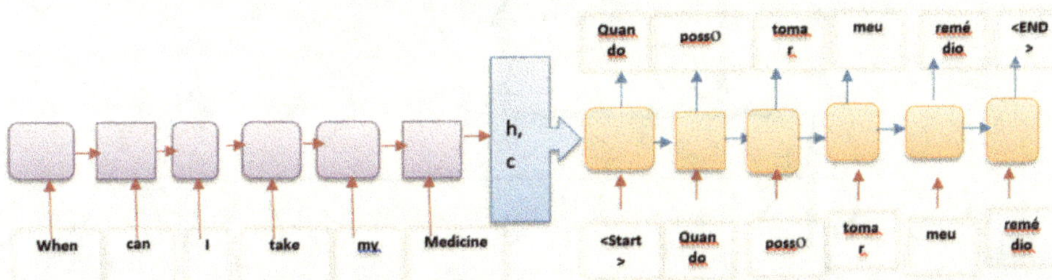

In the following sections, we will explore various neural networks architecture that can be utilized in sequence models.

2.2 Recurrent Neural Networks (RNNs)

RNNs are components of artificial neural networks, equipped with memory and loops for perceiving information in sequences of inputs, the same function is applied to every single input, and the output depends on the computation of the previous time steps. Numerous researchers have utilized different types of neural networks (Zhi et al., 2024; Assayed et al., 2025), however, the hidden states (ht) represents the memory of RNN which store the previous and current input.

Nevertheless, the weight (W) parameter is crucial for the learning. It can be adjusted during the training process, this optimization technique known as back-propagation, which the weight (w) can be fine-tuned better results. Figure 4 depicts the RNN architecture.

Figure 4. RNN architecture using a single activation function (tanh).

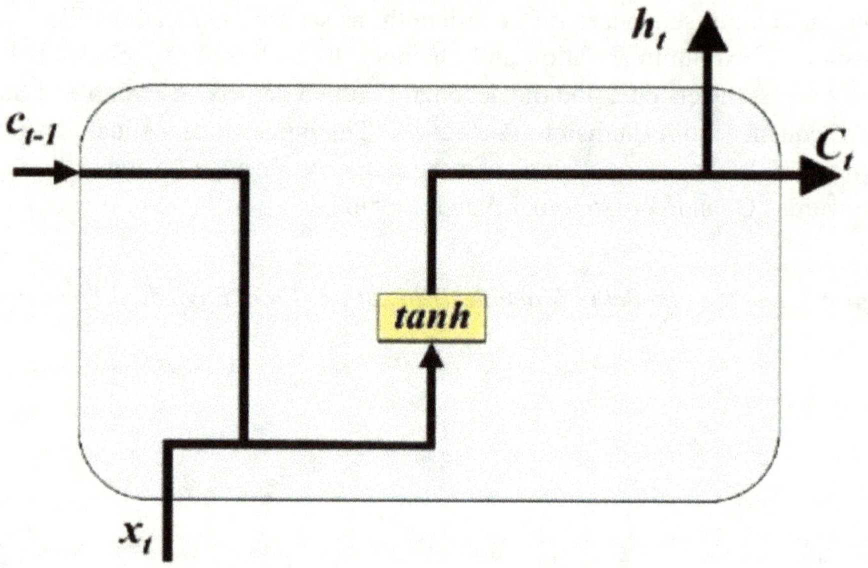

2.3 Long Short-Term Memory (LSTM)

While the RNN consists a single activation layer, the LSTM has a set of activation layers and gates, in order to memorize and capture the dependencies over a long period of time. Though, the cell state is usually referred to the memory of the LSTM and the hidden state in represents the output of the cell state. However, in each time step a calculation is performed by utilizing different components and gates including: the input gate, forget gate and output gate. Figure 5 explains the gates of LSTM.

Figure 5. LSTM architecture illustrating the various gates.

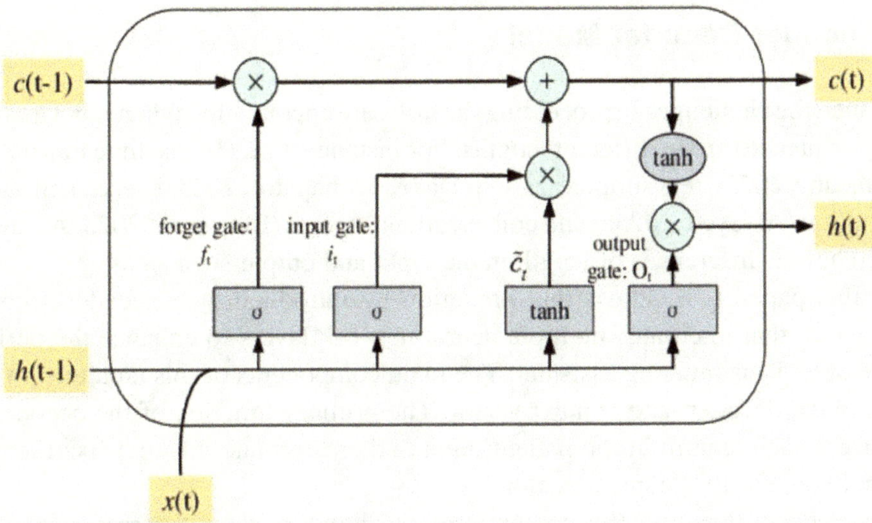

The input gate is responsible to decide which information should be added to the cell state, however, the sigmoid function decides which input value is allowed to be stored into the cell state, as (0) means is not allowed, and (1) it can be passed to the cell state. However, it is represented by using this formula: Input Gate (t) = Sigmoid (Wi * [h(t-1), Xt] + bi). As tanh function gives a weight of the degree of the importance of this value and it's represents by using this formula: Cell State(Ct) = tanh (Wc * [h(t-1), Xt] + bc). On the other side, the forget gate is responsible to decide which information should be reserved in the cell state.

The output gate determines the output, as the Sigmoid function is used to decide which value will be kept. Whereas, the tanh function is used as well to gives the weight to the importance of the value.

2.4 Gated Recurrent Unit (GRU)

The GRU is seen as an alternative to the RNN, with fewer parameters in the training process. This streamlined structure allows it to handle simpler tasks compared to the LSTM model. Interestingly, studies indicate that while the LSTM may outperform the GRU in specific tasks ((Zhang, Zeng, & Starly, 2021) it also requires longer training times due to its higher number of parameters and model complexity. The GRU utilizes two main gates: the reset gate, which manages which data can be discarded, and the update gate, which decides which data to retain from the previous state.

2.5 Encoder-Decoder Model

In fact, the challenges in processing the tasks are encountered when input and the output sequences are in different lengths. For instance, tasks in machine translation (Akhmedov, 2025), text summarization (Das & Mohapatro, 2025) speech and audio recognition (Assayed, 2025a) and conversational agents (Liao et al., 2023; Assayed, 2025b) have a differences of length in the input and output sequences.

In this paper, we address this limitation by introducing an encoder-decoder architecture that integrates multiple neural network layers to enhance the performance of a virtual nursing assistant. The main components of this architecture are the encoder, decoder, and context vector. The primary function of the encoder is to process each feature in the patient input and encapsulate it into a fixed-length vector, known as the “context vector.”

The decoder then uses this context vector as input to generate a response to the patient’s inquiry. Figure 6 below illustrates the use of LSTM within the encoder-decoder architecture

Figure 6. The encoder-decoder architecture for processing patient’s enquiry.

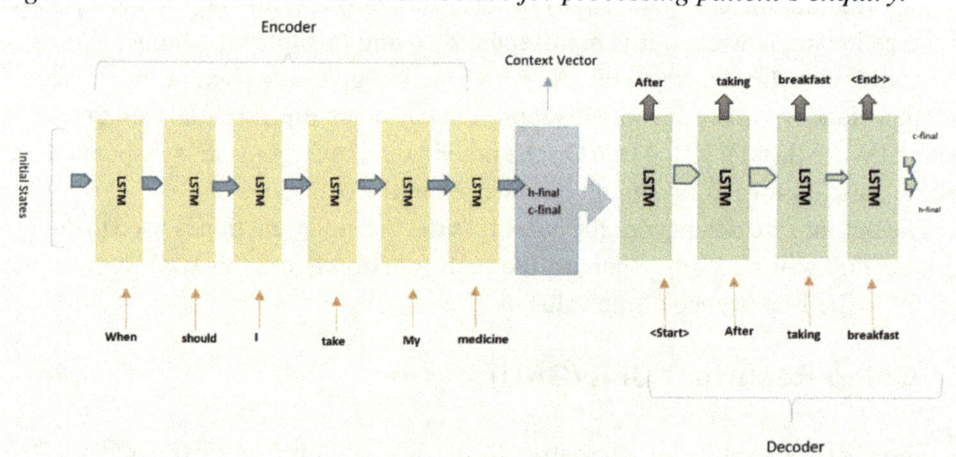

The following steps summarize this process as follows:

1. The cell state and the hidden state are both initiated to (c0, h0).
2. Then, the first word “When” is converted to numerical representation.

3. Next, the LSTM takes the numerical vector "When" with the initial states to process the new values of (c1, h1).
4. The output of the first time step is denoted by the hidden state (h1), which is combined with the new token "should." This resulting output serves as the input for the LSTM in the next step (step 2). The calculation is carried out using the gates and activation functions to obtain the new values of (c2, h2). This process continues until the final token in the sequence is reached.
5. The final values of states are represented with (c-final, h- final), encapsulating all the sequence of the question within a vector. This vector is referred to as the "context vector".
6. The context vector helps the decoder to predict the output sequence from the virtual nursing assistant.

3 RELATED WORK

There have been numerous research experiments applying neural network algorithms in healthcare. However, the research initiatives have varied in their focus. For example, some authors focused on improving the administrative services within hospitals including the implementation of standardization work as well as processing the medical data effectively (Kim & Huh, 2020), while others developed applications to enhance the customer services (Bohr & Memarzadeh, 2020; Assayed, Shieh, & Gupta, 2025) between patients. Additionally, some researches have focused on supporting doctors in disease analysis and predictions (Men et al., 2021; Kumar, U, & Maben, 2025; Assayed, 2025c).

Interestingly, several AI conversational applications have been implemented in hospitals, using the state-of-the-art machine learning models as well as natural Language processing (NLP) techniques. For example, Bharti et al. (2020) designed a multilingual conversational bot as a personal virtual doctor to interact with patients by providing preventive measures and interactive counseling sessions. The authors utilized the Dialogflow conversational API from Google Cloud service. Moreover, Christopherjames et al. [2021] developed a chatbot utilizing the Dialogflow application programming interface (API) to collect patients' health data and depending on data, the chatbot recommends a treatment. Nevertheless, Tripathy, Singh, and Ray (2023) opt for Transformers over seq2seq models. They developed a system to recognize the symptoms for Covid-19 by using transformer and pre-trained systems such as BERT and GPT were fine-tuned with using English dataset to generate responses for Covid-19 which were doctor-like to further solve the problem for medical consultations.

In fact, despite the effectiveness of using the seq2seq models in the conversational applications, but few authors who utilized this architecture in the conversational healthcare models. Boulesnane et al. [2022] developed a medical assistant chatbot specifically for Arabic Algerian speakers, utilizing a limited corpus size of 2,150 medical data to develop a chatbot. This chatbot employed an encoder-decoder architecture with multiple neural network layers including LSTM, BiLSTM and GRU. However, Li et al. [2021] developed a seq2seq based model by using a larger dialogue corpus with 53663 samples, but, this model works only in Chinese healthcare consultation.

In contrast, our proposed conversational AI model is designed for English speakers, utilizing a corpus of 16,412 data points. The dataset encompasses various aspects of medical questions and answers in a conversational format.

4 METHOD

4.1 Data Collection and Preparation

In this study we utilized the MedQud dataset (Miller, n.d.) from Kaggle website. MedQuAD includes 47,457 medical question-answer pairs, which collected from 12 National Institutes of Health websites, including cancer.gov, niddk.nih.gov, GARD, MedlinePlus Health Topics, and more. The collection covers questions about treatment, diagnosis, side effects and more.

4.1.1 Data Cleaning

It's an essential step of processing the data, it includes removing the repetitive words, unnecessary symbols, and fixing the uncompleted. Cleaning the data can improve the reliability of the output.

4.1.2 Lowercasing the Data

In this study we used we used the function lower () from Python libraries to convert the tokens in the English corpus to the lowercase. The consistency of texts can enhance the data processing.

4.1.3 Tokenization

We applied the split() function from python's library to split the texts into tokens and sub-tokens. This function is responsible to convert the texts into understandable format that can be interpreted by machine learning algorithms.

4.1.4 Padding the Data

We used the "padding" augmentation function from the Keras library to standardize the length of all input texts.

4.2 Word Embedding

This technique plays an important role to lower the dimension space in representing the 9,865 tokens. Therefore, we utilized only 50 dimensional vector to represent each word from the input text, as all similar words can closer together. Since word embedding can learn from large size of corpus by using some of neural network models such as Word2Vec, GloVe and FastText.

4.3 Creating Vocabulary list

In this study, we used the Python language to create the vocabulary list from all our corpus. All unique cleaned token words are indexed and saved into the vocab list. However, the vocab size in our data is 9,865 tokens.

4.4 Building the Seq2Seq Model

In reference to the systematic review conducted by Alsayed et al. (2024) several AI models have addressed human well-being using various machine learning techniques and NLP tools. There are several studies utilized the deep learning algorithms including the LSTM and BILSTM. However, in this study we have included the LSTM layer into both components the encoder and the decoder.

The architecture starts with encoding the input of health enquiry into the embedding layer using 50 dimensional vector, then the semantics and the context of the input text is encapsulated into a "context vector". Next, the decoder takes the context vector as input for starting to predict the health response. We integrated the long short-term memory (LSTM) with using 400 units to improve the memory and the performance of the recurrent neural network (RNN) models by addressing the vanishing gradient problem, especially for long sequences. The below Table 1 displays the number of parameters in each layer. The total number of parameters in this model is 5,892,365.

Table 1. The characteristics of the LSTM Model and Number of Parameters in Each Layer.

Layer (Type)	**Output Shape**	**Number of Parameters**
Encoder		
Input (Encoder)	(None, 13)	0
Embedding	(None, 13, 50)	493,300
LSTM (Encoder)	[(None, 13, 400), (None, 400), (None, 400)]	721,600
Decoder		
Input (Decoder)	(None, 13)	0
LSTM (Decoder)	[(None, 13, 400), (None, 400), (None, 400)]	721,600
Dense	(None, 13, 5294)	3,955,865
Total Parameters		**5,892,365**

4.5 Training and Compiling

During training, the model uses the teacher forcing technique, which involves leveraging actual annotated data rather than the predicted output from the previous time step [40]. Essentially, each generated output token is compared with the true token using a loss function. The model was implemented on a device equipped with an Intel i7-1065G7 CPU at 1.30GHz and 16GB of RAM. However, Table 2 presents the results of the training process after completing 120 epochs.

Table 2. Training results after 120 epoch.

Epochs	**Accuracy score**	**Loss**	**Time**
120	0.98%	0.03	4 hours

4.6 Model Implementation

After the model has been trained in the dataset, the model is implemented to predict the unseen data based on the probability of each output token. However, the ROUGE and BLEU metrics use n-gram to compare the generated answer. For example, ROUGE-1, evaluate the individual words in the generated sequence that match words in the reference sequence. Whereas, in ROUGE-L focuses on capturing the longest essential content present in both the generated sequence and the reference answer. In this study, we applied the metric of ROUGE-L with using five unseen questions as depicted in Table 3.

Table 3. Implementing the model with using new five unseen medical questions.

Question	The proposed model prediction	Reference answer
What is the glaucoma disease?	the optic nerve is a bundle of more than 1 million	Glaucoma is a group of eye conditions that damage the optic nerve, often due to increased pressure within the eye, leading to vision loss and potentially blindness
What is high blood pressure ?	high blood pressure is a common disease in which blood flows	High blood pressure, also known as hypertension, is a medical condition characterized by elevated pressure in the arteries, increasing the risk of heart disease and other health complications."
What symptoms of heart attack?	no most heart attack patients do not have all of the symptoms	Symptoms of a heart attack include chest pain or discomfort, shortness of breath, nausea, lightheadedness, and pain or discomfort in other areas of the upper body.
What is diabetes?	diabetes is a disease in which your blood glucose or blood	Diabetes is a chronic condition characterized by high blood sugar levels due to either insufficient insulin production or ineffective use of insulin by the body.
How to prevent symptoms of Peyronie's Disease?	researchers do not know how to prevent peyronies disease	Preventing symptoms of Peyronie's Disease involves avoiding penile injuries and seeking early treatment for any penile curvature or pain.

a. Model Evaluation

In this section, we describe how the evaluation metrics (Recall, Precision, F1-score) are calculated using the ROUGE-L metric. We compared the model's generated answers with the reference answers.

i. Recall

This below metric calculates the matching words between the virtual nursing model's answer and the reference text:

$$= \frac{\text{\#Matching words between model's answer and reference}}{\textit{Total \# ofwords } \text{and } \textit{subwords in the refernce answer}}$$

ii. Precision

The precision metric calculates the matching words between the virtual nursing model's answer and the reference text as depicted in the below formula:

iii. F-score

F1-score metric calculates the quality of the virtual nursing model's answer compared to the reference 's answer as depicted in the below formula:

The table below, Table 4 displays the results of ROUGE-L scores in evaluating the model.

Table 4. The results of ROUGE-L scores in evaluating the model.

	F1-Score	Precision	Recall
What is Glaucoma	0.20	0.33	0.14
What is high blood pressure ?	0.30	0.54	0.21
What symptoms of heart attack?	0.21	0.33	0.15
What is diabetes?	0.27	0.45	0.2
How to prevent symptoms of Peyronie's Disease	0.20	0.33	0.15
Average Metric score	0.24	0.40	0.17

b. Model Design

In Python, we utilized the *Tk* toolkit as it offers a variety of options and features for designing user interfaces. For instance, it provides settings for selecting fonts, colors, labels, and more.

In our proposed model, we opted for a simple, interactive, and user-friendly interface. We selected a blue color scheme, featuring two intuitive text boxes: one for the patient and the other for the virtual nursing assistant as depicted in Figure 7.

Figure 7. The interface of the proposed nursing assistant model.

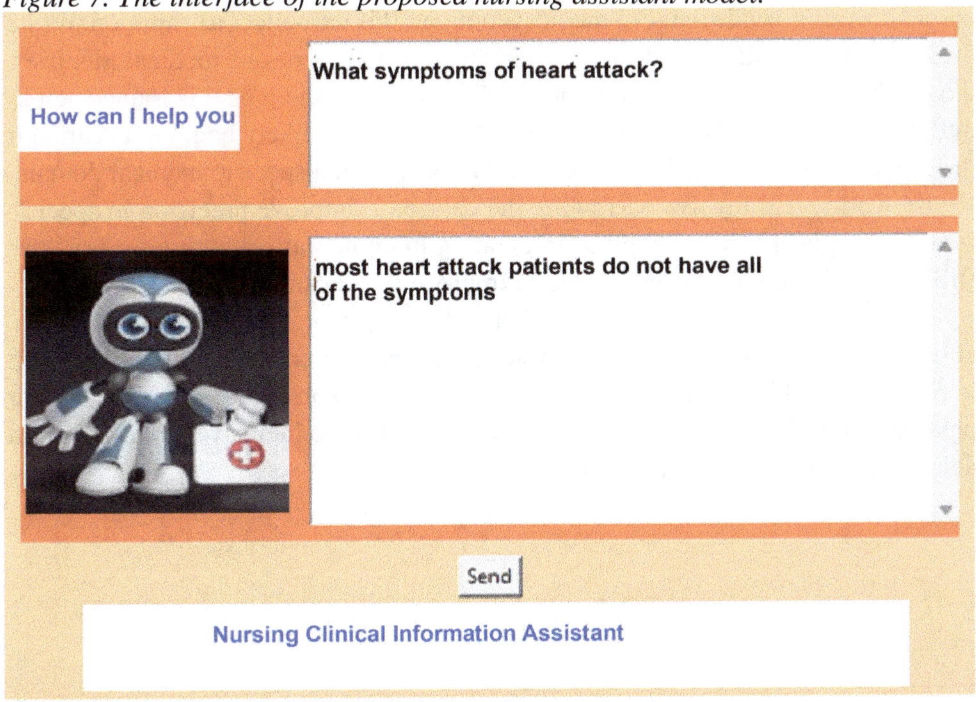

5 CONCLUSION

In the context of healthcare 5.0, a variety of intelligent agents and assistants have been employed within medical service and various health applications. According to the World Health Organization (WHO), health equity is achieved when everyone can attain their full potential for both health and well-being. However, not all individuals can access and afford medical services equally and efficiently. This research aims to develop a virtual nursing assistant using a neural network model to provide individuals with immediate and effective answers to their medical inquiries, employing an affordable sequence-to-sequence (Seq2Seq) architecture integrated with multiple neural network layers. We utilized the MedQud dataset from Kaggle, which includes 47,457 medical question-answer pairs covering topics such as treatment, diagnosis, side effects, and more. The dataset was preprocessed using various Python functions, including cleaning, lowercasing, padding, and tokenization. The sequential model is built using an encoder-decoder architecture, integrated with an LSTM layer. The model's performance was evaluated using the ROUGE-L score, with precision being the most accurate metric compared to recall and F1-score. Since we used a general corpus covering a wide range of medical domains, this introduces a limitation. While the broad dataset allows the model to address various types of medical inquiries, the results may lack domain-specific precision because the model is trained across multiple medical fields. Therefore, the outcomes would likely be more accurate if the model were fine-tuned on a focused dataset within a specific medical domain. Future work could involve narrowing the dataset to improve precision in specialized areas of healthcare as well as integrating more neural network layers such as BiLSTM and attention layer in order to improve the performance

Additionally, the model will be enhanced to incorporate a speech mechanism, allowing users to interact with the system via voice commands. This feature will improve accessibility and usability, especially for patients with limited literacy or physical disabilities, making the conversational AI more inclusive and efficient in delivering real-time medical assistance.

Authorship Contribution Statement: The authors are contributed to the conceptualization, methodology and experiment, analyzing the results and reviewing the entire paper.

Declaration of Competing Interests: The authors have no competing interest.

REFERENCES

Akhmedov, B. A. (2025). Integrating ICT and artificial intelligence in teaching philological disciplines: a focus on machine translation of textual data. *Экономика и социум*, (6-1 (133)), 115-122.

Al Sadi, K., & Balachandran, W. (2023). Prediction model of Type 2 diabetes mellitus for Oman prediabetes patients using artificial neural network and six machine learning classifiers. *Applied Sciences (Basel, Switzerland)*, *13*(4), 2344. DOI: 10.3390/app13042344

Alfakhry, G., Naeem, A., AboHajar, M. B., Alfakhry, A., Mohandes, A. F., Ali, I., Makhoul, E., Ahmed, N., Abla, M. M., Alhomsi, K., & Jamous, I. (2023, January 3). Revealing the significant shortcomings in the learning environment at the three largest medical schools in Syria: What's next? *BMC Medical Education*, *23*(1), 2. DOI: 10.1186/s12909-022-03978-4 PMID: 36597081

Alsayed, S., Assayed, S. K., Alkhatib, M., & Shaalan, K. (2024). Impact of artificial intelligence chatbots on student well-being and mental health: A systematic review. *People and Behavior Analysis*, *2*(2), 1–3. DOI: 10.31098/pba.v2i2.2411

Assayed, S., & Maheshwari, P. (2023). Agent-based simulation for university students admission: Medical colleges in Jordan universities. *Computer Science & Engineering* [CSEIJ]. *International Journal (Toronto, Ont.)*, *13*(1).

Assayed, S. K. (Ed.). (2025a). *Educational Applications of Natural Language Processing, Chatbots, and AI*. IGI Global. DOI: 10.4018/979-8-3373-6791-0

Assayed, S. K. (Ed.). (2025b). *Enhancing student support and learning through conversational AI*. IGI Global. DOI: 10.4018/979-8-3373-3316-8

Assayed, S. K. (2025c). *Transforming healthcare through generative and agentic AI: A systematic review*. In *Proceedings of the 10th International Conference on Information Technology Trends (ITT)* (pp. 124–129). IEEE. DOI: 10.1109/ITT69610.2025.11352935

Assayed, S. K., Alkhatib, M., & Shaalan, K. (2024). Transforming student advising in smart cities: A deep learning conversational AI chatbot. In *Proceedings of the 2024 Mediterranean Smart Cities Conference (MSCC)* (pp. 1–6). IEEE. https://doi.org/DOI: 10.1109/MSCC62288.2024.10696988

Assayed, S. K., Alkhatib, M., Shaalan, K. F., & Alsayed, S. (2025). HSGAdviser: AI speech assistant for enabling sustainable education solutions. In *Proceedings of the 2025 1st International Conference on Computational Intelligence Approaches and Applications (ICCIAA)* (pp. 1–6). IEEE. https://doi.org/DOI: 10.1109/ICCIAA65327.2025.11013058

Assayed, S. K., Shieh, C. S., & Gupta, S. K. (2025). Engineering intelligent healthcare systems: Understanding medical queries with AI and NLP. *Journal of Engineering and Applied Sciences (Asian Research Publishing Network)*, *72*(1), 212. DOI: 10.1186/s44147-025-00800-y

Baidoo-Anu, D., & Ansah, L. O. (2023). Education in the era of generative artificial intelligence (AI): Understanding the potential benefits of ChatGPT in promoting teaching and learning. *Journal of Artificial Intelligence*, *7*(1), 52–62.

Bharti, U., Bajaj, D., Batra, H., Lalit, S., Lalit, S., & Gangwani, A. Medbot: Conversational artificial intelligence powered chatbot for delivering tele-health after covid-19. In2020 5th international conference on communication and electronics systems (ICCES) 2020 Jun 10 (pp. 870-875). IEEE

Bohr, A., & Memarzadeh, K. (2020). The rise of artificial intelligence in healthcare applications. In *Artificial intelligence in healthcare* (pp. 25–60). Academic Press., DOI: 10.1016/B978-0-12-818438-7.00002-2

Boulesnane, A., Saidi, Y., Kamel, O., Bouhamed, M. M., & Mennour, R. (2022, October 12). Dzchatbot: A medical assistant chatbot in the Algerian Arabic dialect using seq2seq model. In *2022 4th International Conference on Pattern Analysis and Intelligent Systems (PAIS)* (pp. 1–8). IEEE. DOI: 10.1109/PAIS56586.2022.9946867

Christopherjames, J. E., Saravanan, M., Thiyam, D. B., Sahib, M. Y., Ganapathi, M. V., & Milton, A. (2021, August 4). Natural language processing based human assistive health conversational agent for multi-users. In *2021 Second International Conference on Electronics and Sustainable Communication Systems (ICESC)* (pp. 1414–1420). IEEE. DOI: 10.1109/ICESC51422.2021.9532913

Das, T. K., & Mohapatro, A. (2025). Text summarization: An application of generative AI. In Vajjhala, N. R., Roy, S. S., Taşcı, B., & Hoque Chowdhury, M. E. (Eds.), *Generative artificial intelligence (AI) approaches for industrial applications* (Vol. 24, pp. xx–xx). Springer., DOI: 10.1007/978-3-031-76710-4_16

Khanna, A., Selvaraj, P., Gupta, D., Sheikh, T. H., Pareek, P. K., & Shankar, V. (2023). Internet of things and deep learning enabled healthcare disease diagnosis using biomedical electrocardiogram signals. *Expert Systems: International Journal of Knowledge Engineering and Neural Networks, 40*(4), e12864. DOI: 10.1111/exsy.12864

Kim, S. K., & Huh, J. H. (2020). Artificial neural network blockchain techniques for healthcare system: Focusing on the personal health records. *Electronics (Basel), 9*(5), 763. DOI: 10.3390/electronics9050763

Kumar, A., U, P. R., & Maben, M. (2025). Heart disease prediction using machine learning algorithms. In *Proceedings of the 2025 Third International Conference on Networks, Multimedia and Information Technology (NMITCON)* (pp. 1–6). IEEE. https://doi.org/DOI: 10.1109/NMITCON65824.2025.11187908

Lee, D., & Yoon, S. N. (2021). Application of artificial intelligence-based technologies in the healthcare industry: Opportunities and challenges. *International Journal of Environmental Research and Public Health, 18*(1), 271. Advance online publication. DOI: 10.3390/ijerph18010271 PMID: 33401373

Li, Y., Wen, G., Hu, Y., Luo, M., Fan, B., Wang, C., & Yang, P. (2021). Multi-source Seq2seq guided by knowledge for Chinese healthcare consultation. *Journal of Biomedical Informatics, 117*, 103727. DOI: 10.1016/j.jbi.2021.103727 PMID: 33713854

Liao, L., Yang, G. H., & Shah, C. (2023, February 27). Proactive conversational agents. In *Proceedings of the Sixteenth ACM International Conference on Web Search and Data Mining* (pp. 1244–1247). ACM. https://doi.org/DOI: 10.1145/3539597.3572724

Mbunge, E., Muchemwa, B., & Batani, J. (2021). Sensors and Healthcare 5.0: Transformative shift in virtual care through emerging digital health technologies. *Global Health Journal (Amsterdam, Netherlands), 5*(4), 169–177. DOI: 10.1016/j.glohj.2021.11.008

Men, L., Ilk, N., Tang, X., & Liu, Y. (2021). Multi-disease prediction using LSTM recurrent neural networks. *Expert Systems with Applications, 177*, 114905. DOI: 10.1016/j.eswa.2021.114905

Miller, J. (n.d.). *MedQuAD* [Dataset]. Kaggle. https://www.kaggle.com/datasets/jpmiller/layoutlm

Nahavandi, S. (2019). Industry 5.0—A human-centric solution. *Sustainability (Basel), 11*(16), 4371. Advance online publication. DOI: 10.3390/su11164371

Noble, S. M., Mende, M., Grewal, D., & Parasuraman, A. (2022). The fifth industrial revolution: How harmonious human–machine collaboration is triggering a retail and service (r)evolution. *Journal of Retailing, 98*(2), 199–208. DOI: 10.1016/j.jretai.2022.04.003

Tripathy, S., Singh, R., & Ray, M. (2023). Natural language processing for COVID-19 consulting system. *Procedia Computer Science, 218*, 1335–1341. DOI: 10.1016/j.procs.2023.01.112 PMID: 36743786

Umamaheswari, S., & Valarmathi, A. (2023, April 21). Role of artificial intelligence in the banking sector. *Journal of Survey in Fisheries Sciences., 10*(4S), 2841–2849.

World Health Organization. (2022). *Regional strategy for fostering digital health in the Eastern Mediterranean Region (2023–2027)* (EM/RC69/8). Cairo: World Health Organization, Regional Office for the Eastern Mediterranean. https://apps.who.int/iris/handle/10665/359945

World Health Organization. (n.d.). *Health equity*. World Health Organization. https://www.who.int/health-topics/health-equity#tab=tab_1

Zhang, J., Zeng, Y., & Starly, B. (2021). Recurrent neural networks with long term temporal dependencies in machine tool wear diagnosis and prognosis. *SN Applied Sciences, 3*(4), 442. DOI: 10.1007/s42452-021-04427-5 PMID: 33855273

Zhi, W., Appling, A. P., Golden, H. E., Podgorski, J., & Li, L. (2024). Deep learning for water quality. *Nature Water, 2*(3), 228–241. DOI: 10.1038/s44221-024-00202-z PMID: 38846520

Ziatdinov, R., Atteraya, M. S., & Nabiyev, R. (2024). The fifth industrial revolution as a transformative step towards Society 5.0. *Societies (Basel, Switzerland), 14*(2), 19. Advance online publication. DOI: 10.3390/soc14020019

Chapter 9

AI for Hospital Administration, Staff Scheduling, and Operational Efficiency:

Transforming Healthcare Operations Through Intelligent Automation

K. Saravanan
http://orcid.org/0000-0002-0672-1568
SRM Institute of Science and Technology, India

M. Sadhasivam
Panimalar Engineering College, India

G. Sumathy
http://orcid.org/0000-0001-6759-5967
SRM Institute of Science and Technology, India

A. Maheshwari
http://orcid.org/0009-0009-7357-8536
SRM Institute of Science and Technology, India

M. G. Dinesh
http://orcid.org/0009-0009-7643-5338
Easa College of Engineering and Technology, India

DOI: 10.4018/979-8-3373-8247-0.ch009

ABSTRACT

Artificial Intelligence (AI) is reshaping hospital administration, workforce management, and operational efficiency by enabling intelligent automation, predictive insights, and data-driven decision-making. This chapter explores the integration of AI technologies including machine learning, deep learning, natural language processing, and reinforcement learning within key hospital operational domains such as administrative workflows, staff scheduling, resource allocation, and performance optimization. It highlights how AI enhances patient flow, reduces delays, improves asset management, and supports real-time operational intelligence. The chapter also discusses challenges related to data privacy, bias, system interoperability, governance, and workforce acceptance. Finally, emerging trends and future research directions, including digital twins, federated learning, and explainable AI, are explored to guide the development of resilient and efficient healthcare operations.

1. INTRODUCTION

1.1 Background and Motivation

The world is experiencing unprecedented pressure on healthcare organizations to provide high-quality and patient-centered care and at the same time streamline the workflow, overcome the workforce shortage, and limit the increasing costs. The hospital, particularly, is a dynamic, and complex system where administrative processes, staffing, patient demand and resources availability and clinical processes must be balanced at any given time. The traditional administrative practices which are typically rooted on manual coordination, pre-set schedules templates, and fragmented information systems are struggling to cope up with the dynamic medical environments of the modern world. As the patient loads, administrative loads, and the wish to be efficient change, the hospitals are turning to digital transformation and automation as the process of simplifying the operations. One of the powerful agents that have made this change possible has been Artificial Intelligence (AI), which supports decisions in real-time, has predictive capabilities and automation options, which can significantly enhance the efficiency of operations(Subramanyam, S. V. 2022). Introducing AI in the hospital management and workforce scheduling can provide hospitals with access to information-based insights and smart applications that can optimize workflow, predict resource demand, reduce bottlenecks, and increase the overall quality of provided services(Bhimavarapu, U. 2026).

1.2 The Evolving Role of AI in Healthcare Operations

In the last few years, AI technologies, including machine learning (ML), deep learning (DL), natural language processing (NLP), and reinforcement learning (RL), have rapidly evolved and infiltrated various spheres of healthcare activity. Even though AI has always been associated with clinical decision support or diagnostic imaging, the utilization of AI in non-clinical operational fields has grown exponentially. The problems that the hospitals are facing presently are: long waiting lines, inefficient resource utilization, overworked administration, inefficient staffing, and uncontrollable flow of patients, which contributes significantly to the quality of services and financial sustainability. The AI solutions address the mentioned problems because they are based on the past and current data to offer the appropriate predictions, propose the most efficient schedules, automate routine tasks, and help the administrators make sensible decisions. The administrative efficiency is also served by the use of intelligent automation, i.e., robotic process automation (RPA), which is applied to automate the workflows according to the rules, i.e., billing, appointment processing, record updates, and claims management(Mohideen, S. K et al., 2026). This transition to operational AI is indicative of a wider trend in healthcare: that of transitioning away from reactive, human-centered decision-making and toward proactive, data-driven, and automated decision-making.

1.3 Importance of AI for Hospital Administration

The hospital administration involves very diverse activities, such as patient registration, scheduling appointments, admission and discharge process, billing and insurance procedures, facility management, supply chains, and inter-clinical and non-clinical unit coordination. These processes are important and at times take a long time and can easily be delayed when done manually. AI can assist the administrators with automation of routine work, lessening of paperwork, and simplification of departmental communication. To illustrate, predictive analytics will help predict patient admissions, manage the bed placement and detect possible workflow disruptions. NLP tools may be used to extract significant information within clinical records or patient communication, enhancing precision and decreasing the administrative load. The AI-based chatbots and virtual assistants could assist patients with booking an appointment, information, and decrease the workload of the front-desk staff. Altogether, AI enhances the accuracy of the administration, minimizes redundancy, and speeds up the working process, leaving employees with more strategic and patient-facing tasks to perform. With the process of hospital digitalization, the importance of AI in administration is likely to grow even further.

1.4 Need for Intelligent Staff Scheduling and Workforce Optimization

One of the most challenging and difficult operational activities in hospitals is staff scheduling. Manual scheduling is challenging and time-consuming because of nurse shortages, patient volumes, and skills requirement variability, regulatory limits, staff preference, and emergency situations. Conventional shift scheduling approaches that are usually tied to preset patterns or hand-made modifications cannot respond to fluctuations in real-time demand and regularly lead to burnout, understaffing, or workload imbalances. The models of AI-based workforce optimization make use of data like past patient demand, seasonal trends, staff availability, skill levels, and real-time capacity to come up with the best schedules that can balance the operational requirements and employee welfare. Patient inflow is predicted by machine learning models, which allows distributing staff proactively. The reinforcement learning techniques are able to adjust the schedule of shifts to the dynamic environment, and learn the most effective strategies. Such smart systems do not only increase the efficiency of hospitals but also make the staff happier, less fatigued, and healthier at workplace. Artificial intelligence enhances the productivity and quality of services of hospitals by changing the staff scheduling as a manual operation to an automated, predictive process.

1.5 Enhancing Operational Efficiency Through Intelligent Automation

Hospitals need to be efficient in their operations to sustain them, promptly offer care to patients, and maximize resource usage. The delays in surgical schedules, overcrowding in the emergency room, long waiting lines, poor inventory control, and equipment inaccessibility are all inefficiencies that directly affect the patient outcomes and satisfaction. The AI technologies can assist in overcoming these operational inefficiencies by offering real-time insights, demand forecasting, workflow automation, and intelligent resources tracking. Predictive models are able to predict the peak times in outpatient departments, which can be used by the hospital to plan on how to change the staff and resources. Laboratory processes, pharmacy and supply chain processes can be optimized using automation tools that minimize delays and wastage. The IoT-based AI systems are capable of monitoring the locations and usage trends of equipment and provide the necessary assets in time. In addition, AI-based operational dashboards give administrators informative insights into the performance of the system to make informed decisions in a short period of time. With the implementation of smart automation into the work processes, hospitals can enhance the throughput, minimize the costs of operations, and increase patient experience considerably.

1.6 Scope, Structure, and Contributions of this Chapter

This chapter presents an in-depth discussion of the AI uses in hospital administration, staff scheduling, and operational efficiency. It discusses the background of AI, recent developments on intelligent automation, applications, challenges, and opportunities in healthcare operations. Subsections that follow provide a systematic discussion of the most important issues: Section 2 expounds on the underlying AI methodologies and intelligent automation technologies applicable in the hospital settings. The third section discusses administrative workflow AI-powered innovations such as patient flow management, billing automation, appointment systems, and supply chain optimization. Section 4 addresses the models of AI-based workforce scheduling and resource allocation, their focus on the optimization techniques, their practical application, and their measurable impact. Section 5 touches on the application of AI on enhancing overall performance of the operations with allusions to predictive analytics, asset management, facility optimization, and real-time decision support. Section 6 summarizes the most challenging issues, including privacy, bias, data integration, interoperability, and ethical issues, and gives the future research directions, including human-AI collaboration and working digital twins. Finally, the 7th section is the conclusion and summation of the transformational potential of AI in changing the operations of hospitals.

2. FUNDAMENTALS OF AI AND INTELLIGENT AUTOMATION IN HEALTHCARE OPERATIONS

2.1 Overview of AI Technologies Relevant to Hospital Operations

Artificial Intelligence evolution is now a critical component of modern healthcare work and offers advanced calculation algorithms that can process complex information, predict events, automate the working process, and support decision-making(Geetha, S et al., 2026). Machine learning (ML), deep learning (DL), natural language processing (NLP), reinforcement learning (RL), and hybrid intelligent systems are some of the AI technologies that are necessary in automating the administrative processes and ensuring that hospitals work efficiently. Machine learning allows systems to learn trends based on the information and extrapolate them to the new situation; it is necessary to predict patient admissions, staff workload, equipment utilization, and operational bottlenecks. Deep learning is a further extension of the ML which applies multi-layered neural networks to identify more complicated relationships in high-dimensional data like patient records, scheduling logs, operational metrics, and sensor feeds. NLP is a process of analyzing unstructured text that can be presented in various forms such as clinical notes, administrative records, patient queries, and communication channels and allows automatic extraction of information, classification, and response generation. Reinforcement learning is an AI paradigm that is based on trial-and-error learning and optimizes the sequential decisions (e.g., staff scheduling, bed allocation, and patient flow routing) through adaptation to dynamically changing environments. All of these technologies are a component of a more intelligent automation system that will restructure the way things work in hospitals to become more efficient and data-driven(Thottempudi, P., & Kumar, V. 2024).

Figure 1. Fundamentals of AI and Intelligent Automation in Healthcare Operations

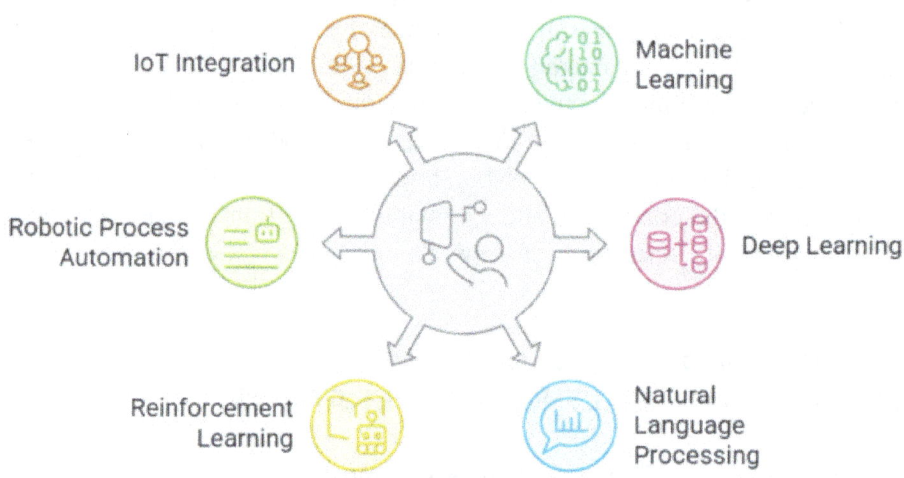

2.2 Machine Learning and Deep Learning Techniques for Predictive Analytics

One of the most effective applications of AI in healthcare operations is predictive analytics, which can be used to help in forecasting and decision-making in regards to patient inflow, resource demand, workflow performance, and operational risks(Badawy, M et al., 2023). The machine learning methods (regression models, decision trees, random forests, gradient boosting, and support vector machines) provide hospitals with opportunities to recognize and model trends in both historical and real-time data. These models enable the administrators to predict the high-activity periods, overflow of the emergency department, seasonal illnesses, or delays in operations, which prepares them better and enhances resource allocation(Asha, R et al., 2026). Deep learning methods, especially recurrent neural networks (RNNs), long short-term memory networks (LSTMs), transformers offer improved time-series forecasting functionality, in terms of long-range dependency and nonlinear patterns(Kumar, V., & Garg, M. L. 2017). As an illustration, big amounts of operational data, including patient arrival times, laboratory turnaround times or average bed occupancy ratios, can be analyzed using DL models to produce highly precise predictions that can be used to make scheduling decisions and operational planning. Moreover, convolutional neural networks (CNNs) are becoming more commonly applied to images and sensor data of a smart hospital environment to maximize the use of assets and safety surveillance. These predictive analytics solutions help hospitals to transform the problem solving mode into the anticipatory mode of operations management(Chahal, A., & Gulia, P. 2019).

2.3 Natural Language Processing for Administrative Automation

NLP is important in the automation of administrative functions which depend on un-structured or semi-structured textual information. Medical records, discharge summaries, appointment requests, insurance forms, patient feedback, and communication logs are some of the text generated in huge volumes in the hospitals(Subramanian, R. S et al., 2026). The NLP algorithms can be used to extract, categorize, and interpret this information automatically. Some of these applications are AI-based chatbots to help patients book appointments, give symptom advice, and ask questions about the administration; automated transcription to help doctors turn their conversations into computer-readable data; and text-mining to analyze patient complaints or feedback on services to determine which parts of the system are causing problems. NLP can also facilitate semantic search in electronic health records (EHRs), which enable administrators and clinicians to find a particular type of information quickly. More sophisticated systems of NLP rely on transformer-based architectures to make context-dependent reasoning and summarization. With these features, NLP can greatly decrease the amount of administrative work, facilitate communication processes, and increase the overall responsiveness of the work of hospitals.

2.4 Reinforcement Learning for Dynamic Decision-Making and Optimization

One of the most appropriate methods in the context of hospital operation is reinforcement learning because it can be used to model dynamic and uncertain environments where decisions would have to be continuously adjusted depending on the feedback. In contrast to the classical ML models which use historical data only, RL is also able to engage with the environment and learn optimal policies over time. The RL can be applied in a hospital environment to optimize staff scheduling with the help of learning their patient demand pattern and dynamically adjusting the staff schedules to minimize crowding, overtime, and fatigue. Patient flow optimization can also be done using RL algorithms. Equally, RL can assist in resource allocation by means of learning the optimal way to assign bed, equipment or operating rooms real time. Such methods as the Q-learning, deep Q-networks (DQN), policy gradient models, and actor-critic models can assist hospital systems with the complex decision making process where multiple interacting components are involved. The continuous and adaptive learning of RL makes it useful in designing intelligent and self-optimizing systems of running a hospital that can change over time as its operational conditions change.

2.5 Robotic Process Automation and Intelligent Automation

Robotic Process Automation (RPA) is another technological force that is applied to healthcare operations to automate repetitive and rule-based administration. RPA systems replicate human behavior by engaging with digital interfaces, data extraction, form filling, record updating, and a series of actions across dissimilar systems. Combined with AI, which creates Intelligent Automation (IA), RPA will be able to perform more complicated tasks that involve decision-making, classification, prediction, or anomaly detection. The AI-powered RPA can be used in the hospital administration to speed up the billing process, claims, appointment reminders, insurance checks, routing of workflow, and reports on compliance. The intelligent automation tools minimize human error, lower the administrative expenses, and improve system reliability by making sure that the tasks are done on time. As an example, an RPA process with AI can detect differences in patient insurance records, check the information with the assistance of the NLP, and forward the unresolved cases to the administrators. An AI and RPA combination will assist the hospitals to transform the manual and paper-based workflow into the automated and scalable processes of the administrative operations that are highly efficient.

2.6 IoT, Sensors, and Data Streams for Real-Time Operational Intelligence

IoT, sensor networks, and smart devices are a combination that has significantly expanded the sphere of AI implementation in hospitals. The existing hospitals are premised on multiple IoT-driven systems such as real-time location tracking systems (RTLS), wearable health monitors, smart beds, automated medication dispensers, RFID-enabled inventory systems, and environmental temperature and air quality sensors. These devices generate a flow of information, which AI can utilize to provide valuable operational information. To use RTLS data as an example, AI models can be used to track the utilization of equipment, reduce the loss of assets, and optimize maintenance schedules. Sensors assist in intelligent control of facilities which is energy saving, and reduces the operating cost. The IoT data would be used together with predictive analytics to forecast equipment breakdown, stock shortage, or inefficient patterns of patient movement. The IoT in conjunction with AI constitutes an operational intelligence system that will be real-time, which will assist in managing the hospital in a manner that is responsive and adaptable.

2.7 Data Requirements, Interoperability, and Digital Infrastructure

The effectiveness of AI within healthcare processes requires the availability of quality information, as well as digital systems, which are interoperable. Hospitals are forced to merge data of different types such as EHRs, HIS systems, workforce management systems, lab information system, IoT sensors, and administrative databases. This requires regular data formats, robust interoperability designs and robust data governance designs. The success of AI models is determined by the quality of data, the cleansing and integration of data provided to them, and thus the quality of the data, its cleaning, and integration is a requirement. Another area that hospitals should invest in includes computational infrastructure, which can be scaled, cloud computing, and edge computing devices, as well as secure data pipelines, to support the use of AI. Additionally, in handling patient and operational data which is sensitive, it is worth ensuring data privacy and compliance with regulations. The digital infrastructure does not only exist to support AI performances but also offers long-run sustainability and scalability of intelligent automation systems.

3. AI FOR HOSPITAL ADMINISTRATION AND WORKFLOW MANAGEMENT

3.1 Transforming Administrative Workflows Through AI

The hospital administration is vast; it involves patient registration and admission, billing, insurance, documentation, and communication, the majority of which are tedious, time-consuming, and prone to human mistakes. These administrative processes have already begun to be automated and provided with intelligent decision support and predictive intelligence through artificial intelligence technologies. Traditional administrative systems tend to be manual data entry, silo based information systems and rigid work process which leads to inefficiencies, bottlenecks and poor service delivery. The AI has the potential to address these inadequacies by integrating the data across departments, automating the routine procedures, and creating actionable insights that will facilitate coordination and responsiveness. The AI-based systems will be capable of analyzing the past trends in the administration, detecting the anomalies, optimizing the workflow processes, and delivering an effective distribution of the work among the administration staff. The features are not only useful in making the work of the hospital easier, but also in lessening the administrative burden, lessening delays, and the overall patient experience. As the healthcare organizations continue to embrace the use of digital tools, AI-based administrative systems are emerging as a critical source of scalability and efficiency of managing hospitals.

3.2 AI-Powered Patient Flow and Bed Management

One of the most difficult and significant hospital administration is patient flow and bed allocation. Poor flow of patients leads to congestion in the emergency departments, queues, inefficiency in delivery of procedures and poor use of hospital resources. Artificial intelligence can be a solution to these issues, as it can anticipate the arrival of patients, the number of beds, and admission, treatment, and discharge flow. Machine learning systems are able to process historical data, seasonality, and real-time data to forecast patient traffic at different touchpoints and allow hospitals to preemptively prepare personnel and resources(Indu, V. T et al., 2026). Predictive models assist administrators to determine the busy times and the expected rate of discharge as well as predict the level of bed occupancy a number of days or even weeks beforehand. Moreover, the AI-based algorithms can dynamically allocate patients to the available beds depending on their acuity level, specialty needs, infection control protocols, and the availability of resources. There are other sophisticated systems that use reinforcement learning to continuously refine the bed allocation strategies depending on the real-time conditions. By automating decisions to do with patient flow, AI greatly decreases congestion, increases bed turnover, improves coordination between departments, and assists in timely provision of care.

3.3 Intelligent Appointment and Scheduling Systems

One of the most visible and patient facing administrative operations of a hospital is appointment scheduling. Conventional schedules are usually characterized by inefficiencies like appointment conflicts, queues, low attendance and underutilization of clinical time. AI-based scheduling systems improve this process with the help of predictive analytics, optimization algorithms, and adaptive adjustments in real-time. Trends in patient behavior (no-shows or cancellations) can be reviewed by machine learning models based on historical appointment information and change the schedule(Prabhu, D et al., 2025). Intelligence systems are capable of proposing the best appointment time according to the preferences of the patient, the availability of the clinician, and future demand. They are able to automate the rescheduling, remind patients of the appointments being smart, and respond to the unforeseen circumstances like the unavailability of the staff or emergency visits. Reinforcement learning is also utilized in advanced systems in order to constantly optimize scheduling schemes and minimize idle time. AI makes appointments more precise, wait time shorter, disruptions minimal, and clinical resources better utilized by developing more efficient scheduling workflows. In the case of patients, AI-assisted scheduling becomes more convenient, transparent, and overall more satisfactory to the healthcare experience.

3.4 Enhancing Billing, Claims Management, and Financial Operations

Some of the most time consuming administrative activities in hospitals are billing and claims management which in most instances entail a lot of paperwork, elaborate regulations and mistakes. AI makes important contributions in these financial processes, as it robotizes the creation of claims, information verification, inconsistency detection, and simplifies submissions. NLP can be used to retrieve pertinent data in medical records, coding systems, and discharge notes that will be used to guarantee proper billing. Machine learning applications are able to find the patterns in claims data to find possible fraud, billing mistakes, or missing documentation when submitting claims(Maithili, K et al., 2024). Robotic Process Automation (RPA) also adds value to efficiency through the repetitive work, including filling the form, transferring the data, reconciling, and tracking the status. These technologies minimize the number of claims rejected, accelerate claims, and enhance revenue cycle management. There are also predictive financial analytics, which are possible with the help of AI and allow hospital administrators to predict the trends of revenue, track cash flow, and detect financial risks. Consequently, financial automation with the help of AI will improve accuracy, compliance, and operational efficiency and decrease the administrative load and financial losses.

3.5 Improving Supply Chain, Inventory, and Asset Management

The supply chain and inventory management are essential in the provision of continuous care. Hospitals have to deal with thousands of vital products - medications and consumables, medical devices and equipment and often in numerous departments. The manual tracking system and the ordering system can easily be affected by stockouts and overstocking as well as wastage and mismanagement. The AI systems can improve the supply chain process by predicting the demand, optimizing inventory, and automating purchasing decisions. Predictive analytics is able to make projections on the usage pattern that is dependent on the patient load, seasonal illness patterns, and past consumption patterns. The machine learning models assist the hospitals in ensuring that they have the right amount of stock which minimizes shortages and wastage. Besides, AI-powered IoT devices and RFID sensors ensure real-time access to the location of inventory, the condition of assets and equipment. Intelligent procurement systems have automated alerts to inform staff when stocks are low or expired, and can re-order supplies when the demand is predicted to be high. AI is also used to detect inefficiencies, supplier delays and any possible disruptions in supply chains. The combination of these capabilities helps to save money, minimise delays in operations and to make sure that the required resources are ready at the moment of need.

3.6 AI-Driven Communication, Documentation, and Information Management

Communication and proper documentation are the core of the work in the hospital. AI can improve these processes by making information exchange between the departments easier and by guaranteeing the uniformity of the documentation practices. Chatbots and virtual assistants with NLP capabilities can process the questions of a patient, a request to book an appointment, or any administrative task, which will alleviate the workload on human employees. Spoken clinical documentation is transcribed into structured text by automated transcription tools and reduces manual input and maintains accuracy. AI-based email triage systems classify messages, rank messages, and automatically route workflows. Also, smart document management software can be used to provide important information on the forms, lab reports, or administration documents and allows to process them much faster and minimize clerical errors. Semantic search tools enable the administrator to find the required documents, clinical guidelines, or patient records in a short period. These communication tools based on AI improve coordination, minimize delays, and further improve the trustworthiness of information exchange in hospitals.

3.7 Case Studies and Real-World Implementations of Administrative AI

The practical use of AI in the management of hospitals shows its practical effect on workflow efficiency, cost reduction, and service quality. A number of hospitals have rolled out AI-based patient flow management systems that minimize overcrowding in the emergency department and enhance the bed turnover. Scheduling solutions based on AI have been demonstrated to reduce the rate of no-show, forecasting patient behavior and sending smart notifications. Healthcare systems with large size have already implemented AI-based billing and coding applications to streamline the claims submissions, leading to quicker reimbursements and reduced errors. The hospitals that use AI-powered inventory systems document a steep decrease in wastage and better availability of resources. In addition, chatbots that are based on AI and are applied to administrative questions can process thousands of interactions every day, decreasing the human workload and enhancing the experience of patients. These real-life cases indicate the relevance of AI in administrative areas and indicate the possibilities of its extensive implementation.

4. AI-DRIVEN STAFF SCHEDULING, WORKFORCE OPTIMIZATION, AND RESOURCE ALLOCATION

4.1 Overview of Workforce Challenges in Modern Hospitals

Workforce management is one of the most complicated and serious operational tasks in hospitals. In most cases, when the uncertainty is high, healthcare institutions have to make sure that they have sufficient staffing levels in various departments such as emergency units, intensive care, surgical theatres, outpatient clinics, and administrative offices. The unpredictable patient flow, understaffing, and skills sets, staff burnout, regulatory requirements, and unexpected emergencies still cause much strain to the scheduling systems. Traditional scheduling incorporates strict templates, manual adjustments, and human-made decisions, an aspect that tend to contribute to poor allocation of resources, overtime, staffing imbalance and burnout. These are compounded by the chronic workforce shortages that are being faced by the healthcare sector in the world, especially in the area of nurses and specialized clinicians. In this regard, AI-powered scheduling and workforce optimization systems have turned out to be powerful means of enhancing efficiency, employee welfare, and quality patient care. The AI systems may be utilized to automatize the complex scheduling processes, predict the staffing needs, and optimize resource utilization with the assistance of predictive analytics, machine learning, and optimization algorithms, and help hospitals to deliver stable and efficient services.

4.2 Predictive Analytics for Forecasting Patient Demand and Workload

The most important point of effective and prompt staffing schedules is the forecast of the patient demand. Predictive analytics models are AI-based in order to predict patient volumes and workload requirements on the basis of previous admission records, seasonal trends, demographic trends, epidemiological variables, and real-time patient flow records. Machine learning algorithms that can be applied to estimate the number of patients to arrive in specific departments or at a specific time are regression models, gradient boosting machines, random forests, and time-series forecasting models. LSTMs and transformer architecture Deep Learning models enhance the accuracy of predictions by learning intricate patterns in data that is multidimensional. These forecasts will help administrators to be prepared in the peak periods, decongest the under staffing in the peak periods and eradicate the over staffing in the slow periods. The predictive models may be particularly useful in the dynamic environment, like an emergency department, intensive care unit, and maternity ward, where the sudden surge in the number of patients can upset the flow. By adding demand forecasts to a scheduling system, hospitals will be in a position to optimize the staff placement, minimize operational bottlenecks and guarantee quality of care reliability.

4.3 Optimization Algorithms for Intelligent Staff Scheduling

One of the factors in the redesign of the staff scheduling is the optimization algorithms based on AI. They are the traditional methods of scheduling that struggle to accommodate such aspects as staff preference, limit of work hours, labor laws, skill-based coverage, and continuity of care principle. Artificial intelligence-based optimization techniques, such as mixed-integer programming, constraint programming, genetic algorithms, simulated annealing, ant colony optimization, and reinforcement learning can be used to design schedules that are optimal in a variety of constraints simultaneously. Such algorithms are going to generate the best or the most optimal staffing schedules that maximize productivity, and ensure that the regulatory compliance and staff availability is in line with the workload forecasts. E.g. genetic algorithms can be applied to create scheduling solutions in repetitive cycles to reduce conflict of shifts and cover more. The constraint programming is carried out in such a manner that ensures schedules based on the nursing ratios and required skills set and equity measures. Reinforcement learning strategies keep enhancing the scheduling techniques through learning processes based on real time responses and performance results. With these sophisticated optimization methods, AI will turn scheduling into a time-consuming, error-prone manual process into a quick, automated, and data-driven one.

4.4 AI for Skill-Based Matching and Shift Allocation

Hospitals require various types of skills, such as specialized physicians, registered nurses, technicians, administrative workers and support workers. The correct balance of skills in every shift is critical to ensuring quality care and efficiency at work. The AI systems will be able to compare the abilities, certification, experience, and competency data of the staff to consider the most suitable shifts. Machine learning models can be used to determine which skill sets are needed in particular units or cases of patients. An example is a case of intensive care unit where a combination of nurses who have ventilator management skills, physicians who are skilled at critical care, and respiratory therapists is needed. The matching algorithms are based on AI, which guarantees that the combination of skill sets is optimal in terms of staffing each shift to minimize gaps in care and enhance the overall efficiency of the workflow. Such systems also take into account the preferences of the staff, the patterns of fatigue, and the past performance records to suggest the assignments that both assist in efficiency and well-being. AI makes the distribution of skills more effective, boosts team efficiency, and minimizes the chances of clinical errors.

4.5 Managing Staff Fatigue, Burnout, and Workforce Well-Being

The stress, fatigue, and burnout among healthcare personnel, particularly front-line employees, are high because of the lengthy working hours, heavy workload, and emotional work pressure. These problems may be worsened by poor scheduling practices which will result in reduced performance, high rates of absenteeism and turnover. The AI-based workforce optimization solutions will integrate the well-being metrics of scheduling to facilitate healthier working conditions. The predictive models have the potential to determine the trends of fatigue based on the duration of shifts, the intensity of workload, the frequency of breaks, and the impact of circadian rhythms. AI systems have the capacity to prescribe rotations of shifts in a manner that reduces the number of sequential night shifts, excessive overtime, and sufficient rest. Moreover, schedules can be adjusted with time by the reinforcement learning algorithms relying on staff feedback, performance indicators, and wellness information. Other sophisticated systems have the sentiment analysis of employee surveys or feedback to comprehend mental workload and stress patterns. Focusing on the well-being of its staff, AI increases the efficiency of operations, as well as job satisfaction, staff retention, and long-term workforce sustainability.

4.6 Real-Time Workforce Management and Dynamic Scheduling

Conventional scheduling systems are not flexible and tend to be very rigid to any unexpected occurrences during operations like sudden increase in inpatient numbers, absence of personnel or emergencies. AI can be used to support dynamic scheduling systems that can rearrange the deployment of staff on-the-fly depending on the prevailing circumstances. Combining the data of EHR systems, patient flow dashboards, IoT sensors, and workforce management systems, AI systems will be able to identify demand fluctuations and automatically suggest the redistribution of staff. As an illustration, when an emergency department gets overwhelmed, AI can propose the shift of the employees working in other units with fewer people or request the on-demand workers. The algorithms of reinforcement learning are especially useful when it comes to dynamic scheduling as they are constantly learning with new data and improving decision-making policies. Mobile applications or digital dashboards can be utilized by hospitals to provide real-time scheduling information to employees to make sure that there is a seamless coordination. Dynamic scheduling minimizes administrative burden, enhances responsiveness to operational disturbances, and helps to make hospitals staffed adequately during the day.

4.7 Resource Allocation Beyond Human Workforce

Although the management of staff is an urgent concern, AI also helps in the allocation of more extensive resources, such as operating rooms, diagnostic equipment, ICU beds and other critical resources. Predictive analytics will be able to estimate the demand of these resources, and it will allow hospitals to allocate them efficiently and prevent the existence of bottlenecks. Optimization algorithms are capable of producing operating room schedules that reduce idle time, minimize surgical delays and match the availability of staff with the availability of surgical teams. Artificial intelligence is able to suggest the allocation of resources among departments depending on patient acuity, estimated admissions, and capacity limitations. Artificial intelligence can be used in intensive care units to aid in triage procedures and bedside placement plans to provide critical patients with timely treatment. The capabilities form an integrated model of human and non-human resource distribution to facilitate the overall hospital performance.

4.8 Real-World Implementations and Impact of AI-Driven Workforce Optimization

Other hospitals and healthcare systems have already implemented AI-based workforce optimization systems and have seen a significant increase in efficiency and workload management. For instance, AI-based nurse scheduling systems have minimized the overtime by estimating the peak patient load and altering shifts. The use of AI-based demand forecasting systems in emergency departments has been associated with decreased waiting time, optimized staff, and patient throughput. Dynamic scheduling systems helped hospitals to alleviate staffing shortages and resiliency during operational wave surges which are hard to forecast. Many healthcare facilities also claim to have seen the satisfaction of the staff increase due to the more balanced and equitable scheduling. Combined, these practical applications depict the groundbreaking potential of AI-based workforce optimization to enhance the efficiency of the operations, reduce burnout, and lead to better patient care outcomes.

5. AI FOR OPERATIONAL EFFICIENCY AND PERFORMANCE OPTIMIZATION

5.1 Importance of Operational Efficiency in Modern Hospitals

Operational efficiency, timely services and cost-efficiency are the main pillars of quality healthcare services provision. Hospitals are complicated systems, and they are made up of units which are interconnected and dependent on one another such as emergency departments, surgical suites, outpatient clinics, laboratories, pharmacies, and administrative offices. The inefficiency in one of the units might cause a ripple effect to the rest of the system resulting in overcrowded waiting rooms, increased procedures, bottlenecks in the diagnostic processes, underutilized resources, and increase in the operational costs. Traditional methods of operations management tend to rely on historical methods, manual coordination, and responsive strategies that are no longer adequate due to the growth in the number of patients, the complexity of care streams, and regulation. The AI has become a game-changer in the provision of operational excellence in hospitals, such as the ability to analyze and detect in large and diverse volumes of data, detect hidden patterns, emulate outcomes, and improve resource distribution. AI helps hospitals transform their reactive and manual procedures into more proactive and data-driven and self-optimizing processes that improve performance and patient experience.

5.2 Predictive Analytics for Workflow Optimization and Capacity Planning

One of the underlying AI capabilities in increasing operational efficiency is predictive analytics. Machine learning should be able to examine historical data, real-time patient flow metrics, seasonal trends, and contextual variables and predict operational trends, including patient arrivals, wait times, diagnostic turnaround times, laboratory workload, and surgical times. As an illustration, time-series models will be able to forecast the maximum outpatient hours, enabling hospitals to assign personnel and resources accordingly. Predictive analytics is becoming increasingly popular in emergency departments to predict a surge and make appropriate changes to the triage or staffing plans. Predictive analytics is also beneficial to capacity planning as it predicts the bed occupancy, ICU demand, and day-to-day admission/discharge trends. These insights will help hospitals to better manage patient flow, decrease congestion, and decrease length of stay. High-end analytics systems enable administrators to model the impact of operational choices, including changing shift schedules or adding new processes to workflows, and then execute them in practice. Predictive intelligence helps hospitals in the provision of resources in the right time and place without delay and enhances the overall fluidity in operations.

5.3 Reducing Waiting Times and Enhancing Patient Throughput

Reduction of waiting time is one operational improvement area of high priority due to the fact that long waiting periods cause low patient satisfaction, anxiety, and stress among the clinical staff. The AI-controlled systems can optimize the flow of patients by detecting the inefficiencies in the care routes and suggesting the interventions to simplify the flow of patients. As an example, AI algorithms can trace the patient journey through registration and triage to diagnosis, treatment, and discharge and identify the bottlenecks in the process, including a slow diagnostic process, poor triage times, or slow specialist appointments. The delay-related information can be obtained with the help of NLP tools through the clinical notes and administrative logs, and the optimization algorithms can suggest workflow changes that can be made to minimize these delays. AI-based queue management systems predict the real-time waiting times and dynamically direct patients to the service units that are less crowded. In radiology and lab departments, AI will be able to prioritize cases in order of urgency, reducing waiting time with patients that are very urgent.

The outcome is a better workflow that is more predictable and easier to manage, enhancing patient and provider experience.

5.4 Optimizing Operating Room Scheduling and Surgical Workflows

One of the most costly and income-generating departments in hospitals, operating rooms (ORs) are also vulnerable to inefficiencies in the form of late start, last-minute cancellations, excessive turnover and uneven use. The use of AI is very beneficial to OR management, especially in predictive modeling, simulation, and intelligent scheduling. Machine learning models have a better ability to predict durations of surgery than conventional estimates, considering patterns of surgeons, patient factors, and complexity levels. Surgical scheduling algorithms have the ability to produce optimal schedule of OR utilization, decrease idle time and pre-operative and post-operative bottlenecks. Reinforcement learning systems are able to adjust the scheduling decision depending on real-time events, e.g. delays or emergency cases. Moreover, AI-based monitoring can be used to monitor the metrics of the OR workflow, including turnover, equipment availability, and staffing, and give recommendations on how to improve them. AI-based OR management improves the level of preparedness, boosts operational efficiency, and patient outcomes by decreasing the number of delays related to surgical operations.

5.5 Intelligent Asset Tracking, Equipment Management, and IoT Integration

The number of equipment and medical devices used in a hospital is enormous, consisting of infusion pumps, wheelchairs, diagnostic equipment, and surgical equipment. Poor monitoring and management of these assets usually results in lost or duplicate purchases, downtime of equipment or patient waiting. The IoT systems with AI functionality can dramatically change the state of asset management as they can give real-time information on the location, condition, and functionality of medical equipment. Sensors or RFID tags built into devices transmit a continuous stream of data to AI algorithms that determine patterns of use, detect anomalies, and anticipate maintenance requirements. The predictive maintenance models are able to predict the failure of equipment even before it happens and this reduces the time associated with the downtime of the equipment. The AI can also be used to optimize the distribution of equipment across the departments according to the forecasted demand to minimize unnecessary transfers and guarantee their availability in time. AI-supported real-time location tracking (RTLS) systems reduce the time of equipment search and loss or theft. Consequently, the intelligent asset management process can lead to a considerable increase in the operational reliability, cost reduction, and responsiveness in the patient care settings.

5.6 AI for Energy, Facility, and Environmental Management

In addition to clinical and administrative processes, AI is also involved in the facility management process, which is the key in the efficiency of the hospital. Hospitals use masses of energy because of massive HVACs, use of medical equipment, lighting and operations of the facilities. AI-supported building management systems process the environmental data, occupancy, temperature variations, and energy consumption trends to maximize the functioning of the facility. Machine learning models can regulate HVAC loads, the intensity of lighting, and energy distribution depending on the real-time data of occupancy, which is gathered by the use of IoT sensors. Energy consumption or equipment malfunction can be identified with predictive analytics, and timely action can be taken. Also, AI helps in controlling infections by monitoring air quality, humidity, and movement in hospital areas to minimize chances of contamination. The smart facility management systems guarantee safe, sustainable, and efficient environment which promotes the operational objectives and minimizes energy expenses.

5.7 Real-Time Operational Dashboards and Decision Support Systems

AI-based dashboard has become a critical asset to hospital administrators that provides real-time data about key performance indicators (KPIs), including patient throughput, staff availability, resource utilization, equipment, appointment adherence rates, and wait times. The dashboards unite the results of many systems EHRs, IoT devices, workforce management applications, scheduling applications, and financial systems and use AI analytics to generate actionable intelligence. The machine learning models indicate deviations to the expected performance, risk factors, and provide recommendations to be taken through quick intervention. As an example, once an emergency department starts displaying the signs of overcrowding, the system can suggest the transfer of employees to other departments or change the triage rules. Scenario planning is also supported using real-time dashboards to simulate the effects of potential interventions and allow the administrators to make informed decisions within a short amount of time. These systems make the operational management more of a proactive, adaptive, and data-driven process as opposed to a reactive process.

5.8 Case Studies and Evidence of Improved Operational Efficiency

A number of hospitals across the world have recorded quantifiable enhancements in the performance of operations following the adoption of AI-based systems. The use of AI surge prediction systems in emergency departments has minimized the wait of patients in the ED through improved staff and resource preparations. When used in OR scheduling, AI-based systems in hospitals are associated with increased OR utilization rates, decreased cancelled surgeries, and decreased turnover times. Asset tracking systems that have been integrated with the IoT have been able to reduce equipment search time by more than 50 per cent and eliminate expensive losses. Medical device predictive maintenance software has reduced downtime and enhanced safety. AI-powered energy management systems have resulted in high energy savings and operating expenses. Also, the patient satisfaction scores in the case of the implemented AI-based queue management systems and real-time navigation tools increased, proving the diverse influence of AI on the efficiency of operations.

6. CHALLENGES, ETHICAL CONSIDERATIONS, AND FUTURE RESEARCH DIRECTIONS

6.1 Data Privacy, Security, and Ethical Concerns

There are significant opportunities associated with the AI use in the hospital administration, staffing, and operational efficiency, yet there are also critical concerns regarding data privacy, security, and ethics. Patient records, administrative data, employee work schedules, financial information, and logs of the operations are very sensitive data that hospitals deal with. This mixture of these unlike types of data into AI-based systems increases the risks of data breach, unauthorized access, and misuse of confidential data. In order to prevent the violation of patient confidentiality and trust in the institution, one will have to make sure that the rules on the protection of data and national health data policies, are adhered to strictly. The AI systems operate on large amounts of operational data as well, which may include personal identifiers, staff performance analytics, or patterns of patient movement, which introduces the problem of surveillance, informed consent, and misuse of insights. Algorithms Ethical issues can be applied even to the field of algorithmic decision-making, where unintelligible algorithms or biased algorithms can negatively affect some groups proportionately more or lead to unequal distribution of resources. To deal with these threats, hospitals must apply strong governance mechanisms, apply encryption policies, and introduce transparency to the development of AI models.

The ethical auditing, the regular control, and the involvement of stakeholders would be necessary to realize the principles of responsible AI ecosystems with the rights of patients and fairness at the center of its focus.

6.2 Algorithmic Bias, Fairness, and Transparency

Algorithms bias is among the most pressing issues of working AI systems that can be provoked by the history or erroneous assumptions or even the unbalanced dataset. Existing disparities can also be further reinforced by the use of AI models trained on biased or partial data, including providing some groups of staff with disadvantaged schedules or distributing resources inefficiently to departments where the training data is not representative. Bias algorithms can be used in hospital administration to distort the behavior of patients, misunderstand performance metrics of the staff, or falsely predict, which can adversely impact the quality of services. To guarantee that AI decision-making is fair, it is necessary to be very strict in detecting bias, use various training datasets, and provide mechanisms to constantly evaluate the models. It is also important to be transparent since stakeholders, such as hospital administrators, clinicians, and staff, need to know how AI systems come up with recommendations or decisions. Explainable artificial intelligence (XAI) methods can assist in interpreting the outputs of models, offering information about the importance of features, and making sure that the process of decision-making is responsible. Hospitals should also put a strong emphasis on fairness and transparency, which relates to integrating ethical principles into the model design and developing a culture of doubt and verification concerning AI tools.

6.3 Integration Challenges with Legacy Systems

Most hospitals are using old infrastructure, such as old electronic health record software, independent scheduling solutions, and disjointed administrative applications, which make integration of AI difficult. Such systems are not readily interoperable, and it is hard to unify streams of data, coordinate workflows, or apply AI-based automation. Data silos are a barrier to the effectiveness of AI by making whole and consistent datasets inaccessible. Moreover, hospitals might not be in a position to upgrade the current systems due to budgetary limitations, workforce, or business interruptions that come with massive technological changes. The introduction of AI to these complex environments is necessitated by strong data integration designs, uniform communication protocols, and application programming interfaces (APIs) designed. The management of change is crucial, because the employees should be trained to be able to use new AI tools. Hospitals will have to implement in phases and focus on high impact use cases and to integrate collaborate with the technology providers. These issues of integration must be addressed to achieve the transformational potential of AI in the operations of the hospital in full.

6.4 Workforce Resistance, Trust, and Human-AI Collaboration

Automation by AI can bring up fears about staff being replaced in the hospital or having more surveillance or lack of autonomy in decision making. Such fears may cause resistance, the unwillingness to use AI tools, or the distrust of algorithmic advice. To successfully integrate AI, it is necessary to create a culture in which personnel do not consider AI as a threat to their jobs. The human-AI collaboration should be highlighted with a particular focus on AI efficiency, administrative load, and allowing staff to perform their work on higher value activities including care-giving, critical decision-making, and interaction with patients. Hospitals should invest in communication strategies that will inform the staff on the possibilities of AI, its limits and the desired advantages. Employees should be provided with digital literacy skills and a sense of security when working with AI-driven systems through training programs. The promotion of collaborative feedback, i.e., human knowledge to enlighten AI models, and vice versa, may help build trust and establish an equal relationship between humans and intelligent systems. Finally, the implementation of AI will be successful in case an environment in which human experience and technological innovation can coexist is created.

6.5 Ensuring Reliability, Robustness, and Safety of AI Systems

The AI systems implemented in the context of hospital operations should be very reliable, strong, and safe because the breakdown of the operation may cause a significant violation or other negative outcomes. As an illustration, failures in predictive demand forecasting can lead to shortage of staff, whereas inaccurate scheduling algorithms can overwork a specific department or undermine the health of staff. To achieve accuracy and reliability in changing hospital settings, AI systems need to be carefully tested, validated and monitored at all times. It has to be resistant to noise, data inconsistencies, and unexpected occurrences. The hospitals should implement the use of fail-safe, which enables human control and overriding in case the AI suggestions are doubtful or unsafe. In addition, AI systems should be flexible to changing operational trends, regulatory reforms, and emerging clinical processes. The version control, regular retraining, and real-time monitoring tools can be used to ensure the relevance and performance of the system. The confidence and the trust that can be promoted and the large-scale implementation of AI into healthcare processes requires the assurance of reliability and safety.

6.6 Regulatory, Governance, and Standardization Gaps

The pace of AI in the medical field has surpassed regulatory standards and regulations, raising ambiguity in the field of implementation, compliance, and responsibility. Most countries are in the process of coming up with AI regulations based on ethical practices, risk classification, data handling, and model validation. Hospitals are struggling to deal with these changing regulatory environments, especially in relation to third-party vendors of AI or cloud services. Governance models need to define the ownership of data, quality assurance, auditability and liability in the event of failure of AI systems. The standardization is necessary to ensure interoperability and to establish benchmarking systems in order to compare AI effectiveness in various institutions. Without standardized measures, it is difficult to compare AI solutions, analyze the performance of the solutions, or even guarantee that the decisions are uniform. Technology developers, policy-makers and healthcare institutions must work together to come up with comprehensive AI governance frameworks that will enable safe and ethical innovation.

6.7 Future Research Directions in AI for Healthcare Operations

The AI in the hospital management and operational management is a rapidly developing field, and several perspectives remain that can be researched. One of the directions is development of human-AI co-operations where human judgement is integrated with automated decision-making to optimize the scheduling, triage, and workflow design. Another new field is the use of digital twins, a virtual model of a hospital setting simulating conditions of operation, testing interventions, and forecasting outcomes. These models will enable the administrators to experiment with the policy changes, staffing or the implementation of new technologies without endangering the reality. The explainable AI-based operational decision support is a pressing research issue, as the transparency and interpretable models are the major factors in establishing trust. Furthermore, federated learning offers a new path in AI training in multiple hospitals without breaking privacy of data and enabling large-scale operation intelligence. Multimodal AI systems based on a combination of visual data, sensor data, administrative records and clinical documentation to form a complete image can also be researched in the future. As smarter, networked ecosystems become the new standard in hospitals, research on AI ethical governance, adaptive automation and contextualized decision-making will become the central focus in defining the future of AI-powered healthcare processes.

7. CONCLUSION

The hospital management system, workforce and efficiency, and operational efficiency are rapidly becoming transformed by Artificial Intelligence, with intelligent automation being introduced to the healthcare environment and data-driven decision support. The implementation of AI is a powerful means of establishing a resolution to the constantly growing complexity, labor deficit, and escalating patient demands in hospitals, with more and more hospitals experiencing difficulties in changing their mode of operation to become more precise, receptive, and sustainable in their day-to-day operations. Being directly related to the workflow efficiency, AI enhances efficiency on all levels of hospital management, such as appointment systems, bed allocation, workforce coordination, and overall use of resources. The chapter mentions the fact that AIs-based solutions do not just make administrative tasks easier but also facilitate the number of bottlenecks, patient flow, and financial and operational planning. As well, the use of IoT tools, real-time dashboards, and AI-powered monitoring solutions enable hospitals to operate in a more visible and flexible state, which would guarantee that they react to the alterations in demand and unexpected malfunctions of the operations in time. This results in improved patient experience in the form of less waiting time, improved care paths, and enhanced reliability of services. However, AI is associated with such concerns as information privacy, algorithmic justice, systemic incorporation, acceptance by the employees, and adherence to the regulations. The best way to address these issues is to ensure that the governance structures are well established, that the algorithms are well designed, that there is continuous supervision and working human-AI models, which are centered around trust and accountability. The operational intelligence of the future lies in future research directions like digital twins, federated learning, and explainable AI that will assist in shifting to more resilient and adaptive healthcare ecosystems. In conclusion, AI is an innovative technology of the modern healthcare process. It assists in making hospitals achieve new standards of efficiency, coordination and quality, as in a responsible and strategic way. Careful automation can help healthcare organizations to create smarter and patient-focused systems, which can meet the future needs that are evolving.

REFERENCES

Asha, R., Sangeetha, J., Adaikkammai, A., Thilagam, T., & Aparna, P. (2026). Machine Learning and Computational Intelligence for Smart Healthcare: Advancing Diagnosis and Treatment. In *Applied AI and Computational Intelligence in Diagnostics and Decision-Making* (pp. 87-110). IGI Global Scientific Publishing.

Badawy, M., Ramadan, N., & Hefny, H. A. (2023). Healthcare predictive analytics using machine learning and deep learning techniques: A survey. *Journal of Electrical Systems and Information Technology*, *10*(1), 40. DOI: 10.1186/s43067-023-00108-y

Bhimavarapu, U. (2026). AI in Healthcare: Automating Hospital Operations for Better Patient Care. In *Evaluation and Assessment of AI-Driven Systems in Hospitals* (pp. 279-306). IGI Global Scientific Publishing.

Chahal, A., & Gulia, P. (2019). Machine learning and deep learning. *International Journal of Innovative Technology and Exploring Engineering*, *8*(12), 4910–4914. DOI: 10.35940/ijitee.L3550.1081219

Geetha, S., Srinidhii, P., & Madhusudanan, J. (2026). Assessment of AI's Impact on Precision Medicine and Personalized Healthcare in Clinical Environments. In *Evaluation and Assessment of AI-Driven Systems in Hospitals* (pp. 139–168). IGI Global Scientific Publishing.

Indu, V. T., Elumalai, M., & Gracious, L. A. (2026). Optimization Algorithms for Machine Learning Model Enhancement in Healthcare. In *AI Model Design and Data Management for Disease Prediction* (pp. 159–192). IGI Global Scientific Publishing.

Kumar, V., & Garg, M. L. (2017, November). Deep learning in predictive analytics: A survey. In *2017 International Conference on Emerging Trends in Computing and Communication Technologies (ICETCCT)* (pp. 1-6). IEEE. DOI: 10.1109/ICETCCT.2017.8280331

Maithili, K., Ponmalar, A., Yamini, B., Karthikeyan, M., Anish, T. P., Maheswari, B., & Subramanian, R. S. (2024). Advances in AI and Machine Learning for Healthcare Informatics. In *Machine Learning and Generative AI in Smart Healthcare* (pp. 1–22). IGI Global. DOI: 10.4018/979-8-3693-3719-6.ch001

Mohideen, S. K., Tamilselvan, L., & Khan, M. W. (2026). AI Integration and Clinical Workflow Optimization in Hospitals. In *Evaluation and Assessment of AI-Driven Systems in Hospitals* (pp. 205–234). IGI Global Scientific Publishing.

Prabhu, D., Tejasri, M. V. S. L., Saratha, B., & Anish, T. P. (2025, April). Future Horizons: Key Trends Shaping the Evolution of Machine Learning. In *2025 8th International Conference on Trends in Electronics and Informatics (ICOEI)* (pp. 1091-1099). IEEE.

Subramanian, R. S., Swetha, M., Krishnaveni, K., Thilagam, T., Saranya, K., Gracious, L. A., & Sudha, K. (2026). Transforming Education with NLP and Machine Learning: Innovations, Applications, and Future Prospects. In *Educational Applications of Natural Language Processing, Chatbots, and AI* (pp. 269-292). IGI Global Scientific Publishing.

Subramanyam, S. V. (2022). AI-powered process automation: Unlocking cost efficiency and operational excellence in healthcare systems. [IJARET]. *International Journal of Advanced Research in Engineering and Technology*, *13*(1), 86–102. DOI: 10.34218/IJARET_13_01_008

Thottempudi, P., & Kumar, V. (2024). The Role of IoT in Modern Healthcare: Innovations and Challenges in Pandemic Era. In *Technologies for Sustainable Healthcare Development* (pp. 57–80). IGI Global. DOI: 10.4018/979-8-3693-2901-6.ch004

Chapter 10
Generative Artificial Intelligence in Smart Nursing:
Transforming Clinical Decision-Making, Patient Care, and Healthcare Workflows

Arun Agrawal
http://orcid.org/0000-0001-7233-6660
Institute of Technology and Management, Gwalior, India

Sagar Kukkamudi
http://orcid.org/0009-0005-6137-6276
Independent Researcher, USA

Swati Harshad Mirlekar
St. Vincent Pallotti College of Engineering and Technology, India

Sudheer Nandi
http://orcid.org/0009-0008-4294-1964
Vels Institute of Science, Technology, and Advanced Studies, Chennai, India

M. Abinaya
http://orcid.org/0009-0000-1144-5177
Erode Sengunthar Engineering College, India

Koppuravuari Gurnadha Gupta
KLEF University, Vaddeswaram, India

Deepak Gupta
http://orcid.org/0000-0003-3929-1362
Institute of Technology and Management, Gwalior, India

ABSTRACT

Generative AI is revolutionizing nursing by enhancing clinical decision-making, patient care, and workflow efficiency. By integrating predictive analytics, person-

DOI: 10.4018/979-8-3373-8247-0.ch010

alized care planning, and real-time decision support, AI enables nurses to deliver proactive, evidence-based, and patient-centered care. Applications include automated documentation, intelligent staffing, remote monitoring, and culturally sensitive patient communication, improving adherence, satisfaction, and safety. Despite its promise, challenges such as data quality, bias, and ethical considerations necessitate careful implementation and workforce training. The future of smart nursing lies in a collaborative approach where human expertise and AI innovation work synergistically to optimize healthcare delivery.

1. INTRODUCTION

The healthcare sector is experiencing a paradigm shift with the current level of technological advancement and the resultant escalating complexity of patient care. One such development is smart nursing, which brings out the paradigm as a requirement of integrating technology and clinical practice and knowledge to improve patient outcomes, enhance, and develop the process of healthcare delivery. Smart nursing is not just an ordinary nursing practice, as it employs real time information, whichever health digital tools, and evidence based decision support to provide the correct, tailored and proactive care. As nurses are at the frontline of treating patients, they are also best placed to benefit and offer towards this change in technology since they have to use clinical judgment, patient needs, and operational needs to balance them continuously (Wang et al., 2024).

Alongside this trend in the field, there is the emergence of artificial intelligence (AI) in medicine. It is already being demonstrated by AI technologies, especially machine learning and predictive analytics, that they can handle large amounts of patient data and extract patterns and assist in clinical decision-making. Early-warning systems that identify patient deterioration, AI-based diagnostic tools that help focus on the imaging data interpretation are just a few of the technologies that started to improve the efficiency and accuracy of clinical workflows. Nonetheless, conventional AI solutions tend to be restricted to recognition and prediction of patterns with references to the past. Although they are helpful, the methods are usually unable to produce new information, respond to complicated situations in clinical settings on the spot, or offer contextually relevant advice to frontline nurses (Fahim et al., 2025).

This weakness has triggered the adoption of generative AI, which is a subset of AI that can generate new content, combine information available on various sources, and make actionable suggestions instead of interpolating the available data. Since statistics and AI can work together in healthcare, AI may be used as an interface to facilitate dynamic clinical decision-making, individualized care planning, and workflow optimization. As an example, an example based on generative AI can be applied when a patient has a combination of electronic health record, lab findings, and real-time vitals, and is proposed specific care intervention, possible complication prediction, or detailed patient education. With its ability to combine data analysis with innovative problem-solving, the generative AI will enable nurses to have tools that can expand their thinking capacity and clinical intuitions, and eventually enable them through more informed and timely interventions (Sam-Oyerinde et al., 2025).

Generative AI is relevant in nursing to an extent which is difficult to overestimate. The workload, documentation, and complicated process of coordinating care is becoming strainer on nurses as they seek to ensure high patient care standards. Generative AI will be a solution since it will decrease the burden of cognitive and administrative activities, enhance clinical accuracy, and allow nurses to concentrate on direct patient care. Besides, it leads to a more patient-centered practice in the sense that the care plans can be designed to suit the medical history, lifestyle, and preferences of the patient so that healthcare delivery is effective and sensitive. AI use in nursing also facilitates the use of evidence-based decision-making because it synthesizes the recent clinical research, guidelines, and institutional protocols into actionable information on the front line caregiver (Rabbani et al., 2025).

This chapter will be used to talk about the generative AI transformative role in intelligent nursing and how it changes key factors in healthcare delivery. To begin with, the chapter sheds light on, the contribution made by AI-based tools towards the enhancement of clinical decision-making since nurses can assess the risks or predict the complications, to say the least, as well as streamline the treatment plans, on a level of accuracy never attainable before. Subsequently, it speaks about the impacts of generative AI on patient care quality and the support of increased patient satisfaction, adherence, and health outcomes that lowers proactive monitoring, personalized communication, and interventions. Finally, the aspect of workflow efficacy is mentioned in the chapter, which reflects how AI makes documentation easier, day-to-day tasks automated, and the content of resources distributed to reduce nurse turnover and offer time to engage with patients directly.

Within the broader context of intelligent nursing, this chapter clearly demonstrates the possibility of generative AI with offering innovative, effectiveness, and increased clinical performance. It also indicates that the AI integration is not oriented towards eliminating the human judgment, but rather oriented at the expansion of the decision-making power of the nurses in an attempt to provide them with safer, more personalized and quality care. Later, with the healthcare systems remaining more active, the numerous opportunities, concerns, and practical implementations of the generative AI in nursing remain more critical to teachers, clinicians, administrators, and policymakers.

Collectively, the convergence of intelligent nursing and the generative AI is a paradigm change in the provision of healthcare. The chapter is an in-depth discussion of how AI-related inventions can assist nurses to make more effective clinical decisions, lead to better patient outcomes and efficiency of the work. Considering the applications that already are already in effect, the practical usages of this aspect of technology and the potential innovative changes of the latter, it lays the groundwork of the further comprehending of how technology and human abilities may find their way to a feasible pattern of introducing smarter, more mindful, and patient-focused healthcare setting.

2. FOUNDATIONS OF GENERATIVE AI IN HEALTHCARE

The use of AI in healthcare has been growing at a heightened pace in the last ten years, with previously rudimentary predictive analytics giving way to generative sides of artificial intelligence. Generative AI, which is a kind of AI that creates innovative content and simulates events and generates actionable information, is a revolutionary one in the current healthcare (within the context of nursing) in its practice. Contrary to the conventional AI systems which mostly process old data and find trends, generative AI has the potential to create information, develop patient-centered research and assist in making decisions dynamically, thereby becoming a fundamental component of intelligent nursing. To be able to implement generative AI in healthcare in a responsible manner, it is important to understand its origins, its specific features, regulations and ethical guidelines applicable to this technology (Selvaraj, 2024).

2.1. Overview of Generative AI

2.1.1. Key Concepts (LLMs, Diffusion Models, Multimodal AI)

The fundamental principle of generative AI is the Large Language Model (LLM) that is trained on large amounts of text-based data to comprehend human language and provide human-like language. LLMs, including GPT and its descendants, can comprehend complicated commands, summarize clinical records, and produce natural-language prompted outputs that are in situational contexts. In healthcare, one of the ways in which LLMs can be useful is creating patient education resources, synthesizing laboratory data, or writing care plans based on the specifics of each patient (Lin and Kuo, 2025).

- Diffusion models, in their turn, are generative models that have been extensively applied in creating high-fidelity images, simulations, or visual data. These models are capable of creating life-like representations of medical images in a clinical environment in order to train or support diagnostic and communicate with a patient. Indicatively, by depicting wound healing in stages, diseases progress, or providing visual sites through which patients can understand their health status, among others, diffusion models can be used to improve not only nurse education but also patient understanding (Kazerouni et al., 2022).

- Multimodal AI is an expansion of generative AI that comprises various forms of data and text, images, audio, and structured patient records to generate insights in detail. To nurses, this implies a synthesis of the lab reports, vital signs data, imaging information, and patient history to come up with recommendations that are accurate, as well as holistic. Multimodal AI allows dynamic synthesis of various inputs so that agile creation of actionable outputs can be produced in real-time, such as patient-specific care guidance or anticipating risk (AlSaad et al., 2024).

2.1.2. Differences from Traditional AI Tools in Healthcare

Conventional AI in health care has been more of prediction or description, which aims at discovering trends in past data. Such systems are good at predicting admissions, identifying unusual lab findings, or identifying the high-risk patients. Although effective, they are simultaneously reactive since they examine what has happened and give out warnings or predictions using previous trends (Seenu & Rani, 2024).

Generative AI, in its turn, is reactive and creative, able to generate new content, to simulate the possible results and to assist with the intricate decision-making. As an illustration, a classic AI device would tell you that a patient has a risk of pressure, ulcers, but generative AI may design an entire preventive care strategy, design educational materials to be given to the caregiver, and even simulate the results of various interventions. Such synthesizing, simulating, and the capacity to generate new solutions are the distinguishing features of the generative AI as a potentially transformative technology in nursing practice (Pramanik et al., 2025).

2.2. Generative AI vs Traditional AI in Nursing

2.2.1. Examples of Predictive vs Generative Capabilities

The conventional predictive AI has been useful in clinical nursing processes. Indicatively, predictive models have the ability to determine at-risk patients of falls or of developing sepsis by analyzing historical vital signs and demographic information. Although useful, these predictions usually go up to the alert level and it is upon the nurses to figure out what to do next in care planning.

These abilities are extended by generative AI which proposes interventions and provides actionable results. The application of a generative AI system to the identical case would suggest personalized plans of preventing falls, create patient education content on the reasons and precautions of safety, and predict the possible consequences of various actions. Correspondingly, predictive AI has an ability to predict chances of patient worsening, whereas generative AI has the possibility to develop an adaptive care map taking into account the stylistic variations in clinical and patient needs and hospital standards (Baig et al., 2024).

2.2.2. Potential for Creating Simulations, Care Plans, and Patient Education Content

One of the most interesting simulations of education and training is the potential of generative AI application in nursing. Virtual patient cases which are developed by artificial means allow nurses to practice tricky decision-making issues in a safe environment where the circumstances are controlled. In this kind of a simulation, it can include moving responses by patients, a variety of clinical presentations and real-time feedback, which help in better critical thinking and development of clinical competence.

It is also possible to be developed through the assistance of generative AI that develops personal care plans incorporating the history of patients, comorbidities, and live clinical information. It is possible to apply this capability to make sure of customized, evidence-based, and adaptable care, reduce errors and enhance patient outcomes. In addition, patient education materials generated in AI presented as discharge instructions to multimedia tutorials could be useful to understand, adhere, and interact, especially when specific to the language, literacy rate, and culture of a patient (Saba and Hadidi, 2025).

2.3. Ethical, Legal, and Regulatory Considerations

Due to the high penetration of generative AI in the nursing practice sphere, there is a need to address ethical, legal, and regulatory challenges to ensure safe, fair, and responsible use of this technology.

- Privacy and consent This is a fundamentals problem due to which AI systems do not generate significant results in the absence of sensitive patient information. The most significant one is to ensure that patient data is anonymous, secure, and shared under informed consent (Nkrumah et al., 2025).

- The other issue that is cardinal is that of bias. The use of trained generative AI models in the healthcare sector has the potential to add to the existence of irrelevant disparities, so it must be specifically considered that minority groups have a low medical-care history. Nurses and organizations will need to sift through AI outputs, and they will also possess systems that will help prevent biased suggestions (Okonji et al., 2024).
- The problem of accountability is a confusing one. The human care practitioners still have a task to make clinical decisions although AI can offer care recommendations or patient education. Liability is supposed to have clear policies and legal framework to be consistent, clear, and trustworthy between the patient and the provider (Bragazzi & Garbarino, 2024).

Regulatory bodies, such as FDA, and other comparable national agencies are given increased concern over AI-based medical software, in which the usefulness of the validation, safety, and clinical effectiveness standards of value. Compliance with these schemes is the solution to the successful application of the generative AI to nursing practice.

The origins of generative AI in the healthcare sector can be traced to its functional peculiarities, disruptive nature, and the need to promote ethical behavior. People should view the process of predicting clinical insights as an opportunity to dwell upon new predictive methods rather than traditional methods of prediction when it comes to generative AI where the nurses can have a chance to improve decision-making processes through the design, simulation, and customization of clinical insights, achieve better patient engagement, and workflow management. Its application must nonetheless be guided with acceptable ethical, legal and regulatory provisions so that it may be well incorporated safely, fairly, and responsibly in clinical practice. Generative AI is not the human judgment alternative, though it is also a powerful reinforcement that accompanies the nursing knowledge of the dynamic healthcare environment.

3. ENHANCING CLINICAL DECISION-MAKING

The nursing practice entails the combination of patient information, clinical knowledge, and experiences to make clinical decisions, which is the central aspect of the art of nursing practice. The increasing complexity of the patient needs, the large number of patients and the dynamic nature of client care in the contemporary healthcare demand a substantial psychological and operational workload on nurses. The issue of generative AI has emerged as a powerful tool to facilitate and inform this decision-making process by providing real-time data, automated guidance and forecasting recommendations. Generative AI enhances the quality of nursing decision-making, its efficiency and formulation of actionable interventions, through the generation of massive amounts of data, simulation of potential outcomes, and better patient outcomes (Watson et al., 2025).

3.1. AI-Assisted Assessment and Diagnosis

3.1.1. Generative AI for Symptom Analysis, Risk Stratification, and Personalized Recommendations

Generative AI may be applied in enabling nurses to come up with finer and holistic assessments of complex clinical data, and generate situation-specific understandings. An AI-based system can be applied to processed and unstructured data, such as lab reports and vital signs, and patient histories and doctor notes, respectively, and identify patterns that can potentially indicate a potential health concern. This allows conducting proper risk stratification, i.e. dividing patients based on the risk of complications and monitoring them respectively and providing interventions in time (Bhuyan et al., 2025).

Moreover, one could create personalized recommendations to the individual patients that would rely on their profile with the assistance of generative AI. The medical history, comorbidities, and along with the addition of the patient demographics and responses to the treatment, AI models can suggest the individualized strategies of care, which ensures higher outcomes. Considering an example,in a patient with chronic heart failure, one can recommend the specific medication regime and diet, as well as the rate of monitoring using generative AI, which will aid in the prevention of rehospitalization and adverse outcomes.

3.1.2. Real-Time Decision Support for Complex Cases

This will require making quick decisions because clinical issues collide with high acuity or complex cases of nurses. Generative AI will complement real time decision making activities by synthesising multi source data and having the ability to provide workable data within a few seconds when an issue arises. An example is rapid creation of a sepsis case, which may be done with the help of AI to identify the tendencies of vital signs, lab tests, and previous interventions and may suggest the recommended rules that will help control fluids and pick antibiotics and check the hours (Cheungpasitporn et al., 2025). Nursing judgment cannot be replaced by such insights, but rather, they can be considered complements of one another, as they contribute an even more qualified perspective that reduces uncertainty and advances evidence-based interventions. Generative AI enhances the security and trustworthiness of clinicians within the complicated care environment by enhancing the rate and correctness of evaluations.

3.3.2. Reduction of Adverse Events through Proactive Care

Generative AI acts as a major participate in the prevention of adverse events as it supports the early detection of adverse situations and the appropriate intervention. The nurse will be able to make an evidence-based approach with the help of the AI-generated guidance that will help minimize the chances of falling, infections, or medication errors (Bugaj et al., 2023). To present the example, in the oncology units, a generative AI can also evaluate neutropenic complications with the assistance of lab trends and treatment courses so that nurses could apply protective measures to protect their patients such as protection isolation or antibiotic prophylaxis. Similarly, the AI-assisted geriatric ward fall risk analysis can generate custom mobility plans, environmental, and teaching resources, lowering the incidence rates.

Preventive treatment can enhance patient security in addition to enhancing performance of nursing procedures. By prioritizing interventions whereby it is most required and prevents its complications at an early phase, nurses can allocate more resources and reduce the costs incurred in the hospital as well as the quality of care overall (Whig et al., 2025).

The technology that can reshape the clinical decision-making process is generative AI which will provide AI-assisted reviews, evidence-based clinical prescriptions, and predictive analytics making the nursing interventions more accurate, timely, and personalized.

3.2. Evidence-Based Care Recommendations

3.2.1. AI-Generated Guidelines Integrating Latest Research and Patient History

Among the strongest uses of generative AI in the nursing field, one can mention the creation of the dynamic, evidence-based care recommendations. The conventional clinical guidelines are generalized and thus a nurse is expected to interpret it and tailor to a specific patient. The present research, clinical procedures, and patient-related data can be synthesized using generative AI to provide individualized recommendations. As an illustration, an AI system can combine new rules on managing diabetes with past blood glucose trends, comorbid conditions, and other lifestyle characteristics of a patient, and propose them with a customized plan of insulin adjustments (Garg, 2025).

The automation of this synthesis process provides generative AI with the ability to ensure that nurses can have current and evidence-based guidance at the point of care. This minimizes the use of memory or literature review, boosts the speed of decision-making, and facilitates the best practices in a variety of clinical settings (Dai and Swaminathan, 2025).

3.2.2. Case Studies Illustrating Improved Clinical Outcomes

Various clinical examples can be used to illustrate how generative AI influences clinical outcomes. According to a hospital study on the post-operative management, AI-inspired decision supports systems offered an individualized monitoring/ intervention regimen to nurses, taking into account the risks of each patient. The implementation also led to a quantifiable decrease in the occurrence of post-operative complications, the reduction of the length of stay at the hospital, and the patient satisfaction. In another study, recommendations on pressure ulcer prevention provided through AI-based systems combined with real-time patient positioning and skin integrity measurements resulted in a reduction of the occurrence of ulcers by a significant percentage. These examples prove that the extent of generative AI does not only elevate the accuracy of nursing interventions but also leads to the improved result of a healthier situation and more efficient utilization of resources available.

3.3. Predictive Analytics & Early Intervention

3.3.1. How Generative Models Can Anticipate Patient Deterioration

One of the focal points in nursing practice is the ability to predict clinical deterioration prior to becoming critical especially in the intensive care unit as well as in high intensity units. Generative AI models are quite efficient in anticipatory analytics, which means defining the early warning signs by simulating patient trajectories in diverse conditions. Based on the trends in the vital signs, lab tests, drug reactions, and past success, AI can provide probabilistic predictions of possible complications, including sepsis, respiratory dysfunction, or heart attacks (Stanford & Sorensen, 2025).

Such predictive insights enable nurses to act in advance and modify care plans, monitor more often or even start preventive treatments before it is too late. It is possible to give the example of a patient presenting with the slight indication of respiratory compromise, where AI-based warnings and intervention recommendations allow taking crucial steps prior to the development of an emergency condition.

3.3.2. Reduction of Adverse Events through Proactive Care

Generative AI plays a central role in the prevention of adverse events since it facilitates timely intervention by helping to detect them early on. With the assistance of the AI-generated guidance, nurses will be able to take evidence-based steps that will help reduce risks of falls, infections, or medication errors (Bugaj et al., 2023). As an example, in oncology units, a generative AI assesses neutropenic complications with the help of lab trends and treatment schedules to enable nurses to use protective measures like protective isolation or antibiotic prophylaxis. On the same note, AI-supported geriatric ward fall risk assessment can produce tailored mobility plans, environmental solutions, and instructional materials, which reduce the incidence rates.

Proactive care can increase patient safety besides boosting the efficiency of nursing processes. By directing interventions where it is most needed and its complications are prevented at an early stage, nurses may better allocate resources, incur lower costs in the hospital, and improve the quality of care on the whole (Whig et al., 2025).

Generative AI is the technology that can transform clinical decision-making by delivering AI-assisted evaluations, evidence-based care recommendations, and predictive analytics enhancing the accuracy, promptness, and customization of the nursing interventions.

4. IMPROVING PATIENT CARE AND ENGAGEMENT

Patient care is not solely about clinical intervention, and among the core issues of positive health impact, communication, engagement, and long-term support should be mentioned. Nurses are very crucial figures in the present day healthcare practices that imply instructing patients to pursue complex treatments, counseling them on their illness disorders, and defining adherence to treatments. However, the increasingly strained requirements, of the nursing profession, and the emergence of patient diversity and complexity, have put noteworthy pressure on the ongoing delivery of especially customized, prompt, and efficient interactions with the patients. Both Generative AI introduces solutions that have the greatest propensity of revolution in this field, in personalized communication, enhanced monitoring, and simplified patient experience and, by extension, as a connecting point between clinical knowledge and patient-centered care (Unanah & Aidoo, 2025).

4.1. Personalized Patient Communication

4.1.1. AI-Generated Patient Education Materials, Discharge Instructions, and Reminders

Generative AI allows nurses to develop individual educational content according to the needs of the patients. An example is the creation of discharge instructions based on a patient-specific diagnosis and medications, comorbidities and literacy level, which AI can generate and offer a clearly viable instruction on how to utilize post-hospital care. Likewise, AI-based prescriptions remind patients to take medicine, see doctors, or change their lifestyle habits so that they can comply with the treatment to lower the risk of complications or readmissions.

In automating these communication functions, nurses will have an opportunity to spend more time and attention to face-to-face interaction with patients as well as convey information to patients in a consistent, accurate, and contextually relevant way. This is not just helpful in promoting compliance but also helps to build the trust of patients since they are made to get the information in a manner and language that is meaningful to their specific situations (Stanford & Sorensen, 2025).

4.1.2. Multilingual and Culturally Sensitive Content Creation

The healthcare systems are becoming more inclusive of heterogeneous populations of patients and thus language and cultural sensitivity are vital in effective care. Generative AI has the potential to generate educational resources and instructions on care in various languages and modify the content to prevent cultural mismatch and conform to the cultural standards and values (Özyurt, 2024). As an illustration, nutritional teaching about diabetic patients can be made according to the traditional food, cultural or religious taboos, making them more relevant and obedient. The AI-enhanced communication benefits healthcare equity by eliminating linguistic and cultural barriers and guarantees that patients understand what is happening and develop trust between healthcare providers and patients.

4.2. Enhanced Monitoring & Follow-Up

4.2.1. Integration with IoT Devices, EHRs, and Telehealth Platforms

Generative AI is able to improve patient care by means of relying on Internet of Things (IoT)-based data and utilizing electronic health records (EHRs) and telehealth. Wearable sensors and home-based devices would enable constant tracking of vital signs, followed by watching AI to identify abnormalities in the regular pattern and give both patients and nurses early warnings. Connecting to EHRs can make AI-generated insights informed by the full medical history and provide more specific and individualized interventions (Kumar and Ganesh, 2024).

Augmented with generative AI, telehealth platforms can make nursing care available to more people than in a hospital environment. As an example, artificial intelligence-based virtual visits may produce summaries, personalized recommendations, and follow-up instructions at once. This type of seamless integration provides continuity of care to a nurse who can intervene proactively and achieve a compatible commitment to the patients even in remote or underserved locations (Sai et al., 2024).

4.2.2. AI-Generated Insights for Long-Term Care Planning

In addition to the acute care, generative AI can be used to assist in the long-term care planning process because of the ability of this technology to examine patient data in a longitudinal setting and predict trends and risks and provide preventive action plans. An example is when used in chronic diseases like heart failure or chronic obstructive pulmonary disease (COPD), AI can forecast when an patient is likely to exacerbate the disease condition under historical conditions and constant monitoring. The nurses are then able to make changes in care plans in advance, make follow-ups, or prescribe lifestyle changes to avoid worsening. The AI can be used to aid more strategic, patient-focused planning by means of long-term care decisions and lessen complications, hospitalizations, and healthcare-related expenses with the help of data-driven insights (Lukkien et al., 2024).

4.3. Patient Experience Optimization

4.3.1. Empathy Simulation and Virtual Health Coaching Using AI

The empathetic attitude to patients and their perceived assistance vary such that patient engagement is greatly shaped. Generative AI provides empathy simulator and virtual health coaching, which increases patient experience and motivation. The chatbots and virtual assistants fueled by AI have the potential to deliver emotionally sensitive responses, promote positive actions, and provide the guidance on dealing with chronic diseases or lifestyle modifications. Although AI does not take the place of human empathy, it supports the nursing care by offering an accessible and non-interrupted support, especially during the non-clinical hours (Morrow et al., 2023).

Virtual health coaching systems are also capable of personalizing the interaction, using a variety of tonal, content, and motivational interventions, depending on patient feedback and engagement behaviour. Such a constant reminder helps patients to keep actively involved in the process to adhere to it and engage in healthier lifestyles (Batra and Dave, 2024).

4.3.2. Impact on Patient Satisfaction and Adherence

It has been shown that a more personalized and AI-driven interaction enhances satisfaction levels in patients and compliance with treatment. Timely, relevant and culturally sensitive information is found to give patients greater confidence in their ability to manage their conditions, less anxiety, and greater perceptions of collaboration with their care team. Adherence is also supported through generative AI, which reminds, instructs and gives immediate instructions, decreases the number of missed appointments, medicine mistakes, and spontaneous readmissions to the hospital (Jain, 2024).

In such a manner of facilitating patient experiences, not only clinical outcomes are improved but the efficiency of healthcare delivery is also boosted by generative AI. Nurses will be able to spend time on complicated clinical processes and direct communication with patients, and AI will take care of the routine communication, monitoring, and educational assistance. Such synergy brings about a more responsive, patient-centered and resilient healthcare environment.

Patient experience can be optimized and personalized since the continuous monitoring and communication with patients become possible with the help of generative AI. Nurses can provide more specific, effective, patient-centered treatment using educational materials based on AI, multilingual content, integration with IoT and telehealths, and caring virtual coaching. Generative AI can bridge the gap in clinical expertise and patient experiences by enhancing adherence, satisfaction, and long-term outcomes and support nurses in addressing the needs of the present healthcare industry, upholding quality, equity, and human-centered care (Selvaraj, 2024).

5. STREAMLINING NURSING WORKFLOW

The working process of nurses is always complicated, and they have to balance their efforts on patient care, recording of clinical facts, interdisciplinary contacts, and operational tasks. Given that healthcare demands are growing, patient complexity is increasing, and administrative overload, time, inefficiency, and workflow impairments that may affect nurses may be distracting direct care (Alshalawi et al., 2024). Generative AI helps in creating strong potential to automated nursing, making the workflow more effective, cost-efficient, minimizing burnout, and allowing nurses to concentrate on clinical judgment and communication with the patient. AI will be the stimulus of a more responsive, intelligent, and sustainable healthcare environment through automation of routine tasks, optimization of organizational time, and the creation of an interdisciplinary environment of work (Tischendorf et al., 2025).

5.1. Automating Routine Tasks

5.1.1. Documentation, Reporting, and Administrative Support

Completion of documentation and administration is one of the longest processes in the nursing practice. Each shift, nurse's waste a significant part of it to input information about patients, work on reports, update electronic health records (EHRs), and meet the regulations. Most of these repetitive tasks could be automated with generative AI which creates the documentation of any accuracy and with the correct context using both structured and unstructured data. An example here is that AI is capable of transcribing and summarizing clinical notes, producing discharge summaries, real-time updates to patient charting and producing the necessary regulatory reports with little to no manual effort (de Paula et al., 2025).

This automation decreases the amount of administration on the side of nurses, yet it does not compromise accuracy and compliance. Efficiency in repeating the tasks would reduce errors and help AI provide timely reports and allow nurses to focus on tasks that demand thinking along with close patient interactions. Moreover, AI-generated notes also enhance the continuity of care because, with the help of automated documentation, they can be standardized and are readily accessible and can be easily integrated across any interdisciplinary team.

5.1.2. Reduction in Nurse Burnout and Increased Time for Direct Patient Care

The decrease of the administrative load has a direct effect on the well-being and job satisfaction of nurses. Burnout is an important issue within medical care, with much attention usually given to it due to the plethora of paperwork, large patient numbers, and workload issues. Generative AI will enable nurses to have more time to engage directly with patients, provide clinical assessment and primary care, which are fundamental aspects of professional nursing satisfaction and patient-centered care by automating routine tasks.

Research has also demonstrated that with the administrative workflow being simplified, nurses will be able to spend more time communicating with patients, administering timely treatments and working with other in-service members, which will lead to a better patient outcome and work retention. Moreover, AI-based assistance may offer reliable support during the entire shift to avoid cognitive overload and make sure that nurses will be able to pay attention to complex decision-making and high-priority clinical work.

5.2. Intelligent Scheduling & Resource Allocation

The proper staffing and distributing of resources is vital in ensuring high quality and safety of care, particularly in the dynamic hospital settings. Conventional configurations are usually based upon fixed or historic-pattern or manually based schedules, which lack in responsiveness to current patient acuity, patient admission, or staff availability conditions. Intelligent scheduling models are provided by generative AI that can be reconfigured to dynamically match the nursing resources with the needs of patients (Ali, 2022).

Through assessing patient acuity, the expected processes, workflow, and nurse skills, the AI can contribute to creating optimal shifts and staffing strategies that guarantee staff to work within the limits of their options, avoid burnout, and cover critical fields. As one example, AI can suggest redistribution of seasoned nurses to the department where the patient risk is high or shift scheduling, which supports the continuity of care in the case of complicated patients. In addition to staffing, AI can also help in the allocation of other resources like medical devices, support staff or telehealth device depending on real time needs of the patient.

This is a data-driven model that guarantees efficiency and responsiveness of care delivery, minimizes delays, limits the number of bottlenecks, and lowers the overall effectiveness of operations. Through the provision of proactive optimization in the allocation of resources, AI helps facilitate safer and more structured and patient-centered conditions in health care settings.

5.3. Interdisciplinary Collaboration

Healthcare provision is based on interdisciplinary practice where nurses, physicians, therapists, pharmacists, and other allied health professionals combine their efforts in delivering seamless care efforts. The lack of communication, incomplete documentation, or those with a slow exchange of information can result in mistakes, unnecessary interference, or poor patient outcomes. Generative AI will be able to serve the purpose of interpreting different fields, bringing together actionable knowledge in real time and spreading across the teams (Tamli and Sain, 2023).

As an example, patient progress can be summarized automatically with AI systems, critical trends revealed, and interventions recommended, and then transferred to the corresponding healthcare professionals. Multimodal AI systems have the ability to combined EHR, lab data, imaging, and wearable information, creating reports that may be read in a straightforward manner by all team members. This will save time and resources devoted to handwork to collate data and will make sure that a decision made is informed by a full, cohesive picture of the situation of the patient.

Moreover, the virtual collaboration tools may be facilitated by generative AI, which allows teams working in various units or facilities to communicate effectively, create plans to organize the interventions, and coordinate further care. Considering this example, AI-generated care summaries and risk analyses can be used in complex surgery cases to direct both the pre-operative and the post-operative care teams, to avoid discordance across disciplines, and continuity of care. Through improving interconnected team communication, AI boosts teamwork, minimizes mistakes, and a culture of coordinated and patient-focused care.

Generative AI can potentially revolutionize the workflow through the automation of sterotypical administrative procedures, optimization of human and resource use and interdisciplinary collaboration. AI lessens documentation and administrational workloads to devote more time to in-patient care, critical thinking, and clinical interventions, burnout decreases, and job satisfaction improves. Smart scheduling is used to fit the needs of patients with the staff knowledge, and the collaboration between teams supported by AI can encourage the flow of information between the healthcare teams. Combined, these innovations produce a more efficient, resilient, and patient-centered nursing setting and show the usefulness of AI as a cognitive, as well as an operational partner in current healthcare.

6. CASE STUDIES AND REAL-WORLD APPLICATIONS

Generative AI is now no longer an imagined idea in healthcare, its applications in nursing are coming to fruition, and as more practical implementations are reflected through quantifiable improvements in patient care, workflow, and clinical decision-making, its role in nursing is being increasingly realized. The case studies also contain useful information about the usability of AI in a transformative way in the practical nursing setting, and they present both successes and failures.

6.1. Hospital & Clinical Implementations

6.1.1. Successful Deployments of Generative AI in Nursing Workflows

The adoption of the generative AI in nursing processes has been successfully implemented in several hospitals across the globe. As one example, a tertiary care hospital deployed an AI-based documentation system, which created an automated system that created patient progress notes, discharge reports, and care plan instructions, but used structured data as input devices, including electronic health records (EHRs) and unstructured nursing observations. This implementation saved about 40 per cent on documentation time as nurses were given an opportunity to spend more time in direct patient care and bedside evaluations.

Generative AI has also been applied in intensive care units (ICUs) where it predicts patient deterioration and suggests intervention plans. It became possible to recommend the interventions in time, be it a change in medications or transfer to a higher level of care, as the AI systems could analyze vital signs and lab outcomes as well as histories of patients and provide recommendations at the right moment. These coverages led to an achievable decrease in the rate of adverse events, such as a 25% drop in ICU rehospitalization rates, which indicate the effectiveness of AI to assist with proactive and data-driven nursing decisions.

6.1.2. Lessons Learned and Metrics of Improvement

The major lessons that were achieved during these implementations include the necessity to prevent the integration of AI tools into the current workflow instead of placing them as independent systems. Hospitals noted that their success with AI was heavily dependent on training and buy-in by the nursing staff; nurses had to learn the output of AI and how to validate it and retain clinical judgment. The metrics of lowered documentation time, the decreased amount of adverse events, better patient outcomes, and a higher level of nurse satisfaction can be taken as the real indicators of the positive influence of AI in practice. As well, these case studies indicate that the constant attention to AI outputs is necessary in order to control and prevent biases, guarantee the correctness of results, and be able to speak of patient safety.

6.2. Innovations in Telehealth and Remote Nursing

Telehealth and remote nursing innovations made possible by generative AI have extended the provision of nursing care by nurses beyond the hospital environment (Azeroual, 2024). Viral care assistants that are powered by AI are now implemented to guide patients in managing chronic conditions, reminders of taking medications, and personalized education. These virtual assistants have the capacity to produce customized recommendations according to the patient health history, recent check-ups, and the habit of life, which is helpful in keeping the nurses in constant contact with patients at a distance (geographically) or confined at home.

Remote patient monitoring solutions that use AI supplement nursing care even more by offering real-time sensor data analysis of wearables, home monitoring devices, mobile health applications, etc. (Agrawal et al., 2024). With generative AI, it is possible to produce alerts, intervention suggestions, and a list of follow-up automatically synthesized on the basis of this information. To illustrate, when dealing with patients whose heart failure, AI systems will be able to identify an early indication of fluid retention, suggest care plans, and notify nurses to enable them to intervene in due time to avoid repeat hospitalization.

These inventions signify that generative AI is not restricted to hospitals, but rather it is an extension of nursing capacity into the home and community of a patient enhancing patient access and continuity of care as well as their patient outcomes. Predictive analytics, individualized advice, and remote surveillance help AI to make healthcare a more connected, responsive and patient-centered ecosystem.

The effectiveness and versatility of generative AI in nursing are demonstrated in hospital applications and telehealth innovations (case studies). Efficient deployments demonstrate apparent workflow enhancements, decrease in patient safety, and clinical decision-making, whereas the lessons learned involve staff training, workflow integration, and ethical supervision. Remote-care AI-supported applications enable proactive interventions, continuous observation, and personalized interaction with patients, which is why the potential of generative AI in radically changing the nursing practice, both in the hospital and community, is enormous.

7. CHALLENGES AND LIMITATIONS

Although the opportunities of generative AI in the context of nursing practice, patient care, and workflow optimization can be seen as quite significant, a variety of challenges and limitations is present when it comes to its adoption. To secure the safe, effective, and sustainable implementation of AI, it is important to address these issues. These obstacles include data quality and integration problems, bias and trust questions and technical and human aspects that might impact the way AI is actually implemented in clinical practice.

7.1. Data Quality and Integration Issues

To produce accurate insights, predictions and recommendations, generative AI is very dependent on quality and exhaustive datasets. Nevertheless, data quality becomes one of the major obstacles in a variety of healthcare systems (Azeroual, 2024). The use of electronic health record (EHR) as one of the main sources of patient data is prone to interoperability difficulties as dissimilar systems may employ diverse formats, standards and terminologies. Such integration deficit may result in decreasing the precision and topicality of the AI-produced results due to the inability to retrieve the entire range of patient information.

Another challenge is to use incomplete datasets. Lack or intermittent data on patient history, drug compliance, or diagnostic outcome may result in erroneous AI guidelines. As an example, the work of a generative AI that forecasts the worsening of a patient might issue false alarms by withholding access to the information that includes the presence of essential laboratory results or comorbidities, which is included in the data. To guarantee successful application of AI in nursing, it is therefore important to ensure that data are complete, standardized, and have interoperability across hospital systems, laboratories, and outpatient clinics.

7.2. Bias, Safety, and Trust Concerns

7.2.1. Addressing AI Biases in Clinical Decisions

One of the biggest issues with AI is bias within systems, especially when the training data utilizes data sets that lack a sufficient number of different patients. When there are no or only a limited number of underrepresented groups in the training data, the AI-produced suggestions might not take into consideration variations in clinical presentation, socio-economic conditions, and cultural requirements. Such biases may cause inequalities in treatment recommendations, misdiagnosis, or missing threats in nursing practice and hence undermine patient safety and equity. The reduction of bias needs to be methodical by regularly reviewing the outputs of the AI, having various and representative training data, and a system to provide control checks by humans to approve recommendations in context.

7.2.2. Ensuring Transparency and Accountability in AI Outputs

Is often a black box Generative AI models have unclear explanations of the underlying reasoning, and their result can be influenced by provided inputs. This obscuration may undermine trust in clinicians and render decision-making to patients, regulatory agencies, or interdisciplinary teams hard to defend. To evaluate the clinical relevance, determine possible errors, and hold accountability, nurses should be aware of the way AI gets to its recommendations. The safety of AI systems, building trust, and professional responsibility in clinical practice is necessary by establishing clear AI systems that offer explainable outputs, audit trails, and decision rationale.

7.3. Technical and Human Factors

7.3.1. Training Nurses to Use AI Tools Effectively

In order to gain a positive outcome in the integration of AI into nursing workflows, sufficient training and digital literacy is necessary. Nurses have to be taught not only how to use AI platforms but also how to analyze AI-created recommendations in a critical manner. The training needs to focus on technical abilities and ethical decision-making, such that the nurses do not become dependent on AI and accept its results blindly. Reported higher rates of adoption and greater effectiveness in the use of AI tools to support patient care has been noted in institutions that offer continuous learning, practical simulations and interdisciplinary AI literacy programs.

7.3.2. Managing Technology Fatigue

Despite the fact that AI could contribute to streamlining working process, technology fatigue among the nurses could appear because of the rise of different digital appliances. The constant alerts, notifications, and novelty of the interface may also cause a high level of cognitive load, the disruption of interaction with the patient, and burnout in cases when these factors are not addressed appropriately. The effective implementation should be incorporated with the design being user friendly, and being compatible with other working processes to bring out priority information in order to minimize unnecessary disturbances. The essential element of the quality of care and well-being of nurses and their quality of care is the combination of automated controls with the help of AI and a human service.

The weaknesses and constraints of generative AI in the nursing profession support the idea of strategic and careful implementation. The low quality of data and the process of its integration are the things which suggest the necessity to possess the interoperable, full, and standard data on healthcare. The bias and safety and trust issues need the constant evaluation, the explainable AI outcomes as well as the human control systems that guarantee the fairness and responsibility. The importance of technical and human training, usability, and workload management has technical and human explanations to ensure that AI did not define the work but helped nurses. They are not a technical requirement, just a fundamental prerequisite to effective and ethical AI insertion. These discoveries and mitigations will allow healthcare institutions to achieve the utmost benefit of generative AI-aided decision-making and improved patient care and simplified work processes without compromising the professional approach, compassion, and human touch that define the nursing practice in the contemporary environment.

8. FUTURE DIRECTIONS

With the further development of generative AI, it will find more clinical uses and applications in nursing and healthcare practice, which has created a scenario where AI will become an integrated partner in clinical decision making, patient care, and workflow optimization. The opportunities of AI to innovate next-generation solutions along with the proactive, predictive, and personalized approaches to nursing leave previously unheard-of prospects of improving healthcare outcomes. Meanwhile, successful integration needs visionary policies and thorough training of the workforce to equip nurses with a clinical environment that is AI-based.

8.1. Next-Generation AI Capabilities

The second avenue of AI in health care is multimodal AI, which incorporates all types of data such as images, written texts about their patients, laboratory tests, and vital signs among others into integrated and usable information sets. The multimodal AI, in contrast to the classic models of AI, utilizes a wide range of data types in parallel, which makes them more reliable, refined, and context-specific.

To nurses, such an ability would translate into better situational awareness and a decision support. As an illustration, a multimodal AI can integrate electronic health record, radiography scan with continuous vital sign monitoring of a patient and predict the change to deterioration and recommend specific interventions. The AI can find subtle relationships between data types that might be overlooked during the traditional workflow in complex scenarios like stroke management or sepsis detection and can provide early warning and evidence-based advice.

In addition to predictive accuracy, next-generation AI can be used to simulate and forecast scenarios, giving nurses an opportunity to understand possible consequences of various interventions in real time. This feature can improve training, get staff ready to when and how rare or high-risk events occur and how staff can make decisions together within clinical teams. In the next generation, these AI models will only be useful in nursing practice as their capacity to adjust to new clinical settings and to develop according to changing data sets will help them become more beneficial as both analytical and creative collaborators.

8.2. Proactive, Predictive, and Personalized Nursing

The future of nursing will shift towards an approach that is proactive, predictive, and personal, and AI is getting chosen as a partner and not a substitute of human judgment. Generative AI may facilitate proactive care where the future complications are predicted and interventions planed based on the individual health characteristics of the patient. As an example, artificial intelligence-based observation arrangements may identify clinical deterioration of heart failure early, plan individual fluid manipulation schedules, and arrange follow-up appointments, and remind nurses of key points in action.

Personalization is not limited to clinical intervention, but also patient involvement and education. AI may produce tailored care maps, culturally relevant learning content, and video-based virtual coaching that can change in line with the literacy status, language, and lifestyle of the patient. AI assist in following instructions, empowerment, and increased health through personalized guidance.

Predictive features also enhance the management of resources enabling nurses and other healthcare organizations to distribute staff, equipment, and time in a more optimal manner. Using predictive modeling is one example: it can predict the number of patients requiring hospitalization, when the workload of a facility is at its peak, and how changes in the nursing staffing can add the greatest value to the provided care with the least risks of nurse burnout. This proactive strategy is what contributes towards a more responsive and resilient medical system that can cope up with dynamic clinical set ups.

8.3. Policy and Education Implications

The ubiquity of generative AI in nursing needs a conscious policy, governance, and education. Regulatory agencies and medical facilities should have clear criteria on AI validation, safety, and accountability so that AI systems are of high quality in clinical, ethical and legal standards. The problem of the privacy of patient data, interoperability, reduction of bias, and the separation of responsibility between human clinicians and AI outputs should be also touched upon by the policies. An open system of governance will be necessary to create confidence between the nurses, patients and the interdisciplinary teams.

The second factor of equal importance is preparing the nursing workforce to work in the AI-enhanced clinical setting. The needs of the AI (AI literacy, data interpretation, ethical) and practical experience with AI tools should be included in education programs. It is possible to make sure that technology does not replace nurses but supplements their professional judgment by learning to be critical of AI outputs. Training through simulation and constant professional development will also be necessary in inspiring the confidence and competence in using AI to provide patient-centered care.

Besides, interdisciplinary education should be established to encourage nurses, physicians, data scientists, and healthcare administrators to work jointly. These initiatives will foster the culture of understanding, as healthcare teams will be able to leverage AI resources and ensure that human-focused care values are preserved.

The vision of the future of smart nursing using generative AI is to create a harmonic interaction between the human and computing powers whereby AI acts as a proactive partner, analyzes multimodal data, predicts clinical events, and designs individual patient care. The next-generation AI devices with improved predictive and generative properties will empower nurses to provide better, more efficient, and personalized care and minimize operational pressure and improve clinical outcomes. To actualize such a vision would take well-developed policy frameworks and regulation, and extensive education and training to equip nurses with an AI-oriented healthcare environment. Through implementing such measures, healthcare organizations will be able to make sure that the integration of AI is ethical, safe, and effective to establish a future whereby smart nursing will utilize technological innovations as well as the experience of human professionals to provide the best care possible to patients.

9. CONCLUSION

Generative AI has established a potential of revolution in nursing transforming clinical decision-making, patient care, and workflow efficiency in a variety of health care settings. Through the enhancement of the cognitive potential of nurses, AI has the capability of making more precise judgments, planning personalized care, and cursory insights that can be utilized to make proactive changes and, eventually, enhance patient outcomes and safety. In the care context, AI-driven tools help to promote personalized communication, culturally aware education, constant monitoring, and virtual mentoring to improve the level of engagement, adherence, and satisfaction. At the same time, AI facilitates the optimization and automation of work processes, such as documentation, staffing and resource use, interdisciplinary work, which reduces the load on the administration and decreases the level of nursing burnout, and helps to allocate more time to direct contact with patients. The achievements mentioned herein highlight the immense advantages of raising the concept of AI into the healthcare system, but it should be offset by the values of human-centered nursing, as empathy, professional judgment, and ethical decision-making processes are priceless in the healthcare context. To be responsible in adopting AI, it is necessary to consider the quality of the data, reduce biases, achieve transparency, and accountability, as well as make sure that AI cannot facilitate but complement clinical skills. No less important is preparing nurses in terms of continuous education and training as well as interdisciplinary cooperation, enabling nurses to properly process AI results, incorporate their suggestions in the process of care delivery, and enjoy both patient and peer trust. The next step in building a smart nursing involves a symbiotic collaboration between human prowess and AI production, where technology will improve efficiency and more accuracy and strengthen patient-centered principles. With the growing adoption of AI by healthcare systems, the necessity to conduct further research, evidenced-based practice, and policy formulation is critical to streamline the results, consider ethical implications, and promote equal access. With a culture of careful, conscientious, and informed adoption of AI, the nursing professionals and medical organizations are able to realize the full capacity of the generative AI to alter the provision of care, enhance clinical practice, and upgrade the overall patient experience.

REFERENCES

Agrawal, A., Soni, R., Gupta, D., & Dubey, G. (2024). The role of robotics in medical science: Advancements, applications, and future directions. *Journal of Autonomous Intelligence*, *7*(3), 1–27. DOI: 10.32629/jai.v7i3.1008

Ali, H. (2022). Reinforcement learning in healthcare: Optimizing treatment strategies, dynamic resource allocation, and adaptive clinical decision-making. *Int J Comput Appl Technol Res*, *11*(3), 88–104.

AlSaad, R., Abd-Alrazaq, A., Boughorbel, S., Ahmed, A., Renault, M. A., Damseh, R., & Sheikh, J. (2024). Multimodal large language models in health care: Applications, challenges, and future outlook. *Journal of Medical Internet Research, 26*, e59505. DOI: 10.2196/59505 PMID: 39321458

Alshalawi, M. A., Almuhlafi, J. M., Alsubiei, S. M., Al-Shamrani, S. E., Alotaibi, M. M., Alenzi, S. M., & Alotaibi, A. H. (2024). The Role Of Clinic Development Strategies In Enhancing Care Coordination And Clinical Workflow: A Systematic Evaluation Of Evidence. *The Review of Diabetic Studies; RDS*, •••, 182–190.

Azeroual, O. (2024). Can generative AI transform data quality? A critical discussion of ChatGPT's capabilities. *Academia Engineering, 1*(4).

Baig, M. M., Hobson, C., GholamHosseini, H., Ullah, E., & Afifi, S. (2024). Generative AI in improving personalized patient care plans: Opportunities and barriers towards its wider adoption. *Applied Sciences (Basel, Switzerland)*, *14*(23), 10899. DOI: 10.3390/app142310899

Batra, P., & Dave, D. M. (2024). Revolutionizing healthcare platforms: The impact of AI on patient engagement and treatment efficacy. [IJSR]. *International Journal of Scientific Research, 13*, 613–624.

Bhuyan, S. S., Sateesh, V., Mukul, N., Galvankar, A., Mahmood, A., Nauman, M., Rai, A., Bordoloi, K., Basu, U., & Samuel, J. (2025). Generative artificial intelligence use in healthcare: Opportunities for clinical excellence and administrative efficiency. *Journal of Medical Systems*, *49*(1), 10. DOI: 10.1007/s10916-024-02136-1 PMID: 39820845

Bragazzi, N. L., & Garbarino, S. (2024). Toward clinical generative AI: Conceptual framework. *JMIR AI*, *3*(1), e55957. DOI: 10.2196/55957 PMID: 38875592

Bugaj, M., Kliestik, T., & Lăzăroiu, G. (2023). Generative artificial intelligence-based diagnostic algorithms in disease risk detection and personalized healthcare procedures. *Contemporary Readings in Law and Social Justice*, *15*(1), 9–26. DOI: 10.22381/CRLSJ15120231

Cheungpasitporn, W., Thongprayoon, C., & Kashani, K. (2025). Artificial intelligence in critical care nephrology: Current applications, emerging techniques, and challenges. *Kidney360.*

Dai, T., & Swaminathan, J. M. (2025). Artificial intelligence and operations: A foundational framework of emerging research and practice. *Production and Operations Management*, 10591478251412943. DOI: 10.1177/10591478251412943

de Paula, P. A. B., Severino, J. V. B., Berger, M. N., Veiga, M. H., Ribeiro, K. D. P., & Loures, F. S.. (2025). Improving documentation quality and patient interaction with AI. *Journal of Medical Artificial Intelligence*, •••, 8.

Fahim, Y. A., Hasani, I. W., Kabba, S., & Ragab, W. M. (2025). Artificial intelligence in healthcare and medicine. *European Journal of Medical Research*, *30*(1), 848. DOI: 10.1186/s40001-025-03196-w PMID: 40988064

Garg, S. (2025). The role of generative AI in personalized medicine and treatment recommendations. *Clinical Medicine and Health Research Journal*, *5*(2), 1214–1227. DOI: 10.18535/cmhrj.v5i02.463

Jain, N. (2024). Revolutionizing patient care: The impact of ChatGPT and generative AI in healthcare. *International Journal of Scientific and Research Publications*, *14*(11), 24–38. DOI: 10.29322/IJSRP.14.11.2024.p15506

Kazerouni, A., Aghdam, E. K., Heidari, M., Azad, R., Fayyaz, M., Hacihaliloglu, I., & Merhof, D. (2022). Diffusion models for medical image analysis. *arXiv preprint arXiv:2211.07804.*

Kumar, M. S., & Ganesh, D. (2024). Improving telemedicine through IoT and cloud computing. *Advances in Engineering and Intelligence Systems*, *3*(3), 123–135.

Lin, C., & Kuo, C. F. (2025). Roles and potential of large language models in healthcare. *Biomedical Journal*, *48*(5), 100868. DOI: 10.1016/j.bj.2025.100868 PMID: 40311872

Lukkien, D. R., Stolwijk, N. E., Askari, S. I., Hofstede, B. M., Nap, H. H., Boon, W. P., & Minkman, M. M. (2024). AI-assisted decision-making in long-term care: Qualitative study on prerequisites for responsible innovation. *JMIR Nursing*, *7*(1), e55962. DOI: 10.2196/55962 PMID: 39052315

Morrow, E., Zidaru, T., Ross, F., Mason, C., Patel, K. D., Ream, M., & Stockley, R. (2023). Artificial intelligence technologies and compassion in healthcare. *Frontiers in Psychology, 13*, 971044. DOI: 10.3389/fpsyg.2022.971044 PMID: 36733854

Nkrumah, I. P., Engmann, F., & Adu-Manu, K. S. (2025). Ethical AI in healthcare: A comprehensive review addressing privacy, security, and fairness.

Okonji, O. R., Yunusov, K., & Gordon, B. (2024). Applications of generative AI in healthcare. *arXiv preprint arXiv:2406.10632.*

Özyurt, S. (2024). AI-assisted English language learning for cross-cultural medical education. *Experimental and Applied Medical Science*, *5*(2), 83–92. DOI: 10.46871/eams.1464830

Pramanik, B., Ghosh, D., Ghosh, D., & Paul, K. (2025). Beyond prediction: How generative AI is creating new healthcare realities. In *Revolutionizing Healthcare 5.0* (pp. 219–233). Springer.

Rabbani, S. A., El-Tanani, M., Sharma, S., Rabbani, S. S., El-Tanani, Y., Kumar, R., & Saini, M. (2025). Generative artificial intelligence in healthcare. *BioMedInformatics*, *5*(3), 37. DOI: 10.3390/biomedinformatics5030037

Saba, D., & Hadidi, A. (2025). Opportunities, challenges, and future directions of generative AI in healthcare. In *Generative Artificial Intelligence in Healthcare* (pp. 276–298).

Sai, S., Gaur, A., Sai, R., Chamola, V., Guizani, M., & Rodrigues, J. J. (2024). Generative AI for transformative healthcare. *IEEE Access : Practical Innovations, Open Solutions*, *12*, 31078–31106. DOI: 10.1109/ACCESS.2024.3367715

Sam-Oyerinde, O. A., Idowu, O. O., & Idowu, O. P. (2025). The future of AI in healthcare. *Modern Technologies in Healthcare*, 290–320.

Seenu, A., & Rani, P. S. (2024). From reactive to proactive: Redesigning patient care pathways. *European Data Science Journal, 2*(1).

Selvaraj, S. (2024). Empowering patients with AI-driven personalized care. *International Journal of Scientific Research, 13*(7), 337–343.

Stanford, M., & Sorensen, Z. (2025). *Integrating generative AI in medical practice.* NuovoNova Ltd.

Tamli, N., & Sain, M. (2023). Exploring innovative strategies for patient-centered care in nursing. *South Asian Journal of Research & Innovation, 10*(1), 19–30. DOI: 10.3126/jori.v10i1.66025

Tischendorf, T., Hinsche, L., Hasseler, M., & Schaal, T. (2025). GenAI in nursing and clinical practice. *Journal of Public Health (Berlin)*. Advance online publication. DOI: 10.1007/s10389-025-02523-z

Unanah, O. V., & Aidoo, E. M. (2025). AI technologies to reduce disparities in healthcare. *World Journal of Advanced Research and Reviews*, *25*(2), 2643–2664.

Wang, B., Shi, X., Han, X., & Xiao, G. (2024). The digital transformation of nursing practice. *Frontiers in Medicine*, *11*, 1471527. DOI: 10.3389/fmed.2024.1471527 PMID: 39678028

Watson, A. L., Bond, C., Aveyard, H., Smith, G. D., & Jackson, D. (2025). Generative AI at the Bedside: An Integrative Review of Applications and Implications in Clinical Nursing Practice. *Journal of Clinical Nursing*, jocn.70151. DOI: 10.1111/jocn.70151 PMID: 41293898

Whig, P., Dutta, P. K., Yathiraju, N., Bhattacharya, P., & Sharma, S. (2025). Transforming healthcare operations with generative AI. In *Revolutionizing Healthcare 5.0* (pp. 289–308). Springer.

Chapter 11
Generative AI-Driven Telehealth and Smart Patient Engagement in Nursing

Vipin Tyagi
http://orcid.org/0000-0003-4994-3686
Jaypee University of Engineering and Technology, Guna, India

ABSTRACT

Generative AI is transforming smart nursing by enhancing telehealth delivery, virtual nursing assistants and AI supported patient engagement. This chapter examines how generative AI technologies support nurses in providing personalized, continuous and responsive care beyond traditional clinical settings. The chapter also explores AI driven patient engagement strategies that promote adherence, self management and real time monitoring through conversational and remote care platforms. Ethical and practical challenges including data privacy, transparency, algorithmic bias, trust and equitable access are critically analyzed within a human centered design framework. By emphasizing collaboration between nurses and intelligent systems this chapter shows how generative AI can augment professional judgment, strengthen therapeutic relationships and contribute to safe effective and compassionate healthcare delivery in smart nursing environments.

EXECUTIVE SUMMARY

The rapid increase in use of telehealth services has transformed healthcare delivery by providing remote, continuous and technology-supported care. Within

DOI: 10.4018/979-8-3373-8247-0.ch011

this evolving digital background, generative artificial intelligence is providing support in smart nursing services by helping in clinical workflows, enhancing patient engagement and strengthening decision making in virtual care. This chapter examines the integration of generative AI into telehealth from a nursing point of view, focusing on virtual assistants, AI supported patient engagement systems and workflow integration.

The chapter shows that telehealth can be used as the foundational infrastructure for smart nursing, proving its role in expanding access, continuity of care and efficiency in the context of workforce shortages and increasing chronic diseases. Generative AI technologies are also reviewed that can be used to extend traditional telehealth capabilities through conversational interaction, automated documentation, adaptive clinical decision support and personalized guidance to patients. A comparative analysis of conventional and generative AI based telehealth systems shows how intelligent automation can change nursing roles from simple task execution toward cognitive supervision and clinical judgment.

Key applications such as virtual nursing assistants for symptom triage, care coordination, follow up and patient education, as well as AI-supported patient engagement systems that promote self-management, adherence and continuous monitoring are discussed. The chapter emphasizes that these systems should be used as a support to human centered care, rather than a replacement for nursing expertise. Technical architectures, evaluation metrics and quantitative performance indicators are discussed to support safe, effective and scalable implementation in nursing practice.

Ethical, legal and governance considerations are discussed that include data privacy, transparency, bias mitigation, accountability and alignment with regulatory frameworks such as HIPAA and GDPR. The chapter concludes by outlining practical implementation guidelines, workforce training requirements and future research directions, underscoring the central role of nurses in shaping responsible and sustainable adoption of generative AI in telehealth.

1. INTRODUCTION

With increasing use of telehealth and artificial intelligence as an important component of modern care delivery, digital transformation in healthcare has accelerated at a fast speed. Among healthcare professionals, nurses have primary responsibility of interaction with patients, coordination of care and health education. Integration of generative artificial intelligence into telehealth systems has changed the way of delivery and monitoring of nursing care and experience of patients. Generative AI-based systems, including large language models and conversational agents, are being used in the development of virtual assistants, clinical decision support and patient engagement systems. The aim of development of these technologies is not to replace nurses but to support them in providing help in their expertise, improve efficiency and enhance the quality of patient-centered care.

Telehealth has evolved from basic video consultations to comprehensive digital care ecosystems that include remote monitoring, automated assessment of issues and continuous patient communication. Within these ecosystems, generative AI enables dynamic interaction, personalization and adaptive learning that were not possible through conventional rule-based systems. For nursing practice, new opportunities and challenges related to workflow design, ethical responsibility, data governance and professional identity have emerged. According to recent research, AI-enabled telehealth is able to improve care accessibility, clinical efficiency and patient engagement across multiple domains, including nursing practice, chronic disease management, and decentralized care delivery (Amjad et al., 2023; Rossi & Rehman, 2025).

This chapter examines the role of generative AI in telehealth, virtual nursing assistants and AI-supported patient engagement. Current applications, technologies required for implementation, advantages for nursing practice and the ethical and regulatory requirements that must be addressed to ensure safe and equitable adoption are discussed in this chapter. By showing the use of generative AI within a human-centered nursing framework, this chapter shows that smart nursing innovation should be used as a supporting technique in nursing practice.

In this chapter, generative AI is used to refer specifically to foundation language models which are capable of producing new text, dialogue, or summaries, distinguishing them from rule-based or purely predictive clinical decision support tools.

2. TELEHEALTH AS A FOUNDATION FOR SMART NURSING

Telehealth refers to the delivery of healthcare services through digital communication technologies that enable clinical interaction without the need for physical co-presence. These technologies are video conferencing platforms, mobile health applications, remote monitoring devices and secure messaging systems. In the field of nursing services, telehealth has become a basic infrastructure for smart care services. It has increased the reach of clinical services across geographical, temporal and logistical boundaries. This transformation is very useful in healthcare systems facing workforce shortages, aging populations and increasing occurrence of chronic disease. Telemedicine has also expanded its access to critical care globally, particularly in resource-limited setup, reinforcing its importance as foundational infrastructure for smart nursing models (Ganapathy et al., 2022; Ndirangu-Mugo et al., 2022).

For nursing professionals, telehealth has expanded the scope and flexibility of their practice. Nurses can evaluate disease symptoms, functional status and care needs through remote discussion and digital observation. Using multimedia tools, patient education can be provided in real time or asynchronously. Chronic disease management programs can utilize telehealth for long-term monitoring, medication adherence and lifestyle change. Post-discharge follow up is possible through telehealth that enables early identification of complications and reduces avoidable readmissions by providing nursing care remotely beyond hospital.

Experimental research shows that telehealth supportive nursing in various clinical applications is effective. Telehealth has the ability to improve access to care for patients in rural and underserved communities where access to healthcare facilities is poor and travel is difficult. Telehealth reduces delay in assessment and providing support and thus contributes to improved clinical outcomes and satisfaction among patients. According to research, telehealth facilities can improve access to medical care, reduce hospital readmissions and enhance patient satisfaction, particularly in rural and underserved populations (Dorsey & Topol, 2016). For nurses, these outcomes support the importance of telehealth as a tool for proactive and preventive care rather than reactive service. Research conducted in remote and underserved regions further indicates that AI-supported telehealth models are able to improve continuity of care and service reach, especially where traditional healthcare access is difficult (Rintyarna et al., 2023; Witkowska-Zimny, 2025).

Empirical nursing-focused evidence supports these outcomes. A randomized controlled experiment conducted by Totten et al. (2016) showed that nurse-led telehealth support significantly reduced hospital readmissions and improved chronic disease self-management outcomes. In a similar way, a multicenter evaluation of virtual nursing follow-up programs showed reductions in emergency admissions in the range of 15–30%, alongside improved patient-reported satisfaction and continuity of care (Kruse et al., 2017). These results prove that telehealth services, guided by nurses are able to produce measurable clinical and operational benefits beyond theoretical efficiency gains.

The COVID-19 pandemic accelerated the evolution of telehealth. Public health restrictions and infection control concerns necessitated rapid adoption of virtual care across almost all healthcare settings. Video consultations, remote assessment of diseases and digital documentation was learned by the nurses quickly. This transition from traditional health systems into virtual system was quick and it showed the adaptiveness of health systems. This also showed the limitations of existing telehealth facilities. To overcome these issues, need of more intelligent and responsive telehealth systems was observed. Requirement of these systems was their capability of supporting complex nursing workflows. With the help of generative AI, many of these challenges can be addressed by enabling automation of routine tasks, natural language interaction and adaptive decision support. AI –based telehealth systems are able to process large amount of patient related data and adjust available responses as per requirement.

In smart nursing environments, telehealth platforms integrated with AI provide useful clinical support. At the same time such platforms should be able to preserve professional autonomy. AI-based systems can identify high risk and provide alert. This will provide support to nurses so that they can decide about urgency requirement of patients. Symptom reports submitted through online platforms can be analyzed and can be used to generate structured summaries from these reports. Structures summaries generated in this way are able to provide support in efficient assessment and decision making.

It is important to note that generative AI-based tools are accurate and efficient but cannot replace human judgment or relational care. These factors are main parts of nursing services. AI-based systems functions as a cognitive support tool that provide support in clinical reasoning and reduces administrative burden. With the help of AI-based systems, repetitive tasks such as data collection, documentation and routine communication can be automated. This will result in time saving and nurses can devote more attention to complex clinical evaluation, ethical deliberation and therapeutic activities. In this way, telehealth supported by generative AI becomes not only a technological convenience but a foundational element of smart nursing. By using AI-based systems care quality and professional sustainability will enhance.

While telehealth services provide the structural foundation for smart nursing, their full potential is realized only when AI-based systems are integrated into implementation. Traditional telehealth is not able to address the growing complexity of nursing workflows, personalization needs and continuous patient engagement. In the following section, it has been discussed that how generative AI technologies can be used to support telehealth capabilities and enable more adaptive, efficient and context aware nursing care.

3. GENERATIVE AI TECHNOLOGIES IN NURSING CARE

There is a technological shift from conventional telehealth to AI-based smart telehealth system in the area of nursing. At the core of generative AI are deep learning architectures trained on extensive corpora of text and domain-specific data. Transformer-based models are mostly used due to their ability to capture long-range dependencies and semantic relationships in language. In nursing applications, these models are often fine-tuned on clinical guidelines, patient education materials and de-identified health records to ensure relevance and accuracy. While computational processes involved are complex, their practical value lies in enabling systems that can understand and generate human-like language in clinical settings.

Generative AI technologies are used in telehealth platforms, virtual assistants and clinical support tools in the area of nursing care. One useful application is conversational interfaces that are used to interact directly with patients. Using these interfaces, patients can get follow-up questions; provide symptom clarifications to be used in decisions. These systems can also respond to patient issues using natural language. Traditional systems used in the process are based on decision trees, while generative AI systems are able to handle ambiguity, variations in expressions and incomplete information more effectively. This capability is particularly important in nursing practice, as description provided by the patients is generally subjective and contains contextual elements that are not capable of classification. In recent reviews, the growing role of machine learning and generative AI in evidence-based telehealth, enabling adaptive decision support and personalized smart care pathways is shown (Christopoulou, 2024; Ramkumar et al., 2020).

To compare various dimensions of traditional telehealth models with generative AI-based systems, Table 1 shows a structured comparison across key functional, clinical and governance dimensions.

Table 1. Comparison of traditional telehealth systems and generative AI-based telehealth

Dimension	Traditional telehealth systems	Generative AI-based telehealth systems
Core functionality	Video calls and secure messaging for remote consultations	Conversational interaction automated summarization and adaptive decision support
Data handling	Manual entry of patient information by nurses	Automated pre-visit data collection and synthesis from patient inputs
Patient assessment	Structured questionnaires and clinician led interviews	AI-assisted symptom interpretation and risk prioritization
Documentation	Manual documentation during or after encounters	Real time transcription and AI generated draft clinical notes
Personalization	Limited personalization based on predefined templates	Dynamic personalization using patient history behavior and preferences
Workflow efficiency	High administrative burden and task fragmentation	Reduced documentation load and streamlined workflow integration
Clinical decision support	Rule-based alerts and static protocols	Context aware generative recommendations with nurse oversight
Patient engagement	Episodic interaction during scheduled visits	Continuous engagement through AI-based follow ups and reminders

continued on following page

Table 1. Continued

Dimension	Traditional telehealth systems	Generative AI-based telehealth systems
Nurse role	Primary executor of all assessment and documentation tasks	Clinical decision maker supported by AI-assisted cognitive tools
Scalability	Limited by staff availability and manual processes	Improved scalability through intelligent automation
Ethical oversight	Primarily policy based governance	Embedded ethical safeguards human override and auditability

Another important requirement of a nursing care system is decision support that can be implemented by use of generative AI. Using AI-based systems symptoms provided by patients, their vital signs and available historical data can be analyzed. Based on this analysis potential concerns can be suggested and the ways to avoid these can be provided. Generative AI based models can integrate multiple data sources and generate contextualized recommendations, which is not possible in deterministic systems. For example, an AI-based system may identify patterns, indicating risk of deterioration. At the same time, relevant psychosocial factors reported by the patient can also be analyzed. This information can be used in providing nursing clinical reasoning without replacing professional decisions. Advanced applications now include AI-driven ill-health detection and remote risk stratification integrated with telemedicine workflows, supporting early intervention and nurse-led care planning (Badola et al., 2024).

Personalization information availability is possible in generative AI technologies. In patient information and engagement, AI-based systems can provide personalized information related to individual health conditions, literacy levels and cultural background. Technical information can be provided based on complexity and format as per patient preferences and responses. For nurses, this capability will increase the effectiveness of counseling and at the same time consistency is ensured with evidence based practice.

AI-based technologies in field of telehealth provide a number of advantages. But at the same time, these systems have certain limitations and risks. Outputs of probabilistic models are not accurate and hence may vary. In nursing, safety of patients is very crucial; therefore there is a need of human intervention. It also shows limitations of using AI-based systems. Generative AI-based systems should not be used as independent decision makers in clinical cases. These can be used as supportive tools only along with nurse led care models.

Bias is another critical concern in AI-based systems. Generative AI models learn from historical data that may reflect existing inequities in healthcare delivery. Without careful investigation and evaluation, these biases can affect AI-based decisions. As a result, patient assessment and engagement will be biased. Therefore nurses should be trained properly so that they are able to recognize such risks and make correct decision.

Transparency and explainability are also important for ethical use of generative AI in nursing care. Deep learning based models are basically complex; research is being conducted to develop user interfaces that provide information into how recommendations are generated. For nurses understanding the underlying principle behind outputs of AI-based systems supports trust and accountability. Clear documentation of AI-based processes is also necessary for legal and professional standards.

In summary, generative AI technologies are useful tools that have the capability of enhancing telehealth and smart nursing practice. By enabling conversational interaction, efficient documentation, adaptive decision support and personalized patient engagement these systems provide support to nursing expertise. However careful integration with ethical governance and continuous human interaction is required for their effective implementation. When designed keeping in mind, nursing values and professional standards, generative AI can help in providing a safer, more responsive and more sustainable healthcare delivery.

In Figure 1, a conceptual framework for integrating generative AI into telehealth nursing practice is provided.

Figure 1. Conceptual framework for integrating generative AI into telehealth nursing

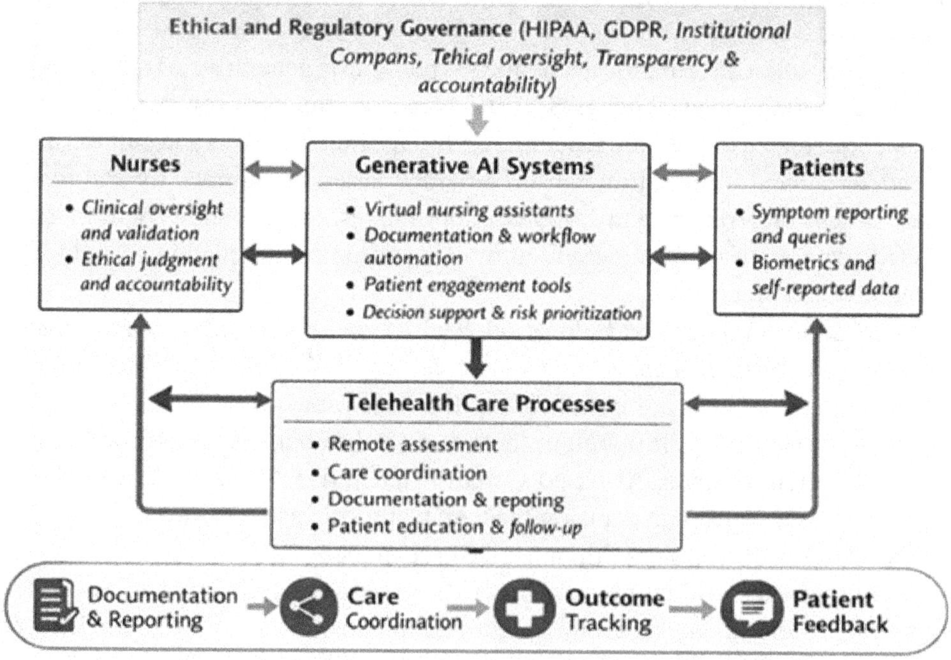

Figure 1 shows the key components involved in integrating generative AI into telehealth nursing practice. Information flows from telehealth interactions, remote monitoring devices and digital communication platforms into generative AI systems that analyze inputs and generate structured summaries and recommendations. The role of the nurses is very important as they have to review these AI generated outputs, validate their clinical relevance and integrating them to take any decision for planning of care. Nursing responsibility includes interpreting AI suggestions, identifying contextual nuances and ensuring that decisions align with clinical standards and patient values. Ethical oversight is embedded through transparency mechanisms, human supported capabilities and accountability structures that prevent autonomous AI driven decision making. Overall, the framework shows a step by step interaction in which data processing and automation are used to support rather than replace, professional nursing care.

4. VIRTUAL NURSING ASSISTANTS AND CLINICAL SUPPORT SYSTEMS

Virtual nursing assistants are developed using AI-based techniques. These virtual assistants are able to provide support through continuous interaction, assistance across telehealth and smart care environments. These systems function as digital intermediaries between patients and healthcare providers. Using these systems, scalable and responsive care can be provided while maintaining nurse supervision. In current telehealth models, virtual nursing assistants are commonly used as initial point of contact tools. These tools support nursing workflows rather than replace human care.

From a functional perspective, virtual nursing assistants perform a range of tasks including collecting patient symptoms, screening medication, reminders, appointment coordination and delivery of instructions. These tasks are traditionally time intensive for nurses but are essential to maintain care quality and continuity. By automating routine interactions, virtual assistants allow nurses to provide more time to complex assessment, clinical reasoning and therapeutic engagement.

In clinical contexts, virtual nursing assistants can support examination by collecting patient reported symptoms and contextual information prior to nurse review. Using conversational interfaces, these systems guide patients through structured yet flexible dialogues that capture relevant data while adapting to individual responses. Nurses then receive synthesized summaries that highlight key concerns and potential risks. This approach improves efficiency while preserving professional control over clinical decisions (Bickmore et al., 2018; Laranjo et al., 2018). Nursing-focused scoping reviews confirm that AI-assisted telehealth systems are able to enhance clinical documentation, triage accuracy and workflow efficiency when combined with professional supervision (Choi et al., 2023; Rutledge & Gustin, 2021). Specialized implementations of generative AI have also been done in oncology telemedicine, where conditional generative adversarial networks support personalized cancer pain management and remote symptom monitoring under clinician supervision (Cascella et al., 2023).

Case Study 1: Virtual Nursing Assistant in Chronic Disease Management

Large healthcare organizations such as Mayo Clinic and Kaiser Permanente have implemented AI-supported virtual assistants to augment nursing care in chronic disease management programs. At Mayo Clinic, conversational AI tools are being used to support symptom monitoring, patient education and follow up communication for patients with chronic conditions. In these systems, nurses review AI-generated summaries before clinical action. Similarly, Kaiser Permanente has deployed AI-enabled digital assistants within its telehealth infrastructure to assist with symptom intake; appointment preparation and post visit follow up, while maintaining nurse supervision for clinical decisions. These systems are used to collect data reported by patients through natural language interaction and transform unstructured inputs into structured summaries aligned with nursing assessment workflows. Nurses have the responsibility of validating information, identifying requirements and providing personalized clinical guidance. By applying such measures, improved workflow efficiency and patient engagement is observed, while continuing the role of nurses as supervisors of AI-supported care.

Quantitative evaluations of virtual nursing assistant system implementation further validate their clinical utility. In a large-scale implementation study, AI-assisted symptom intake systems reduced nurse documentation time by approximately 28% while maintaining clinical safety through compulsory nurse validation checkpoints (Jiang et al., 2017). Importantly, no increase in adverse events was observed in the study, showing that generative AI can safely augment nursing workflows when implemented under structured supervision models.

Virtual nursing assistants also play a role in monitoring and follow up care. In chronic disease management, these assistants can prompt patients to report symptoms, vital signs or adherence behaviors on a regular basis. Generative AI enables these systems to adjust follow up questions and instructions based on patient responses and historical patterns.

In hospital and post acute environment, virtual nursing assistants support care coordination by facilitating communication among patients, nurses and other healthcare professionals. For example, automated updates and reminders can reinforce discharge instructions and follow up appointments. Nurses remain responsible for oversight but benefit from improved continuity and reduced communication gaps.

Natural language generation and understanding models form the conversational core of virtual nursing assistants. These models are often transformer based architectures trained on large scale language data and fine tuned on healthcare specific corpora. Their function is to interpret patient input generate context appropriate responses and manage dialogue flow. In nursing applications domain adaptation and clinical validation are essential to ensure safe and relevant outputs.

Retrieval augmented generation models are increasingly employed to improve factual accuracy and explainability. In this architecture, generative models are coupled with external knowledge bases such as clinical guidelines or institutional protocols. When generating responses the system retrieves relevant information and conditions its output on verified sources. This approach reduces hallucination risk and supports evidence based nursing practice.

Multimodal generative models represent an emerging category particularly relevant to remote monitoring and telehealth. These models integrate text speech and sensor data such as vital signs or wearable device outputs. By combining modalities the system can generate more comprehensive assessments and personalized feedback. For nurses this enables richer situational awareness but also introduces complexity in validation and interpretation.

Reinforcement learning components may be used to optimize interaction strategies over time. In virtual nursing assistants reinforcement learning algorithms adjust conversational flows and engagement strategies based on feedback such as patient adherence completion rates or nurse evaluations. Ethical constraints and human oversight are essential to ensure that optimization aligns with care quality rather than purely efficiency metrics.

While virtual nursing assistants offer substantial benefits their deployment in nursing care requires careful attention to safety and reliability. Generative AI systems can produce plausible but incorrect responses if not properly constrained. In nursing contexts such errors could have significant consequences. Therefore virtual nursing assistants must operate within clearly defined scopes of practice and escalate complex or ambiguous situations to human nurses.

Validation and testing processes should involve nursing professionals throughout development and deployment. Continuous monitoring of system performance is necessary to identify drift errors or unintended behaviors. Feedback mechanisms that allow nurses to correct or flag AI outputs contribute to system learning and accountability.

Transparency is critical for both nurses and patients. Virtual nursing assistants should clearly communicate their role as supportive tools and disclose when interactions are automated. Patients should be informed about data use and have access to human support when needed. Nurses must retain authority over clinical decisions and documentation.

The integration of virtual nursing assistants reshapes nursing roles and responsibilities. Nurses increasingly function as supervisors of digital care processes in addition to direct care providers. This shift requires new competencies in evaluating AI outputs managing exceptions and ensuring ethical use. Rather than diminishing professional identity virtual nursing assistants can elevate nursing practice by reducing administrative burden and enabling focus on advanced clinical reasoning and patient relationships. However this outcome depends on governance models that recognize nursing expertise and involve nurses in system design and oversight.

In conclusion virtual nursing assistants represent a critical application of generative AI in telehealth and smart nursing. Through careful technical design, human centered integration and ethical governance these systems can enhance care delivery while preserving the central role of nursing judgment and compassion.

Similar decentralized architectures using federated learning have been proposed to strengthen data privacy while supporting scalable virtual health systems, reinforcing nurse supervision in distributed telemedicine environments (Bruggen & Sah, 2025).

5. AI-SUPPORTED PATIENT ENGAGEMENT IN SMART NURSING CARE

The quality of health outcomes and satisfaction of patients depends on patient engagement in telehealth services. Patients can be engaged in making decisions about their health and managing the requirements accordingly. Using telehealth this engagement of patient can be increased by permitting anytime interaction. Use of generative AI in area of telehealth will help in further increasing the interaction. Use of generative AI in telehealth will provide personalized adaptive support and scalable engagement.

AI-supported patient engagement techniques promote adherence, self management and continuous care. This is provided through conversational interfaces and personalized messaging facility. Research has shown improvements in patient satisfaction and engagement when such systems are carefully designed and supervised (Laranjo et al., 2018). These systems can be integrated into telehealth platforms and mobile health applications. In this way, these systems can interact with patients through conversational interfaces, reminders, guidance modules and feedback mechanisms. For nurses, AI-based engagement tools increase the reach of care while maintaining professional oversight and accountability. Large language model-based telehealth platforms further improve patient connectivity and engagement by providing user-focused interactions aligned with human-centric care delivery principles (Chaturvedi et al., 2025; Kwan, 2024).

Personalized service is another contribution provided by use of generative AI in patient engagement. Traditional systems in the area of digital health tools provide standardized content only. This is not aligned with individual patient requirements, their preferences or literacy levels. Generative AI systems have the ability to modify communication style, language complexity and guidance based on individual patient profiles and interaction history. For example, a patient having chronic conditions may be provided adaptive self management guidance that will change as their condition changes. Nurses can review and guide these patients ensuring requirement of clinical plans and patient values.

Conversational engagement is also important in providing telehealth services. Using Generative AI, natural language interaction is possible. Using this interaction in natural language, human conversation is similar to human interaction. It allows patients to ask questions, express concerns and receive timely responses. This capability is very useful for such patients who may feel hesitant to contact healthcare providers for minor concerns. AI-supported engagement can provide comfort and guidance while escalating issues that require human involvement. Role of nurses is very critical in supervising these interactions and responding to escalated cases.

Monitoring and feedback loops are also an important aspect of AI-supported engagement activities. Patients can report their symptoms, medication adherence and lifestyle behaviors through digital interfaces. Generative AI –based systems analyze these inputs and generate summaries, alerts or personalized feedback. Nurses can review these results and provide support wherever necessary. This continuous engagement model helps in early detection of problems and proactive nursing care.

Case Study 2: AI-supported Patient Engagement in Telehealth Follow-Up

In the United Kingdom, AI driven patient engagement platforms such as Babylon Health (eMed) and Ada Health have been integrated into National Health Service telehealth pathways to support symptom assessment and patient guidance. These systems use generative and probabilistic AI models to engage patients through conversational interfaces collect symptom information and provide evidence based recommendations, with escalation pathways to nurses and clinicians when risk thresholds are observed. Nurses use AI generated summaries to prioritize follow up, verify clinical relevance and coordinate care interventions. By its use, increased accessibility to health guidance and improved triage efficiency, particularly in primary care and remote settings was observed. Importantly, NHS governance frameworks require transparency, human oversight and clinical accountability, ensuring that

AI supported engagement complements professional nursing practice rather than replacing direct care relationships.

Despite these benefits, AI supported patient engagement has several challenges that require careful management. Over automation may risk depersonalization if patients perceive interactions as impersonal or intrusive. Nurses have the responsibility of balancing automatic engagement with meaningful human contact particularly for patients with complex emotional or social needs. Clear boundaries and escalation pathways are essential to maintain therapeutic relationships.

All patients don't have equal access to digital technologies. Sometimes access to digital technologies is available but they don't feel comfortable with AI-based interaction. Therefore equity is important in telehealth services. Strategies for engagement should be planned in such a way that these strategies are inclusive and adaptable to diverse populations. Again the responsibility lies with nurses to identify barriers and promote patient centered design that accommodates varying needs and preferences. AI-supported telehealth has also shown clinical value in mental health contexts, where virtual engagement platforms complement conventional care by improving access, follow-up, and continuity of psychological support (Morrish et al., 2024).

5.1 System Architecture for AI-supported Patient Engagement

From a technical point of view, AI-based patient engagement systems depend on layered architectures. These architectures combine data collection, data processing, intelligence layer and user interface components. This layered architecture will support development of systems which are reliable, safe and scalable systems and support nursing practice.

At the data layer, patient generated data is collected from input sources. These sources may be telehealth interactions, mobile applications, wearable devices and electronic health records. Types of data may be text, speech, vital signs and behavioral metrics. Secure data handling and compliance with privacy regulations need to be considered at this layer.

The data received is analyzed at the processing layer. Steps in this layer are natural language preprocessing, signal normalization and data validation. In nursing applications, this layer may also include rule based filters that identify urgent symptoms requiring immediate attention to human clinicians.

Multimodal models may be used to integrate text and physiological data to generate context aware feedback. Further, reinforcement learning may be used to optimize involvement strategies over time based on nurse and patient feedback.

The application layer connects AI capabilities to nursing workflows and patient interfaces. This layer provides interaction tools such as dashboards to review patient engagement, report summaries etc.

The governance layer access controls and performance monitoring. This layer contains audit logs. It also ensures ethical use, accountability and compliance. This includes audit logs, access controls, performance monitoring and mechanisms for human override.

The success of AI-based systems in telehealth depends on system design, ethical governance and active nurse involvement.

5.2 Quantitative Evaluation Metrics and Performance Indicators for AI-based Patient Engagement

Evaluation of the effectiveness of AI-based patient engagement systems in smart nursing should be done before implementation. For this purpose quantitative metrics can be used. These metrics should evaluate the system for clinical quality, patient experience and operational performance of the system. Systems used in healthcare must account for safety, equity and professional accountability. Nurses play a central role in interpreting these metrics and utilize the results in improvement of the services.

One primary category of evaluation metrics relates to patient engagement outcomes. These metrics are used to check the extent to which patients actively interact with AI-based systems. Common metrics in this category are engagement frequency, response completion rate, session duration and adherence to recommended use. These metrics are based on changes in symptom severity, rates of hospital readmission, emergency department utilization and disease specific clinical markers. Process and efficiency metrics evaluate the impact of AI-based engagement on nursing workflows. For this, time spent on documentation, number of patient interactions per nurse and frequency of escalations requiring human intervention can be observed. Accuracy and safety metrics are used to check the reliability of AI-based system outputs. Continuous monitoring of these indicators will help in identifying in system usefulness.

Patient experience can be used to check effectiveness of the system. Satisfaction surveys may support trust measures and perceived usefulness scores, capture patient perspectives on AI-based engagement. High satisfaction combined with positive clinical and efficiency outcomes strengthens the case for integration into nursing practice.

Key performance indicators, interpretable for clinical stakeholders are provided below.

Let N represent the total number of enrolled patients and T represent the observation period in weeks.

Patient engagement rate represents average engagement intensity across the population

$$E = (1 / N) \times \Sigma\ (I\ / T) \quad (1)$$

, where I represents the total number of completed interactions by patient i during period T.

Interaction completion ratio $C = \Sigma\ R\ / \Sigma\ P$ (2)

, where R is the number of responses submitted by patient i and P is the number of prompts issued. Values closer to 1 indicate high responsiveness.

Clinical escalation accuracy that indicates clinical relevance and safety $A = TP / (TP + FP)$ (3)

, where TP represents true positive AI escalations validated by nurses and FP represents false positives.

False negative rate $FNR = FN / (FN + TP)$ (4)

, where FN represents clinically significant events not flagged by the AI system. For patient safety, FNR should be minimized.

Nursing workload reduction $W = (D_0 - D_1) / D_0$ (5)

, where D_0 is baseline documentation time per encounter and D_1 represents documentation time with AI assistance. This ratio quantifies efficiency gains.

Equity performance index $Q = 1 - (\sigma_E / \mu_E)$ (6)

, where σ_E is the standard deviation of engagement rates across demographic subgroups and μ_E is the mean engagement rate. Higher values show more equitable engagement distribution.

In applied clinical setup, these metrics have been operationalized in pilot implementations. For example, an AI-supported telehealth follow-up program for heart failure patients reported a nursing workload reduction (W) of 0.32, corresponding to a 32% decrease in documentation time, while maintaining a false negative rate below 5% for clinical escalation events (Sendak et al., 2020). Such applications prove that the proposed formulas are not theoretical abstractions but reflect validated performance indicators used in real-world nursing practice.

Numerical values obtained through these metrics, along with qualitative nursing judgment and ethical reviews should be used to check effectiveness of the system.

5.3 Ethical Analysis of AI-based Patient Engagement Systems

Ethical issues are main concern in adoption of AI-based patient engagement systems. These systems are used to directly interact with patients and hence shape perceptions of care, responsibility autonomy and trust. These should be evaluated under the framework of nursing ethics.

Autonomy is a central ethical principle in engagement of patients with AI-based systems. AI-based systems must respect patient choice and interact responsibly. This is ethical responsibility of nurses to ensure that engagement strategies are supportive rather than directive. Patients should be able to opt out or adjust interaction preferences.

AI-based systems should support transparency. Patients should know very clearly that how their data will be used. Transparency of the system will bring honesty and respect in AI-based communication. In patient engagement systems, other significant factors are: Data privacy and confidentiality. As conversational logs, symptom reports and behavioral data may contain personal details about patients. Strong encryption, access controls and data minimizations are required to ensure data privacy and confidentiality.

A system should be free of bias and show fairness. If an engagement system is trained on limited or unrepresentative datasets, it may not cover certain populations effectively or may misinterpret cultural specific inputs of health and illness. As a result, care and engagement may be biased. Therefore for ethical deployment system performance need to be evaluated across diverse patient groups and nurses should be actively involved in identifying and addressing disparities.

Another ethical issue related to AI-based systems in nursing is responsibility and accountability, which must be defined very clearly. Emotional and relational ethics are also important in this area. There is a possibility of patients' emotional dependence on AI-based systems, if communication with such systems is frequent and personalized. Although loneliness and anxiety can be reduced by such systems, but these cannot replace human relationships. It is the responsibility of nurses to ensure that AI-based engagement complements the relationship and not a substitution of human relationships.

Finally ethical governance requires continuous supervision rather than one time approval. As AI-based systems learn and adapt their behavior may change over time. Ongoing monitoring audit mechanisms and ethical review processes are required to ensure alignment with nursing values and patient welfare. Inclusion of nurses in governance structures strengthens ethical accountability and professional authenticity. For a responsible AI-based patient engagement, quantitative evaluation and ethical analysis are important components.

5.4 Formal Evaluation Framework for AI-supported Patient Engagement

A structured evaluation framework is required for systematic assessment of AI-based patient engagement system in smart nursing. This framework should be able to integrate clinical effectiveness, operational performance, patient experience and ethical safeguards. Table 2 presents an evaluation framework for AI-based systems implementation in smart nursing.

Table 2. Evaluation framework for AI-based systems in smart nursing

Evaluation domain	Metric category	Indicator definition	Measurement method	Nursing relevance
Patient engagement	Engagement intensity	Mean number of patient system interactions per week	Interaction log analysis	Indicates sustained participation and usability
	Completion rate	Percentage of prompted interactions completed by patients	Prompt response ratio	Reflects relevance of AI-based engagement
Clinical outcomes	Readmission rate	Percentage of patients readmitted within 30 days	EHR outcome comparison	Measures effectiveness of post discharge engagement
	Symptom escalation accuracy	Concordance between AI-flagged alerts and nurse validated concerns	Nurse review audit	Supports patient safety and early intervention
Workflow efficiency	Documentation time reduction	Average reduction in nurse documentation time per encounter	Time motion studies	Indicates workload reduction and sustainability
	Escalation frequency	Proportion of AI interactions requiring nurse intervention	System logs	Reflects appropriateness of automation scope
Safety and reliability	False negative rate	Missed clinically significant events identified retrospectively	Incident review	Critical for risk management
Equity and fairness	Differential engagement rate	Engagement variation across demographic groups	Stratified data analysis	Identifies disparities in access and usability
Patient experience	Satisfaction score	Mean patient satisfaction rating	Standardized surveys	Reflects trust and acceptability
Ethical governance	Override utilization	Frequency of nurse override of AI outputs	Audit trail analysis	Indicates alignment with clinical judgment

This framework will provide help in continuous monitoring and iterative improvement of the system. It is important to note that these metrics should not be interpreted in isolation. Results of these metrics should be combined with nursing leadership and interdisciplinary governance teams within clinical realities and ethical priorities and then implemented.

5.5 Mapping Ethical Principles to Regulatory Standards

Alignment between professional ethics of nursing and regulatory frameworks governing health data and digital care is required for effective implementation of AI-based system in nursing. Table 3 maps key ethical principles to HIPAA and GDPR to support compliance oriented system design and evaluation.

Table 3. Mapping of ethical principles with HIPAA and GDPR

Ethical principle	Nursing interpretation	HIPAA alignment	GDPR alignment	Practical implication
Autonomy	Respect for patient choice and informed participation	Right to access and amend records	Lawful basis and consent requirements	Patients control engagement preferences and data use
Transparency	Honest disclosure of AI use and data handling	Notice of privacy practices	Articles 12 to 14 transparency obligations	Clear communication of AI-based interactions
Privacy and confidentiality	Protection of sensitive patient information	Privacy Rule and Security Rule	Articles 5 and 32 data protection	Secure storage encryption and access control
Accountability	Clear responsibility for care decisions	Covered entity responsibility	Controller and processor obligations	Human oversight and auditability
Fairness and non discrimination	Equitable care delivery across populations	Indirect through enforcement guidance	Article 5 fairness principle	Bias monitoring and inclusive system design
Data minimization	Collection limited to care relevant information	Minimum necessary standard	Article 5 data minimization	Avoid unnecessary data capture
Right to explanation	Ethical duty to explain care processes	Not explicit but supported by patient rights	Articles 15 and 22	Explainable AI outputs for nurses and patients

It can be observed from this mapping that ethical nursing principles and regulatory compliance are complementary to each other. If nurses are involved in compliance and governance processes, then it will strengthen ethical integrity as well as legal adherence.

6. INTEGRATION OF GENERATIVE AI INTO NURSING WORKFLOWS

Successful implementation of generative AI techniques in telehealth services depends on performance of the system and integration of these systems in regular nursing workflows. Integration of workflows decides the utility of AI-based systems. It should not be implemented in such a way that it is felt like burden on users. If technologies are not integrated correctly in existing systems then these may increase load and disrupt communication. A well designed and context aware AI-based systems in telehealth can streamline clinical processes, reduce duplication of effort and enhance decision making without compromising patient safety or professional autonomy.

Despite their potential, generative AI systems introduce significant implementation barriers. Initial implementation costs are related to infrastructure upgradation, licensing fees, cybersecurity costs, and continuous training programs, which may disproportionately affect resource-constrained healthcare organizations. It has been observed that upfront costs and unclear return on investment remain major obstacles to AI adoption in nursing environments. Additionally, staff resistance, often driven by concerns about job displacement, workflow disruption, and increased surveillance has been identified as a critical socio-organizational challenge requiring planned change management strategies. Latest reviews emphasize that successful AI-telemedicine integration depends on aligning technical innovation with nursing governance, regulatory compliance and workforce readiness (Rossi & Rehman, 2025).

Interoperability with existing electronic health record (EHR) systems represents another major constraint. Many generative AI tools operate as external platforms, leading to fragmented data flows, duplicated documentation and increased cognitive burden for nurses when integration is not seamless. Furthermore, regulatory uncertainty surrounding liability, AI-generated documentation and cross-border data processing complicates adoption, particularly as frameworks governing clinical AI continue to evolve (Topol, 2019). These realities necessitate a cautious, phased implementation approach rather than a rapid, large-scale implementation (Adler-Milstein & Huckman, 2013).

Nursing workflows in telehealth are basically complex and multitasking. Nurses have to manage many responsibilities such as remote patient assessment, clinical documentation, care coordination, patient education and emotional support on routine basis. At present, these activities are done using different online platforms and within a limited time. Using generative AI will help in reorganizing this workflow by shifting certain preparatory and administrative tasks upstream or into the background where they can be handled asynchronously.

One of the most important integration points is pre-appointment data preparation. AI-based systems can collect and provide structured patient information before scheduled telehealth visits. Using conversational natural language interfaces, these systems can guide patients through symptom reporting, medication reconciliation and articulation of concerns in their own words. Generative models then transform these unstructured input into clinically relevant summaries aligned with nursing assessment frameworks. At the time of appointment, a synthesized overview of patient status, key risks and priority questions which supports more focused and meaningful interaction is available.

It has been shown in various studies that AI-based documentation is able to reduce administrative work and cognitive load when combined with manual supervision and appropriate governance structures (Topol, 2019). In telehealth, this documentation has to be done along with patient interaction. Generative AI systems can support real time transcription of audio or video consultations followed by automated summarization into structured summary. These summaries may include patient information and follow up recommendations mapped to standardized terminologies. Earlier telehealth systems were dependent on manual data entry, different platforms for different activities and static clinical protocols that were difficult to adapt to changing patient needs. Generally such systems use large language models, trained on clinical corpora, combined with speech recognition modules and contextual prompts. The nurse has the responsibility for accuracy completeness and clinical judgment while AI-based systems increase efficiency. It has been observed that AI-assisted documentation can reduce time spent on charting and allow nurses to devote effort toward patient-related activities (Topol, 2019).

AI-based systems are also useful in distributed telehealth models. Generative AI systems can continuously combine data from remote monitoring devices, patient messages and clinical updates to generate dynamic care summaries. These summaries can help in solving serious issues and emerging risks.

Equally important is the alignment of generative AI tools with nursing decision making processes. Adaptive interfaces that learn from nurse feedback can improve relevance over time and further increase trust through collaborative interaction.

Certain organizational factors also play important role in success of workflow integration. Before implementation, nurses should be provided adequate training so that they are able to understand AI capabilities, limitations and appropriate use cases.

In summary, integration of generative AI into nursing workflows is a socio technical challenge that extends beyond model accuracy. Careful implementation is required to task sequencing information. When integration is well designed, generative AI can reduce administrative burden, enhance situational awareness and support high quality telehealth nursing care. But if not integrated properly, it may increase workload on nurses and decrease trust. Future smart nursing systems must therefore prioritize workflow compatibility as a central design principle. Figure 2 shows a workflow model for AI-supported telehealth nursing practice, showing how virtual intake nurse assessment clinical decision support and patient engagement are sequentially integrated.

Figure 2. Workflow model

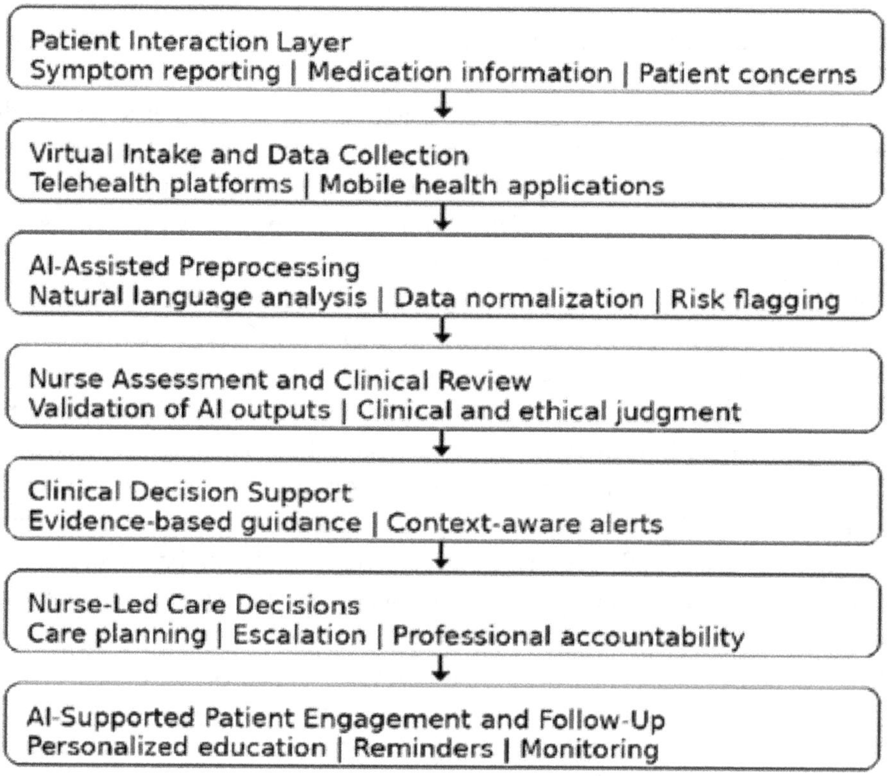

In Figure 2, a sequential workflow model showing AI-supported virtual intake, nurse assessment, clinical decision support and patient engagement integration within telehealth nursing practice is shown. The workflow begins with patient generated virtual data collection and AI-assisted preprocessing, followed by nurse review and clinical interpretation of synthesized information. Information flows bidirectionally, allowing nurses to refine AI inputs, correct inaccuracies and influence downstream recommendations. Nurses have their responsibility at each stage, particularly in validating assessments, prioritizing care needs and managing clinical escalation. Ethical oversight is maintained through pre-defined checkpoints, role boundaries and governance mechanisms that ensure role of AI in nursing decision making rather than substituting professional decisions. The model shows how workflow integration enhances efficiency while preserving accountability and patient safety.

In Figure 2, each stage corresponds to different nursing competencies, including interpretation of AI-generated summaries, critical evaluation of decision support outputs and ethical supervision of automated patient engagement. The workflow shows that how AI functions upstream and downstream of nurse decision making.

Simulation based training can be used to train nurses to prepare them for smart nursing environments. Nurses can be trained on evaluating AI-generated summaries, interpret and make decisions. Collaboration has to be established among nurses, physicians, IT professionals and administrators through training programs. For nurses this collaboration will increase confidence in communicating with technical teams and analyzing the needs of nurses in system design and evaluation.

Leadership development is essential to sustain smart nursing initiatives. Nurse leaders increasingly participate in technology selection policy development and governance structures related to AI. Training pathways should therefore prepare nurses for leadership roles in digital transformation by addressing topics such as change management health informatics, regulation and ethical oversight.

Finally, lifelong learning is a core requirement of smart nursing. Generative AI-based technologies change at fast speed. Therefore fixed training becomes obsolete. There is a need that institutions should support continuous training through modular training resources, communities of practice and access to updated guidelines. Encouraging practice around AI use will provide support to nurses in continuously refine their skills and adapt to new tools while maintaining patient centered care.

Finally, by providing nurses with conceptual understanding, practical skills, ethical awareness and leadership capacity, educational systems can ensure that smart nursing is implemented with professional judgment and concerned care.

6.3. Impact on Patient Experience and Therapeutic Relationships

Use of generative AI in telehealth and patient engagement systems has positive impact on patient experience and quality of therapeutic services. Since beginning, nursing care is defined by relational engagement having trust, empathy and mutual understanding. With the increased use of AI-based tools such as virtual assistants, automatic messaging systems and intelligent triage, concerns arise regarding the effectiveness of such intelligent systems in the effective care.

According to research related to patient experience, timely access to information and consistent communication is very important in determining satisfaction of patients. Another important factor to be considered is perceived quality of services.

Generative AI can positively affect these dimensions by increasing responsiveness and continuity of care.

Figure 3 shows an ethical governance framework that surrounds the implementation of generative AI techniques within smart nursing environments. Core components include data privacy safeguards, transparency measures, accountability structures and equity focused controls that guide system design and use. Information flows between AI systems, nursing supervision processes and organizational governance bodies to enable continuous monitoring, auditability and corrective action. Nursing responsibility within this model involves supervising AI- supported interactions, identifying ethical risks and advocating for patient centered and equitable care practices. Ethical oversight is operationalized through audit trails, clear lines of responsibility and alignment with regulatory requirements such as HIPAA and GDPR. The model emphasizes that ethical governance is an ongoing process that evolves alongside AI system learning and adaptation.

Figure 3. Ethical governance model for generative AI in smart nursing.

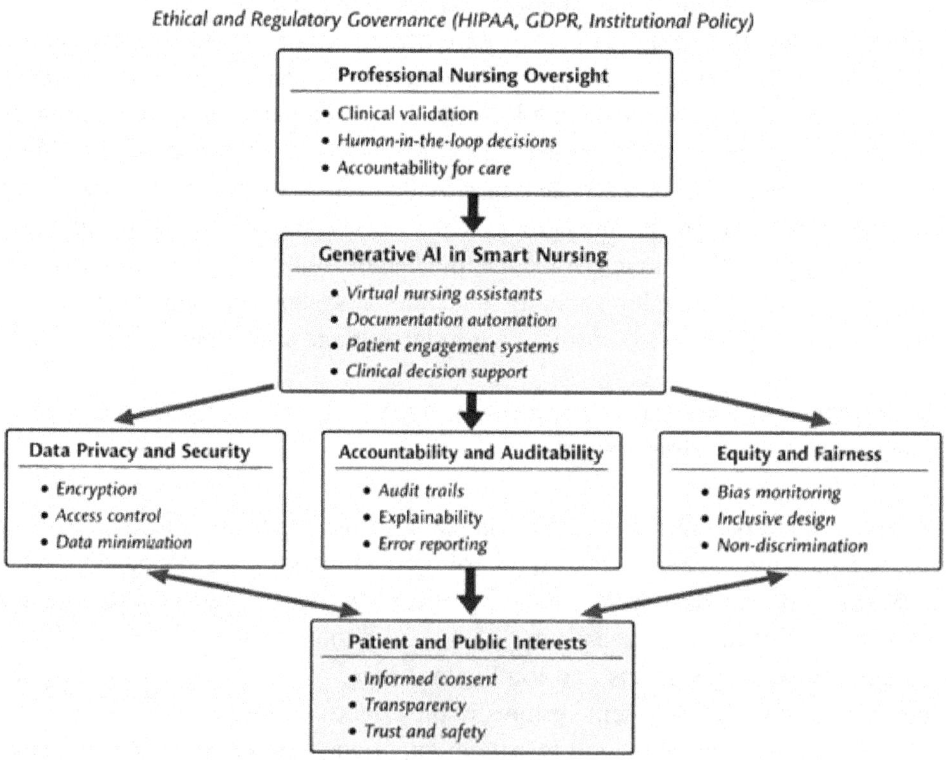

From a nursing perspective, the impact of AI on therapeutic relationships is determined by how well technology aligns with professional values. When AI reduces administrative burden and frees time for meaningful patient interaction, nurses may be better able to engage empathetically and attentively. Opposite to this, if a systems increases monitoring or force rigid interaction protocols then it may constrain relational practice and generate moral distress.

Cultural sensitivity should also be considered while implementing telehealth. Generative AI systems used for patient engagement should be able to respect linguistic, cultural and social differences of patients. Role of nurses is important in evaluating and adapting AI-supported communication to ensure cultural correspondence and relational authenticity.

In conclusion, the impact of generative AI on patient experience and remedial relationships depends on the way, governance is designed and how practice is done. If properly integrated, AI-based systems can enhance responsiveness, continuity and support. These systems can also preserve the central role of human care. By maintaining nurse views, prioritizing transparency and respecting the relational foundation of nursing practice, AI-based systems can contribute to patient experiences that are both technologically advanced and deeply humane.

Generative AI also reshapes professional identity by placing nurses as supervisors of intelligent systems rather than passive users of technology. This shift requires advanced competencies in critical appraisal, ethical reasoning and clinical judgment. When appropriately governed, AI-supported practice can strengthen professional expertise by enabling nurses to focus on complex decision-making and relational care. However, without conscious educational and governance strategies, there is a risk of deskilling and reduction in professional confidence, showing the need for theory-informed implementation models.

6.4 Practical Guidelines for Implementing Generative AI in Telehealth Nursing

Effective implementation of generative AI in telehealth nursing requires a structured, human centered approach. Organizations should begin with readiness assessments that evaluate clinical needs, digital infrastructure, data governance capacity and workforce preparedness. Clear use cases aligned with nursing workflows should be defined to avoid unnecessary automation and workflow disruption.

Training programs are essential to equip nurses with the knowledge required to interpret AI outputs, recognize limitations and exercise appropriate clinical judgment. Education should address ethical responsibilities, bias awareness and escalation protocols. Governance frameworks must establish accountability, define scopes of AI use and ensure continuous performance monitoring with mechanisms for human override.

Pilot testing, followed by phased deployment, allows refinement based on nurse feedback and patient outcomes. Ongoing evaluation using clinical, operational and equity focused metrics supports safe scaling. By prioritizing nurse involvement at every stage, generative AI systems can be integrated in ways that enhance efficiency while preserving patient centered and ethical nursing care.

6.5 Nursing Theory Integration and Professional Identity

The integration of generative AI into telehealth nursing practice must be grounded in established nursing theories to preserve professional identity and epistemic integrity. According to Watson's Theory of Human Caring, relational presence, empathy and intentionality as core components of nursing practice. When generative AI systems reduce administrative work and support informational continuity, they can indirectly enhance capacity of nurses to engage in caring relationships rather than detract from them.

Benner's Novice-to-Expert framework provides a critical view for understanding how AI influences clinical expertise development. While AI-supported decision supports may assist trainee nurses by providing support in assessment and prioritization, there is a risk that overdependence could reduce practical learning if thoughtful judgment is not done actively. Therefore, AI outputs must be considered as provisional inputs requiring interpretation, contextualization and validation by nurses at all skill levels.

From a person-centered care perspective, generative AI should be evaluated based on its ability to support individualized care planning, shared decision-making and respect for patient values. Nursing supervision ensures that algorithmic recommendations remain subordinate to holistic assessment, thereby reinforcing rather than reducing nursing independence and professional judgment.

7. FUTURE RESEARCH

Advances in generative AI techniques and their use in telehealth and patient engagement systems is increasing but still a significant research gap exists. These gaps should be addressed to ensure that smart nursing in telehealth become useful with professional accountability and ethics. Main areas for further research in this area are:

- research in interdisciplinary areas with a long term involvement

- use of explainable AI
- study of cognitive load and decision quality
- Human-AI interaction focused on nursing practice
- concerns related to equity and bias in AI-based nursing care systems
- assess impact of generative AI-based systems in access, quality and outcomes across diverse patient populations

In conclusion, the future research related to use of generative AI in smart nursing is broad and multidisciplinary. By combining experimental techniques, technical innovation and ethics, researchers can provide support in implementation of safe, effective and human centered integration of AI into nursing practice.

8. CONCLUSION

Generative AI has significant potential to transform telehealth and smart nursing practice by enhancing virtual care delivery, patient engagement and clinical workflow efficiency. Through applications such as virtual nursing assistants, AI-supported patient engagement systems and intelligent documentation tools, these technologies can reduce administrative work and support more proactive, continuous and personalized nursing care.

The successful adoption of generative AI technologies depends on careful integration within nursing workflows, strong ethical governance and sustained professional oversight. Nurses play a central role in supervising AI systems, validating outputs, addressing bias and maintaining therapeutic relationships. When designed and implemented through a human centered view, generative AI functions as a supportive tool that can strengthen, rather than diminish, nursing expertise.

Despite its promise, generative AI also presents some limitations related to accuracy, transparency, equity and evolving regulatory requirements. Continuous evaluation, interdisciplinary collaboration and adaptive training are therefore essential. Looking forward, responsible innovation guided by nursing values can ensure that generative AI contributes to more accessible, equitable and high quality healthcare delivery while preserving the foundational principles of compassionate and ethical nursing practice.

REFERENCES

Amjad, A., Kordel, P., & Fernandes, G. (2023). A review on innovation in healthcare sector (telehealth) through artificial intelligence. *Sustainability (Basel)*, *15*(8), 6655. Advance online publication. DOI: 10.3390/su15086655

Badola, A., Chauhan, R., Bhatt, C., Devliyal, S., Kumar, G., & Pillai, R. (2024). Deep learning–based frailty detection in conjunction with telemedicine. In *Proceedings of the 2024 IEEE 9th International Conference for Convergence in Technology (I2CT)* (pp. 1–7). IEEE. DOI: 10.1109/I2CT61223.2024.10544058

Benner, P. (1984). *From novice to expert: Excellence and power in clinical nursing practice.* Addison-Wesley. DOI: 10.1097/00000446-198412000-00027

Bickmore, T. W., Trinh, H., Olafsson, S., O'Leary, T. K., Asadi, R., Rickles, N. M., & Cruz, R. (2018). Patient and consumer safety risks when using conversational assistants for medical information. *Journal of Medical Internet Research*, *20*(9), e11510. DOI: 10.2196/11510 PMID: 30181110

Bruggen, S., & Sah, V. (2025). AI-driven virtual health systems integrating federated learning for decentralized telemedicine. Journal of Nano Molecular Intelligence and Virtual Health Systems. DOI: 10.70023/nmivhs.251101

Cascella, M., Scarpati, G., Bignami, E., Cuomo, A., Vittori, A., Di Gennaro, P., Crispo, A., & Coluccia, S. (2023). Utilizing an artificial intelligence framework (conditional generative adversarial network) to enhance telemedicine strategies for cancer pain management. *Journal of Anesthesia, Analgesia and Critical Care*, *3*(1), 104. Advance online publication. DOI: 10.1186/s44158-023-00104-8 PMID: 37386680

Chaturvedi, U., Chauhan, S. B., & Singh, I. (2025). The impact of artificial intelligence on remote healthcare: Enhancing patient engagement, connectivity, and overcoming challenges. *Intelligent Pharmacy*, *3*(5), 323–329. DOI: 10.1016/j.ipha.2024.12.003

Choi, J., Woo, S., & Ferrell, A. (2023). Artificial intelligence–assisted telehealth for nursing: A scoping review. *Journal of Telemedicine and Telecare*, *31*(1), 140–149. DOI: 10.1177/1357633X231167613 PMID: 37071572

Christopoulou, S. (2024). Machine learning models and technologies for evidence-based telehealth and smart care: A review. *BioMedInformatics*, *4*(1), 42. Advance online publication. DOI: 10.3390/biomedinformatics4010042

Dorsey, E. R., & Topol, E. J. (2016). State of telehealth. *The New England Journal of Medicine*, *375*(2), 154–161. DOI: 10.1056/NEJMra1601705 PMID: 27410924

Ganapathy, K., Haranath, S. P., Baez, A. A., & Scott, B. K. (2022). Telemedicine to expand access to critical care around the world. *Critical Care Clinics*, *38*(4), 809–826. DOI: 10.1016/j.ccc.2022.06.007 PMID: 36162912

Jiang, F., Jiang, Y., Zhi, H., Dong, Y., Li, H., Ma, S., Wang, Y., Dong, Q., Shen, H., & Wang, Y. (2017). Artificial intelligence in healthcare: Past, present and future. *Stroke and Vascular Neurology*, *2*(4), 230–243. DOI: 10.1136/svn-2017-000101 PMID: 29507784

Kruse, C. S., Krowski, N., Rodriguez, B., Tran, L., Vela, J., & Brooks, M. (2017). Telehealth and patient satisfaction: A systematic review and narrative analysis. *BMJ Open*, *7*(8), e016242. DOI: 10.1136/bmjopen-2017-016242 PMID: 28775188

Kwan, H. Y. (2024). User-focused telehealth powered by LLMs: Bridging the gap between technology and human-centric care delivery. In *Proceedings of the International Conference on Cognitive Computing and Artificial Intelligence* (pp. 187–191). IEEE. DOI: 10.1109/CCAI61966.2024.10603150

Laranjo, L., Dunn, A. G., Tong, H. L., Kocaballi, A. B., Chen, J., Bashir, R., Surian, D., Gallego, B., Magrabi, F., Lau, A. Y. S., & Coiera, E. (2018). Conversational agents in healthcare a systematic review. *Journal of the American Medical Informatics Association : JAMIA*, *25*(9), 1248–1258. DOI: 10.1093/jamia/ocy072 PMID: 30010941

Morrish, D., Zayat, N., & Hoskins, I. A. (2024). Use of telehealth as an adjunct to conventional mental health care. *Obstetrics and Gynecology Clinics of North America*, *52*(1), 67–79. DOI: 10.1016/j.ogc.2024.09.006 PMID: 39880567

Ndirangu-Mugo, E., Barros, L. M., Mutwiri, B. D., Shumba, C. S., Waweru, B., & Siika, W. W. (2022). Current state of critical care nursing worldwide. *Critical Care Clinics*, *38*(4), 657–693. DOI: 10.1016/j.ccc.2022.06.014 PMID: 36162904

Ramkumar, P., Kunze, K., Haeberle, H., Karnuta, J., Luu, B., Nwachukwu, B., & Williams, R. (2020). Clinical and research medical applications of artificial intelligence. *Arthroscopy*. Advance online publication. DOI: 10.1016/j.arthro.2020.08.009 PMID: 32828936

Rintyarna, B., Insantuan, O., Widiawati, I., & Purwoko, R. (2023). Telehealth in remote areas: A new artificial intelligence–based model. *The International Journal of Science in Society*, *5*(4), 243–254. Advance online publication. DOI: 10.54783/ijsoc.v5i4.782

Rossi, M., & Rehman, S. (2025). Integrating artificial intelligence into telemedicine: Evidence, challenges, and future directions. *Cureus*, *17*, e90829. Advance online publication. DOI: 10.7759/cureus.90829 PMID: 40988810

Rutledge, C., & Gustin, T. (2021). Preparing nurses for roles in telehealth: Now is the time! *Online Journal of Issues in Nursing*, *26*(1). Advance online publication. DOI: 10.3912/OJIN.Vol26No01Man03

Sendak, M. P., Gao, M., Brajer, N., & Balu, S. (2020). Presenting machine learning model information to clinical end users with model facts labels. *NPJ Digital Medicine*, *3*(41), 41. Advance online publication. DOI: 10.1038/s41746-020-0253-3 PMID: 32219182

Topol, E. (2019). *Deep medicine: How artificial intelligence can make healthcare human again*. Basic Books.

Topol, E. (2019). High-performance medicine: The convergence of human and artificial intelligence. *Nature Medicine*, *25*(1), 44–56. DOI: 10.1038/s41591-018-0300-7 PMID: 30617339

Totten, A. M., Womack, D. M., Eden, K., McDonagh, M., Griffin, J., Grusing, S., & Hersh, W. (2016). Telehealth: Mapping the evidence for patient outcomes from systematic reviews. Europe PMC (PubMed Central). https://europepmc.org/article/MED/27536752

U.S. Department of Health and Human Services. (2013). *HIPAA privacy rule*.

Watson, J. (2008). *Nursing: The philosophy and science of caring* (Rev. ed.). University Press of Colorado.

Witkowska-Zimny, M. (2025). Telemedicine/telehealth in smart hospital care. In *Smart hospital technologies* (pp. 251–264). DOI: 10.1016/B978-0-443-34226-4.00013-7

Chapter 12
Generative Artificial Intelligence in Advanced Clinical Nursing:
Ethics, Education, and Clinical Judgement

Hasan H Alsararatee
http://orcid.org/0000-0003-4252-8201
Northampton General Hospital, UK & Buckingham New University, UK

ABSTRACT

This chapter explores the implications of generative artificial intelligence for advanced clinical nursing practice, with a focus on clinical judgement, professional education, leadership, and ethical governance. The chapter per the authors critically explores how generative artificial intelligence is being integrated into healthcare systems and its potential role in supporting clinical reasoning, documentation, care coordination, and educational practice within advanced nursing roles. Drawing on international research evidence and national and global policy frameworks, the chapter evaluates both the opportunities and limitations of AI-enabled nursing practice. Particular attention is given to challenges related to automation bias, data governance, equity, and professional accountability, alongside the absence of nursing-specific regulatory guidance. The chapter concludes by offering evidence-informed recommendations to support responsible, human-centred adoption of generative artificial intelligence while safeguarding professional judgement, patient safety, and public trust.

DOI: 10.4018/979-8-3373-8247-0.ch012

GENERATIVE ARTIFICIAL INTELLIGENCE AND THE TRANSFORMATION OF ADVANCED CLINICAL NURSING PRACTICE

The widely used of artificial intelligence (AI) within the healthcare sector has become a defining feature of modern service transformation, as its extending the technological innovation into professional identity, clinical reasoning, and ethical accountability (Poalelungi et al., 2023). Recently, attention has increasingly shifted from the rule-based AI models towards the generative AI (GenAI) to produce a new generative outputs such as text and clinical notes, as well as some simulated scenarios through complicated pattern recognition (World Health Organization (WHO), 2021). This shift has significant implications for nursing, particularly for whose roles require complex decision making (Buchanan et al., 2020).

In fact, the healthcare system is currently under pressure from workforce shortages, rising patient awareness and with increasing expectations of efficiency and documentation quality (Raghavan, 2025). In addition, more stress was resulting from the COVID-19 pandemic and its ongoing impact on workforce capacity and population health needs (Organisation for Economic Co-operation and Development, 2023). For example, in the United Kingdom (UK), these pressures are extensively documented within national workforce and digital transformation strategies for improving productivity and care coordination while maintaining patient safety (NHS England, 2025a; NHS England, 2025b). National policy in England has clearly promoted advanced practice as a way for workforce sustainability and service redesign (NHS England, 2025c). This integration of GenAI within these roles therefore raises questions that extend beyond functional efficiency to include how professional judgement is formed and governed within such advanced practice.

While early primary studies suggest that AI tools may help medical professionals with clinical documentation, the majority of this context is medically or technically oriented, with limited attention to particularly nursing-specific implications (Topol, 2019; Kelly et al., 2019). There are limited research studies exploring the impact of GenAI in shaping the advanced clinical reasoning as well as the regulatory expectations. Accordingly, this gap is particularly concerning given the rapid commercial deployment of GenAI tools within healthcare environments. Since in an international level, global policy bodies have begun to articulate principles for the ethical governance of AI in health.

Interestingly, that WHO has emphasised the need for human-centred AI that promotes transparency, accountability, equity, and patient safety, while explicitly cautioning against the uncritical adoption of opaque or poorly regulated systems (WHO, 2021). These principles align closely with nursing values, yet their translation into advanced nursing practice remains uneven. Professional nursing organisations have acknowledged the importance of digital competence and informatics capability, but explicit guidance on generative AI within clinical nursing contexts is still emerging (International Council of Nurses, 2021).

Clinical decision-making in nursing has long been conceptualised as a complex, situated process involving the integration of empirical evidence, patient narratives, professional experience, and ethical reasoning (Thompson and Dowding, 2009). On the other side, Generative AI tools, work through statistical and prediction formulas rather than understanding, producing outputs that may appear authoritative without auditing it through the moral agency (Floridi et al., 2018). For example, in UK, the professional accountability for nursing practice is clearly articulated by the Nursing and Midwifery Council, whose Code places explicit responsibility on registrants for clinical decision-making, record keeping and patient safety (Nursing and Midwifery Council, 2018).

Furthermore, the education represents a domain in which generative AI (GenAI) intersects with advanced nursing practice. For example, postgraduate nursing education increasingly incorporates digital technologies, simulation as well as blended learning for workforce development and lifelong learning (Da Silva Tiago and Mitchell, 2024). Generative AI offers new possibilities for personalised feedback, simulated clinical encounters, and structured reflective learning. However, emerging literature highlights risks relating to academic integrity, superficial engagement with complex material, and over-reliance on automated outputs, particularly at postgraduate level where critical thinking and epistemic reflexivity are central learning outcomes (Ajjawi et al., 2024). However, concerns regarding data governance, consent, algorithmic bias are not abstract technical issues but have direct consequences for patient safety and equity (Zhang and Zhang, 2023). Since the evidence from health informatics research demonstrates that AI tools can be trained on unreliable datasets that may disproportionately affecting marginalised populations (Obermeyer et al., 2019).

This chapter is situated within such intersecting clinical, educational as well as ethical debates. In this we adopt a nursing-centred perspective that conceptualises using the GenAI as a socio-technical intervention that reshapes professional practice and the accountability structures, rather than as a neutral efficiency tool. By integrating empirical literature, national and international policy frameworks, and professional standards. Moreover, this chapter seeks to provide a critical yet practice-informed analysis on engaging the AI responsibly within advanced nursing roles.

GENAI AND CLINICAL DECISION-MAKING IN NURSING

Clinical decision-making is one of the core of advanced nursing practice and that represents the most professionally sensitive domains that are affected by using

GenAI (Alruwaili et al., 2025). Previous decision support systems were relied on only rule-based, the GenAI algorithms, are capable of synthesising large volumes of unstructured dataset and producing a narrative output like typical a clinical reasoning. Thus, the advanced clinical nursing decision-making is widely recognised as a non-linear process that integrates biomedical data, patient experience, related awareness information, as well as professional judgement (Barnard, 2019).

Interestingly, the nursing literature has consistently demonstrated that clinical decisions are shaped not only by evidence and guidelines but also by experiential knowledge, situational awareness, and ethical sensitivity developed through practice experience. GenAI systems, by contrast, derive outputs from statistical correlations within training data rather than from embodied clinical experience or moral reasoning.

On the hand, the Large Language Models (LLMs) have demonstrated the potential in summarising patients' histories with synthesising it from electronic health records (EHRs) (Nazi and Peng, 2024. However, early evaluations suggest that artificial intelligence-assisted summarisation may improve information retrieval and reduce time spent navigating fragmented records (Kelly et al., 2019). Though, the translation of these capabilities into safe nursing practice is far from straightforward. A central risk associated with AI-supported diagnostic reasoning is automation bias, particularly when they appear convincing or aligning with existing expectations (Subasri et al., 2025). Evidence from human factors research demonstrates that even experienced clinicians may defer to automated recommendations, especially under conditions of time pressure or cognitive fatigue (Goddard et al., 2012).

Furthermore, the clinical documentation represents another domain in which GenAI is increasingly promoted as a solution to professional workload pressures (Assayed, 2025; Pelletier et al., 2025). Nurses, particularly those in advanced roles, spend substantial proportions of their working time on documentation, audit, and reporting, often at the expense of direct patient care. Documentation burden has been widely identified across international health systems as a contributor to clinician burnout, reduced job satisfaction, and workflow inefficiency, with excessive time spent on administrative tasks associated with electronic health records linked to increased burnout among healthcare professionals (Wu et al., 2024; Apathy et al., 2022). Generative AI tools capable of drafting clinical notes, discharge summaries, and referral letters are therefore framed as mechanisms to enhance productivity and standardisation (Stanford and Sorensen, 2025).

The Nursing and Midwifery Council Code makes explicit that registrants are personally responsible for the content and accuracy of records of the tools that used to generate them (Nursing and Midwifery Council, 2018). Thus, applying GenAI within the clinical summarisation also raises epistemic concerns regarding what information is prioritised and what is omitted (Barak-Corren et al., 2024). AI algorithms especially in using Transformer technology operate through probabilistic weighting of patterns within data, which may privilege biomedical indicators over psychosocial factors that are central to nursing assessment. Infact, there is emerging evidence that using Ai algorithms in clinical summarisation can underrepresent social determinants of health and contextual complexity, particularly when these all are less consistently with the structured data fields (Obermeyer et al., 2019).

Moreover, communication in healthcare is not limited to the transfer of information; it involves shared understanding, professional judgement and ethical reflection, consistent with the NMC Code's emphasis on clear, compassionate and person-centred practice (NMC, 2018). The question of accountability is particularly salient when generative AI influences clinical decisions. Not like the traditional decision support tools, generative systems often lack transparency regarding how outputs are produced, a characteristic commonly described as the black box problem. This opacity challenges established norms of clinical governance, which rely on traceability, justification, and peer review. International policy frameworks, including those articulated by the WHO, emphasise the importance of explainability and human oversight in artificial intelligence-supported healthcare (WHO, 2021).

Since, the GenAI models are trained on historical datasets that may reflect an inequity in healthcare access. In reference to to different research studies that are demonstrated that AI algorithms that are used in health system management have reproduced racial and socioeconomic biases that are leading to differential treatment recommendations (Obermeyer et al., 2019). For advanced nursing practice, which is explicitly aligned with principles of equity and patient advocacy, uncritical use of such systems risks perpetuating structural injustice.

According to the Topol Review highlighted that digital tools should augment rather than just replace the human expertise which can that enable clinicians and all medical professionals to understand the limitations as well as the capabilities of AI (Topol, 2019).

APPLICATIONS OF GENERATIVE AI IN ADVANCED AND SPECIALIST NURSING ROLES

Advanced and specialist nursing roles have expanded significantly across healthcare systems in response to workforce shortages, increasing clinical complexity, and policy-driven service redesign (Kelly et al., 2025). In the UK, advanced practitioners are expected to work autonomously across clinical assessment, diagnosis, treatment, and leadership domains, as articulated within the Multi-professional Framework for Advanced Practice in England (NHS England, 2025c). The introduction of generative AI into these roles must therefore be examined not as a generic technological intervention, but in relation to the specific cognitive, ethical, and organisational responsibilities that characterise advanced nursing practice. One area in which generative AI is increasingly proposed is acute and urgent care, where advanced nurse practitioners frequently manage undifferentiated presentations under conditions of time pressure and diagnostic uncertainty. Studies in emergency and acute medicine indicate that AI and clinical decision support systems can enhance information synthesis, prioritisation, and workflow optimisation under conditions of high data volume and cognitive load, supporting clinicians with triage, disease risk prediction, and rapid decision-making in emergency departments (Amiot and Potier, 2025; Farrokhi et al., 2025; Ip et al., 2024). However, the majority of these studies focus on physician decision-making or system-level optimisation rather than nursing-specific applications. Where nursing roles are included, the evidence suggests that AI may assist with triage documentation and clinical summarisation (Siira et al., 2025), but does not replace the need for expert clinical assessment and judgement (Longoni et al., 2019).

For advanced nursing practitioners, diagnostic reasoning involves more than pattern recognition. It requires interpretation of symptom narratives, assessment of risk in context, and negotiation of uncertainty with patients and multidisciplinary teams. Generative AI systems may offer probabilistic differential diagnoses based on symptom clusters, yet these outputs are derived from aggregated data rather than from individualised clinical encounters. Research in diagnostic safety indicates that over-reliance on algorithmic suggestions may reduce diagnostic vigilance, particularly for atypical presentations or rare conditions (Alharbi et al., 2025). This is particularly relevant for nursing practice, where patients may present later in illness trajectories or with socially mediated barriers to care that are not readily captured by algorithmic models. In the management of long-term conditions, advanced nursing roles frequently involve complex decision-making across pharmacological management, self-management education, and coordination of multidisciplinary care. Digital health innovations, including mobile health and telehealth platforms, have been widely implemented for chronic disease management and significantly support continuity of care, patient monitoring, and engagement in self-management behaviours across conditions such as diabetes and cardiovascular disease (Pong et al., 2024). However, systematic reviews indicate that evidence for artificial intelligence-driven decision support in long-term condition management remains heterogeneous and context-dependent, with limited high-quality studies demonstrating sustained clinical benefit (Jiang et al., 2017). For advanced nursing practitioners, this underscores the need for cautious integration of generative artificial intelligence, ensuring that algorithmic outputs complement rather than displace relational and educational aspects of care.

Care coordination and multidisciplinary communication represent further domains in which generative AI may influence advanced nursing practice (Wangpitipanit et al., 2024). Advanced practitioners often act as clinical integrators, synthesising information across professional boundaries and facilitating continuity of care. Artificial intelligence-generated summaries and handovers may improve standardisation and reduce information loss during transitions of care, a persistent patient safety concern (Marshall et al., 2025). However, Qualitative and sociotechnical research on clinical handover emphasises that safe information transfer depends on shared situational awareness, context-sensitive interpretation of information, and collective professional judgement, rather than mere completeness of data alone (Sujan et al., 2014; Eggins and Slade, 2015). Generative AI systems, which prioritise efficiency and pattern consistency, may struggle to capture these relational and contextual dimensions. In specialist nursing roles, such as oncology, frailty, palliative care, and mental health, the ethical implications of generative AI become particularly asserted. These fields involve complex value-laden decisions, prognostic uncertainty, and emotionally charged conversations. Evidence from palliative and end-of-life care research highlights the centrality of human presence, narrative understanding, and moral sensitivity in clinical decision-making (Alanazi et al., 2024). While generative AI may assist with symptom documentation or guideline synthesis, there is limited evidence to support its use in ethically complex decision-making contexts. Indeed, concerns have been raised that algorithmic framing of prognosis or treatment options may inadvertently narrow conversations or reinforce biomedical priorities at the expense of patient values (Floridi et al., 2018).

From an organisational perspective, generative AI is often promoted as a tool to enhance productivity and address workforce pressures. NHS England has explicitly linked digital innovation to workforce sustainability and service efficiency (NHS England, 2020a). However, organisational research cautions that technological interventions introduced without attention to professional roles and workflows may generate unintended consequences, including work intensification and erosion of professional autonomy (Greenhalgh et al., 2017). For advanced nursing roles, which are already subject to role ambiguity and variable recognition across organisations, the uncritical adoption of generative AI risks further destabilising professional boundaries and expectations. Leadership and governance responsibilities are integral to advanced and consultant nursing roles, particularly in relation to quality improvement, patient safety, and service development. Policy frameworks at both national and international levels emphasise the need for clinical leadership in digital transformation. The WHO global strategy on digital health explicitly identifies the importance of professional engagement and governance in AI adoption (WHO, 2021). Advanced nursing leaders are therefore positioned not only as users of generative AI but as key stakeholders in its evaluation, implementation, and oversight. This requires critical engagement with evidence, rather than acceptance of vendor-driven narratives regarding efficiency and innovation.

Despite growing enthusiasm for GenAI, there remains a lack of robust nursing-led empirical research studies in evaluating its impact on advanced practice outcomes. Some reviews of AI in healthcare highlight methodological limitations such as small sample sizes, limited consideration of professional and ethical dimensions (Nagendran et al., 2020). For advanced nursing practice, this evidentiary gap is significant. Decisions regarding adoption are often made at organisational or policy levels without sufficient attention to how generative AI (GenAI) reshapes the clinical work as well as the patient experience. The European Union AI Act proposes risk-based regulation, classifying clinical AI systems as high-risk technologies requiring rigorous oversight (European Commission, 2021).

GENERATIVE AI IN NURSING EDUCATION AND PROFESSIONAL DEVELOPMENT

Nowadays, the national and international policy frameworks consistently emphasise the importance of advanced education and reflective competence for nurses who operating at higher levels of autonomy (NHS England, 2025c; International Council of Nurses, 2021). Generative AI (GenAI) is increasingly being integrated within the higher education environments, including postgraduate health programmes using tools for supporting content generation, simulation as well as for academic writing (Preiksaitis and Rose, 2023). However, the pedagogical implications of generative AI (GenAI) are particularly in relation to advanced practice education, where the development of critical reasoning, epistemic judgement as well as ethical reflexivity is paramount (Astbury et al., 2025).

Simulation-based education represents one of the most frequently cited areas of potential benefit. High-fidelity simulation is well established as an effective pedagogical approach in advanced nursing education, supporting the development of clinical reasoning, communication skills, and confidence in managing complex scenarios (Cant and Cooper, 2017). Recent empirical research comparing AI-enhanced virtual reality simulations with traditional simulation modalities found that AI-VR environments including the metaverse tools offer learners immersive and intuitive practice experiences that support engagement and perceived realism in clinical training contexts, complementing simulation pedagogy and contributing to learner confidence and skill development (Harder, 2025). Reflective practice is another domain in which generative AI is increasingly utilised. Reflection is a cornerstone of advanced nursing education and professional regulation, underpinning revalidation, supervision, and continuous professional development (Nursing and Midwifery Council, 2019). Generative AI tools capable of prompting reflective questions or summarising learning experiences are often marketed as supports for reflective learning. While such tools may assist learners in structuring reflections, educational research cautions that automated reflection risks promoting formulaic responses rather than deep critical engagement (Ryan, 2013). In terms of the assessment, the capacity of generative AI (GenAI) produce coherent academic text has raised significant concerns regarding authorship, originality, and the validity of assessment outcomes (Da Silva Tiago and Mitchell, 2024). While some argue that AI should be integrated transparently as a learning tool, others caution that its use risks masking deficits in understanding, particularly in advanced programmes where students are expected to demonstrate independent critical analysis. Professional regulators and educational bodies have begun to respond to these challenges. In the UK, the Quality Assurance Agency and Higher Education (2023) has issued guidance emphasising the need for clear policies on AI use, academic integrity, and assessment design. However, there remains limited profession-specific guidance addressing how generative AI should be used within advanced nursing education. This absence is problematic, given that advanced practice programmes are explicitly linked to regulatory recognition, credentialing, and patient safety. Without clear guidance, there is a risk of inconsistent practice across institutions, potentially undermining the credibility of advanced nursing qualifications. However, systematic reviews of digital decision support tools indicate that access to information alone does not reliably translate into improved clinical practice, particularly when tools are not embedded within reflective and supervised learning processes (Ivers et al., 2012). For advanced practitioners, the risk is that generative AI may encourage passive consumption of synthesised information rather than active engagement with primary evidence. Since, understanding the information always depends on the accuracy of AI and Natural Language processing (NLP) models (Assayed et al., 2025).

However, accessing to generative AI (GenAI) tools is uneven across institutions and regions, reflecting broader digital divides within higher education as well as within different healthcare systems (UNESCO, 2023). Accordingly, there is a risk that differential access to advanced educational technologies may exacerbate existing inequalities in educational attainment and professional progression.

Internationally, policy bodies have emphasised the need for digital literacy as a core professional competence for healthcare practitioners. The WHO global strategy on digital health explicitly identifies education and workforce development as critical enablers of ethical and effective AI adoption (WHO, 2021). There is also a need to consider the impact of generative AI on professional identity formation. Advanced nursing education is not solely about knowledge acquisition but about the development of professional confidence, leadership identity, and moral agency. Sociological research on professional education highlights that identity formation occurs through struggle with uncertainty, feedback from peers and mentors, and engagement with complex practice dilemmas (Trede et al., 2012). Over-reliance on generative AI risks smoothing these productive tensions, potentially producing practitioners who are technically competent but less comfortable with ambiguity and ethical complexity.

From a governance perspective, nurse educators and academic leaders bear responsibility for ensuring that generative AI is integrated into education in ways that align with professional standards and public trust. This requires explicit policies on acceptable use, transparent communication with students, and assessment strategies that prioritise reasoning processes over polished outputs. Emerging research on assessment design in the age of generative AI emphasises that adopting strategies such as interactive oral assessments, case-based evaluations, and tasks requiring higher-order reasoning can mitigate risks to academic integrity by foregrounding skills that are less susceptible to automated generation and require demonstration of authentic learner understanding (Nikolic et al., 2025). Such approaches align well with advanced nursing education, which values professional articulation and clinical justification.

ETHICAL, LEGAL, AND PROFESSIONAL CONSIDERATIONS IN THE USE OF GENERATIVE AI IN ADVANCED NURSING PRACTICE

Ethical nursing practice is grounded in respect for autonomy, justice, and accountability. These principles are articulated consistently across professional codes, including the Nursing and Midwifery Council Code in the UK and the International Council of Nurses Code of Ethics (Nursing and Midwifery Council, 2018; International Council of Nurses, 2021). Generative AI (GenAI) introduces ethical tensions across each of these domains, particularly in relation to transparency, bias, and responsibility for decision-making.

Thereby, Transparency is a core ethical requirement in healthcare, supporting patient trust as well as professional accountability. However, generative AI systems are widely characterised by algorithmic opacity, commonly referred to as the black box problem (Floridi et al., 2018). In advanced nursing practice, where practitioners are expected to articulate and defend their clinical decisions to patients, colleagues, and regulators, reliance on non-explainable systems poses a fundamental ethical dilemma. The WHO explicitly cautions that AI systems used in healthcare must be explainable and subject to meaningful human oversight, particularly where clinical decisions carry significant risk (WHO, 2021). In fact, bias and equity represent further ethical challenges, as substantial empirical evidence shows that AI systems trained on historical healthcare data can reproduce and amplify existing structural inequalities, including racial, gender, and socioeconomic bias, with models often misestimating risk and disadvantaging marginalised groups (Obermeyer et al., 2019; Colacci et al., 2025). Such biases are not only technical artefacts but reflect broader inequities embedded within health systems. For nursing, a profession with a long-standing commitment to advocacy and social justice, the ethical implications are substantial. Advanced practitioners frequently care for populations experiencing health inequities, and algorithmically biased outputs may distort risk assessment, treatment recommendations, or access to services. Ethical practice therefore requires not only awareness of bias but active resistance to its normalisation through technological mediation.

In UK, patient data use is governed by data protection legislation, including the UK General Data Protection Regulation and the Data Protection Act 2018, which impose strict requirements for lawful processing, minimisation, and security; however, empirical analysis indicates that legal and information governance frameworks face challenges in the context of AI-mediated health data use, with concerns about data privacy, oversight, and compliance when deploying generative AI tools across clinical environments (Jones et al., 2023; Tung, 2025). Consent represents a related ethical issue. Ethical consent in healthcare requires that patients understand how their data are used and how decisions affecting their care are made. Where generative AI contributes to clinical decision-making or documentation, patients may be unaware of its involvement. The WHO and UNESCO both emphasise that transparency regarding AI use is essential to maintaining public trust (WHO, 2021; UNESCO, 2023). In advanced nursing practice, failure to disclose the use of generative AI may undermine ethical obligations to honesty and respect for persons, particularly in contexts involving vulnerability or diminished capacity.

Professional accountability remains a defining concern, So the regulatory frameworks are explicit that responsibility for clinical decisions cannot be delegated to technology. The Nursing and Midwifery Council Code states unequivocally that registrants are accountable for their actions and decisions, including those supported by digital systems (Nursing and Midwifery Council, 2018). This point is echoed internationally, with regulatory and policy bodies consistently asserting that AI must augment rather than replace human judgement (WHO, 2021). For advanced nursing practitioners, whose roles involve diagnostic authority and independent prescribing, the legal implications of AI-supported errors are significant. Current legal frameworks offer limited clarity regarding liability when harm arises from decisions influenced by generative artificial intelligence, placing practitioners at potential risk. At a policy level, international regulatory responses to AI in healthcare are evolving but remain uneven. The European Union AI Act proposes a risk-based regulatory approach, categorising clinical AI systems as high-risk technologies subject to stringent oversight, transparency requirements, and post-market monitoring (European Commission, 2021). While this framework offers important safeguards, it does not explicitly address profession-specific issues related to nursing scope of practice, accountability, or education. In the UK, AI governance is currently fragmented across regulatory bodies, with limited nursing-specific guidance on generative systems (NHS England, 2025d). This regulatory ambiguity places a disproportionate burden on individual practitioners and organisations to interpret ethical and legal responsibilities.

Sociological research indicates that public trust in healthcare professionals is sensitive to perceptions of technological over-reach and depersonalisation of care (Greenhalgh et al., 2017). The uncritical adoption of generative artificial intelligence, particularly in contexts that involving sensitive communication or ethical complexity, risks can affect negatively this trust. Advanced nursing practitioners, as visible clinical leaders, play a crucial role in mediating the relationship between technological innovation and public confidence.

PREPARING NURSE LEADERS FOR AI-ENABLED HEALTHCARE

The integration of GenAI within healthcare domain necessitates a reconceptualization of leadership within advanced nursing practice (Sullivan et al., 2024). Nurse leaders, particularly those who are operating at advanced and consultant levels, are increasingly expected to shape the digital transformation while a safeguarding the patient safety and ethical integrity. National and international policy consistently positions clinical leadership as a critical enabler of safe and effective digital innovation, yet practical evidence suggests that many healthcare leaders feel underprepared to govern AI technologies in practice (Topol, 2019; WHO, 2021, NHS England, 2025d). This preparedness gap is especially consequential for nursing, given the profession's central role in care delivery and public trust. Advanced nursing leadership encompasses responsibility for clinical governance, workforce development, quality improvement, and service redesign.

Digital literacy is frequently cited as a prerequisite for effective leadership in technologically mediated healthcare (Campanozzi et al., 2023). However, policy and scholarly literature increasingly emphasise that digital literacy extends beyond functional competence to include critical appraisal, ethical reasoning, and understanding of data governance (WHO, 2021).

Workforce implications are another critical leadership consideration, as GenAI is often framed as a solution to workload pressures (Cohran, 2025); however, organisational and sociotechnical studies caution that technological interventions frequently redistribute rather than reduce work, creating new forms of cognitive burden and supervisory labour as clinicians are required to interpret, verify, and manage complex system outputs (Sutton et al., 2020; Borycki et al., 2023; Sittig and Singh, 2010). Professional development and capability building are central to sustainable leadership in AI-enabled healthcare. The Topol Review highlighted the need for structured education and training to support clinicians in understanding and using AI responsibly (Topol, 2019). However, evidence suggests that existing leadership development programmes rarely address AI explicitly, particularly from a nursing perspective (Car et al., 2019). For advanced nursing leaders, this represents a gap in preparation that risks leaving strategic decisions to technical or managerial actors without sufficient clinical insight. Leadership development must therefore integrate AI literacy with nursing ethics, regulation, and professional identity.

Research on digital health implementation highlights the importance of clinical leadership in mediating these relationships and ensuring that patient care priorities remain central (Sendak et al., 2020). Nurse leaders are uniquely positioned to advocate for nursing perspectives within these collaborations, particularly in relation to holistic assessment, continuity of care, and patient experience. Failure to assert this leadership risks marginalising nursing contributions in AI-driven service redesign. From a policy perspective, international frameworks increasingly recognise the importance of leadership in ethical AI governance. The WHO and UNESCO both emphasise that healthcare leaders must be accountable for ensuring that AI aligns with human rights, equity, and professional values (WHO, 2021; UNESCO, 2023). However, these frameworks remain largely aspirational and do not provide detailed guidance for profession-specific leadership roles. In the absence of such guidance, nurse leaders must exercise interpretive judgement, balancing innovation with caution and professional responsibility.

Public trust is an additional dimension of leadership responsibility. Nursing's social contract is predicated on ethical conduct, transparency, and patient advocacy. Evidence suggests that public confidence in AI in healthcare is contingent on perceptions of professional oversight and accountability (Longoni et al., 2019). Nurse leaders, as visible representatives of the profession, play a key role in communicating how generative AI is used, how risks are managed, and how patient interests are protected. This communicative function is integral to maintaining trust in increasingly technologised care environments.

FUTURE DIRECTIONS AND PRACTICE RECOMMENDATIONS FOR GENERATIVE AI IN ADVANCED NURSING

The future integration of GenAI within advanced nursing practice must be approached as a careful and evidence-informed process rather than just as technological progression. For advanced nursing practice, future directions must therefore prioritise professional governance, ethical integrity as well as patient-centred outcomes over technological novelty.

There is a clear need for nurse-led research programmes that evaluate GenAI systematically within advanced practice contexts. Such research should employ mixed methods designs that capture both quantitative and qualitative methods of practitioners and patients. International policy bodies, including the WHO, have explicitly called for context-sensitive evaluation of digital health interventions, recognising that technological effectiveness is shaped by organisational culture and professional practice (WHO, 2021). While existing regulatory and policy frameworks increasingly articulate high-level ethical principles for artificial intelligence, these instruments offer limited operational clarity for practitioners, particularly in relation to professional accountability, scope of practice, and clinical governance. This limitation is evident internationally, where organisations such as the WHO and UNESCO emphasise transparency, human oversight, and ethical use of AI but stop short of providing profession-specific guidance for nursing practice (WHO, 2021; UNESCO, 2023).

Practice recommendations must emphasise that GenAI should augment, not replace, professional judgement. Evidence from human factors research demonstrates that clinicians are susceptible to automation bias, particularly when systems are perceived as authoritative (Goddard et al., 2012). To mitigate this risk, advanced nursing practice should adopt explicit principles of human-in-the-loop decision-making, ensuring that practitioners retain responsibility for interpreting, validating, and contextualising AI outputs. Organisational policies should mandate critical review of generative outputs and prohibit unsupervised reliance on automated recommendations for diagnostic or treatment decisions. Education represents a further critical area for future development. Advanced nursing curricula must incorporate AI literacy as a core component of professional preparation. However, as emphasised by UNESCO and the WHO, digital literacy must encompass ethical reasoning, critical appraisal, and understanding of data governance, rather than narrow technical competence (UNESCO, 2023; WHO, 2023). Educational programmes should therefore address generative AI explicitly as an object of critique, enabling advanced practitioners to interrogate its limitations, biases, and implications for professional identity.

Practice recommendations should also address organisational readiness. Evidence from implementation science demonstrates that digital interventions are more likely to succeed when aligned with existing workflows, values, and governance structures (Greenhalgh et al., 2017). Healthcare organisations seeking to deploy generative AI must therefore invest in clinical engagement, training, and evaluation rather than relying on vendor-driven implementation. Advanced nursing leaders should be centrally involved in procurement and implementation decisions, ensuring that nursing priorities and patient safety considerations are embedded from the outset.

Equity must remain a guiding principle in future AI adoption. Empirical evidence demonstrates that algorithmic systems can exacerbate existing health inequalities when trained on biased datasets or deployed without consideration of social context (Obermeyer et al., 2019). Future practice recommendations should require equity impact assessments for generative AI tools, with explicit evaluation of differential effects across patient populations. For advanced nursing practice, this aligns with professional commitments to advocacy and reduction of health disparities. The International Council of Nurses has called for stronger nursing involvement in digital health governance, recognising the profession's central role in patient care (International Council of Nurses, 2021). Advanced nursing leaders and researchers should therefore engage with international networks to shape ethical standards, share evidence, and influence global AI policy.

In practical terms, the responsible future use of GenAI in advanced nursing practice can be summarised through some recommendations. First, adoption should be evidence-led with keep evaluating it continuously. Second, governance structures must define accountability explicitly and ensuring the responsibility remains with clinical practitioners. Third, patient involvement and transparency should be part of the implementation strategies in order to maintain the trust along with maintaining the nursing values.

CONCLUSION

While early primary studies suggest that AI tools may help medical professionals with clinical documentation. There are limited research studies exploring the impact of GenAI in shaping the advanced clinical reasoning as well as the regulatory expectations. The most published papers are about medically or technically oriented. However, integrating empirical literature, national and international policy frameworks, and professional standards on engaging the AI responsibly within advanced nursing roles can add value to the clinical professional as well as to the leaders and decision makers within the health service domain. Therefore, this chapter expose readers to different aspect of generative AI (GenAI) tools in advanced and specialist nursing roles as well as highlighting the impact of embedding ethical, legal, and professional considerations within the the clinical practitioners.

Reflective questions

- How might GenAI reshape clinical decision-making in advanced nursing practice without undermining professional judgement and accountability?

- In what ways could reliance on GenAI alter the ethical foundations of nursing, particularly in relation to patient trust, transparency, and equity?

- How prepared are advanced practitioners and nurse leaders to critically appraise, govern, and challenge artificial intelligence-generated outputs in complex clinical environments?

- What risks arise if GenAI is adopted in nursing practice without profession-specific regulatory guidance and robust clinical governance?

- How can nursing education and assessment be redesigned to preserve professional integrity and authentic competence in the context of GenAI?

- What leadership responsibilities do advanced practitioners hold in ensuring that AI enhances, rather than diminishes, person-centred and compassionate care?

REFERENCES

Ajjawi, R., Tai, J., Dollinger, M., Dawson, P., Boud, D., & Bearman, M. (2024). From authentic assessment to authenticity in assessment: Broadening perspectives. *Assessment & Evaluation in Higher Education, 49*(4), 499–510. DOI: 10.1080/02602938.2023.2271193

Alanazi, M. A., Shaban, M. M., Ramadan, O. M. E., Zaky, M. E., Mohammed, H. H., Amer, F. G. M., & Shaban, M. (2024). Navigating end-of-life decision-making in nursing: A systematic review of ethical challenges and palliative care practices. *BMC Nursing, 23*(1), 467. DOI: 10.1186/s12912-024-02087-5

Alharbi, T. A. F., Rababa, M., Alsuwayl, H., Alsubail, A., & Alenizi, W. S. (2025). Diagnostic challenges and patient safety: the critical role of accuracy: a systematic review. *Journal of Multidisciplinary Healthcare, 18*, 3051–3064. DOI: 10.2147/JMDH.S512254

Alruwaili, A. N., Alshammari, A. M., Alhaiti, A., Elsharkawy, N. B., Ali, S. I., & Elsayed Ramadan, O. M. (2025). 'Neonatal nurses' experiences with generative AI in clinical decision-making: A qualitative exploration in high-risk NICUs'. *BMC Nursing, 24*(1), 1–20. DOI: 10.1186/s12912-025-03044-6

Amiot, F., & Potier, B. (2025). Artificial intelligence and emergency medicine: Balancing opportunities and challenges. *JMIR Medical Informatics, 13*(1), e70903. DOI: 10.2196/70903

Apathy, N. C., Rotenstein, L. S., Bates, D. W., & Holmgren, A. J. (2022). Documentation dynamics: Note composition, burden, and physician efficiency. *Journal of the American Medical Informatics Association : JAMIA, 29*(3), 674–685.

Assayed, S. K. (2025, November). Transforming Healthcare through Generative and Agentic AI: A Systematic Review. In *2025 10th International Conference on Information Technology Trends (ITT)* (pp. 124-129). IEEE. DOI: 10.1109/ITT69610.2025.11352935

Assayed, S. K., Shieh, C. S., & Gupta, S. K. (2025). Engineering intelligent healthcare systems: Understanding medical queries with AI and NLP. *Journal of Engineering and Applied Sciences (Asian Research Publishing Network), 72*(1), 212. DOI: 10.1186/s44147-025-00800-y

Astbury, H., Fortune, E., Dal Ponte, C., Lyons, K., & Shaw, L. (2025). Generative artificial intelligence for teaching and assessment in health professions education: A scoping review. *Nurse Education in Practice*, •••, 104697.

Barak-Corren, Y., Wolf, R., Rozenblum, R., Creedon, J. K., Lipsett, S. C., Lyons, T. W., Michelson, K. A., Miller, K. A., Shapiro, D. J., Reis, B. Y., & Fine, A. M. (2024). Harnessing the power of generative AI for clinical summaries: Perspectives from emergency physicians. *Annals of Emergency Medicine*, *84*(2), 128–138. DOI: 10.1016/j.annemergmed.2024.01.039

Barnard, J. (2019). *Clinical decision-making by acute medicine advanced nurse practitioners*. Sheffield Hallam University.

Borycki, E. M., & Kushniruk, A. W. (2023). Health technology, quality and safety in a learning health system. *Healthcare Management Forum*, *36*(2), 79–85. DOI: 10.1177/08404704221139383

Buchanan, C., Howitt, M. L., Wilson, R., Booth, R. G., Risling, T., & Bamford, M. (2020). Predicted influences of artificial intelligence on the domains of nursing: Scoping review. *JMIR Nursing*, *3*(1), e23939. DOI: 10.2196/23939

Campanozzi, L. L., Gibelli, F., Bailo, P., Nittari, G., Sirignano, A., & Ricci, G. (2023). The role of digital literacy in achieving health equity in the third millennium society: A literature review. *Frontiers in Public Health*, *11*, 1109323. DOI: 10.3389/fpubh.2023.1109323

Cant, R. P., & Cooper, S. J. (2017). Use of simulation-based learning in undergraduate nurse education: An umbrella systematic review. *Nurse Education Today*, *49*, 63–71. DOI: 10.1016/j.nedt.2016.11.015

Car, J., Sheikh, A., Wicks, P., & Williams, M. S. (2019). Beyond the hype of big data and artificial intelligence: Building foundations for knowledge and wisdom. *BMC Medicine*, *17*(1), 143. DOI: 10.1186/s12916-019-1382-x

Cohran, A. (2025). *Impact of integrating generative artificial intelligence into organizational processes on individual performance*. Benedictine University.

Colacci, M.. (2025). Sociodemographic bias in clinical machine learning models: A scoping review. *Journal of Clinical Machine Learning*, *12*(4), 1–15.

da Silva Tiago, R., & Mitchell, A. (2024) 'Integrating digital transformation in nursing education: best practices and challenges in curriculum development', in *Digital transformation in higher education*, Part B. Bingley: Emerald Publishing Limited, pp. 57–101.

Eggins, S., & Slade, D. (2015). Communication in clinical handover: Improving the safety of patients. *Journal of Health Services Research & Policy*.

European Commission. (2021) *Proposal for a regulation laying down harmonised rules on artificial intelligence (Artificial Intelligence Act)*. Brussels: European Commission. Available at: https://eur-lex.europa.eu/legal-content/EN/TXT/?uri=CELEX%3A52021PC0206 (Accessed: 2 January 2026).

Farrokhi, M., Fallahian, A. H., Rahmani, E., Aghajan, A., Alipour, M., Khouzani, P. J., Hezarani, H. B., Sabzehie, H., Pirouzan, M., Pirouzan, Z., & Dalvandi, B. (2025). Current applications, challenges, and future directions of artificial intelligence in emergency medicine: A narrative review. *Archives of Academic Emergency Medicine*, *13*(1), e45.

Floridi, L., Cowls, J., Beltrametti, M., Chatila, R., Chazerand, P., Dignum, V., Luetge, C., Madelin, R., Pagallo, U., Rossi, F., Schäfer, B., Valcke, P., & Vayena, E. (2018). AI4People: An ethical framework for a good AI society. *Minds and Machines*, *28*(4), 689–707. DOI: 10.1007/s11023-018-9482-5

Goddard, K., Roudsari, A., & Wyatt, J. C. (2012). Automation bias: A systematic review of frequency, effect mediators, and mitigators. *Journal of the American Medical Informatics Association : JAMIA*, *19*(1), 121–127. DOI: 10.1136/amiajnl-2011-000089

Greenhalgh, T., Wherton, J., Papoutsi, C., Lynch, J., Hughes, G., Hinder, S., Fahy, N., Procter, R., & Shaw, S. (2017). Beyond adoption: A new framework for theorizing and evaluating nonadoption, abandonment, and challenges to the scale-up, spread, and sustainability of health and care technologies. *Journal of Medical Internet Research*, *19*(11), e8775. DOI: 10.2196/jmir.8775

Harder, N. (2025). Comparing artificial intelligence-enhanced virtual reality and traditional simulated patient learning: Perceptions of realism and educational impact. *Journal of Nursing Simulation*, *19*(1), 1–10.

International Council of Nurses. (2021) *The ICN code of ethics for nurses*. Geneva: International Council of Nurses. Available at: https://www.icn.ch/sites/default/files/inline-files/ICN_Code-of-Ethics_EN_Web.pdf (Accessed: 2 January 2026).

Ip, W., Xenochristou, M., Sui, E., Ruan, E., Ribeira, R., Dash, D., Srinivasan, M., Artandi, M., Omiye, J. A., Scoulios, N., & Hofmann, H. L. (2024). 'Hospitalization prediction from the emergency department using computer vision AI with short patient video clips', *npj. Digital Medicine*, *7*(1), 371.

Ivers, N., Jamtvedt, G., Flottorp, S., Young, J. M., Odgaard-Jensen, J., French, S. D., O'Brien, M. A., Johansen, M., Grimshaw, J., & Oxman, A. D. (2012). Audit and feedback: Effects on professional practice and healthcare outcomes. *The Cochrane Library*, *2012*(7), 6. DOI: 10.1002/14651858.CD000259.pub3

Jiang, F., Jiang, Y., Zhi, H., Dong, Y., Li, H., Ma, S., Wang, Y., Dong, Q., Shen, H., & Wang, Y. (2017). Artificial intelligence in healthcare: Past, present and future. *Stroke and Vascular Neurology*, *2*(4), 230–243. DOI: 10.1136/svn-2017-000101

Jones, M. C.. (2023). Navigating data governance associated with real-world health data: Legal and information governance structures in the UK. *BMJ Open*, *13*(10), e069925. DOI: 10.1136/bmjopen-2022-069925

Kelly, C. J., Karthikesalingam, A., Suleyman, M., Corrado, G., & King, D. (2019). Key challenges for delivering clinical impact with artificial intelligence. *BMC Medicine*, *17*(1), 195. DOI: 10.1186/s12916-019-1426-2

Kelly, S., Pryor, C., Stephens, M., & Heaslip, V. (2025). Exploring the presence and impact of advanced nursing roles in care homes and charitable organisations: An international systematic scoping review. *Journal of Advanced Nursing*, jan.70212. DOI: 10.1111/jan.70212

Longoni, C., Bonezzi, A., & Morewedge, C. K. (2019). Resistance to medical artificial intelligence. *The Journal of Consumer Research*, *46*(4), 629–650. DOI: 10.1093/jcr/ucz013

Marshall, N., Carsey, E., Chen, P., Bain, A., Bernard, P., & Patton, L. (2025). 'Pediatric nurses' perceptions of the quality and usefulness of clinical summaries: Surgeons versus generative AI'. *Journal of Pediatric Surgical Nursing*, *14*(4), 126–131. DOI: 10.1177/23320249251362849

Nagendran, M., Chen, Y., Lovejoy, C. A., Gordon, A. C., Komorowski, M., Harvey, H., Topol, E. J., Ioannidis, J. P., Collins, G. S., & Maruthappu, M. (2020). Artificial intelligence versus clinicians: Systematic review of design, reporting standards, and claims of deep learning studies. *BMJ (Clinical Research Ed.)*, •••, 368. DOI: 10.1136/bmj.m689

Nagendran, M., Chen, Y., Lovejoy, C. A., Gordon, A. C., Komorowski, M., Harvey, H., Topol, E. J., Ioannidis, J. P., Collins, G. S., & Maruthappu, M. (2020). Artificial intelligence versus clinicians: Systematic review of design, reporting standards, and claims of deep learning studies. *BMJ (Clinical Research Ed.)*, •••, 368. DOI: 10.1136/bmj.m689

Nazi, Z. A., & Peng, W. (2024). Large language models in healthcare and medical domain: A review. *Informatics (MDPI)*, *11*(3), 57. DOI: 10.3390/informatics11030057

NHS England. (2025a) *The NHS long term plan*. London: NHS England. Available at: https://www.gov.uk/government/publications/10-year-health-plan-for-england-fit-for-the-future (Accessed: 2 January 2026).

NHS England. (2025b) *Data saves lives: reshaping health and social care with data.* London: NHS England. Available at: https://www.england.nhs.uk/digitaltechnology/data-saves-lives/ (Accessed: 2 January 2026).

NHS England. (2025c) *Multi-professional framework for advanced practice in England.* London: NHS England. Available at: https://advanced-practice.hee.nhs.uk/multi-professional-framework-for-advanced-practice/ (Accessed: 2 January 2026).

NHS England. (2025d) *Transformation Directorate: artificial intelligence – information governance guidance.* Available at: https://transform.england.nhs.uk/information-governance/guidance/artificial-intelligence/ (Accessed: 2 January 2026).

Nibbelink, C. W., & Brewer, B. B. (2018). Decision-making in nursing practice: An integrative literature review. *Journal of Clinical Nursing, 27*(5–6), 917–928. DOI: 10.1111/jocn.14151

Nikolic, S., Ros, M., Al-Abdeli, Y. M., & Fairweather, H. (2025). Beyond assessment security: A critical policy analysis of four alternative strategies to uphold academic integrity and adopt the GenAI transformation of teaching and learning for an accredited engineering degree. *STEM Education, 5*(4), 564–586. DOI: 10.3934/steme.2025027

Nursing and Midwifery Council. (2018) *The Code: professional standards of practice and behaviour for nurses, midwives and nursing associates.* London: Nursing and Midwifery Council. Available at: https://www.nmc.org.uk/standards/code/ (Accessed: 2 January 2026).

Obermeyer, Z., Powers, B., Vogeli, C., & Mullainathan, S. (2019). Dissecting racial bias in an algorithm used to manage the health of populations. *Science, 366*(6464), 447–453. DOI: 10.1126/science.aax2342

Organisation for Economic Co-operation and Development. (2023). *Health at a Glance 2023: OECD Indicators.* OECD Publishing., DOI: 10.1787/7a7afb35-

Pelletier, J. H., Watson, K., Michel, J., McGregor, R., & Rush, S. Z. (2025). Effect of a generative artificial intelligence digital scribe on pediatric provider documentation time, cognitive burden, and burnout. *JAMIA Open, 8*(4), ooaf068. DOI: 10.1093/jamiaopen/ooaf068

Poalelungi, D. G., Musat, C. L., Fulga, A., Neagu, M., Neagu, A. I., Piraianu, A. I., & Fulga, I. (2023). Advancing patient care: How artificial intelligence is transforming healthcare. *Journal of Personalized Medicine, 13*(8), 1214. DOI: 10.3390/jpm13081214

Pong, C., Tseng, R. M. W. W., Tham, Y. C., & Lum, E. (2024). Current implementation of digital health in chronic disease management: A scoping review. *Journal of Medical Internet Research*, *26*, e53576. DOI: 10.2196/53576

Preiksaitis, C., & Rose, C. (2023). Opportunities, challenges, and future directions of generative artificial intelligence in medical education: A scoping review. *JMIR Medical Education*, *9*, e48785. DOI: 10.2196/48785

Raghavan, S. (2025). Global advancements in international nursing science and healthcare innovation: Trends, challenges, and future directions. *Journal of Comprehensive Nursing Research*, *1*(2).

Sendak, M. P., D'Arcy, J., Kashyap, S., Gao, M., Nichols, M., Corey, K., Ratliff, W., & Balu, S. (2020). A path for translation of machine learning products into healthcare delivery. *EMJ Innov*, *10*, 19–00172.

Siira, E., Johansson, H., & Nygren, J. (2025). Mapping and summarizing the research on AI systems for automating medical history taking and triage: A scoping review. *Journal of Medical Internet Research*, *27*, e53741. DOI: 10.2196/53741

Sittig, D. F., & Singh, H. (2010). A new sociotechnical model for studying health information technology in complex adaptive healthcare systems. *Quality & Safety in Health Care*, *19*(Suppl 3), i68–i74. DOI: 10.1136/qshc.2010.042085

Stanford, M., & Sorensen, Z. (2025). *Integrating generative AI in medical practice: enhancing patient care and diagnostics with agentic AI systems*. NuovoNova Ltd.

Subasri, V., Baghbanzadeh, N., Celi, L. A., & Seyyed-Kalantari, L. (2025). Potential for near-term AI risks to evolve into existential threats in healthcare. *BMJ Health & Care Informatics*, *32*(1), e101130. DOI: 10.1136/bmjhci-2024-101130

Sujan, M. A., Spurgeon, P., Inada-Kim, M., Rudd, M., Fitton, L., Horniblow, S., Cross, S., Chessum, P., & Cooke, M. (2014). Clinical handover within the emergency care pathway and the potential risks of clinical handover failure (ECHO): Primary research. *Health Services and Delivery Research*, *2*(5), 1–144. DOI: 10.3310/hsdr02050

Sullivan, D., Hall, V. P., & Morrison, J. (2024). Navigating the future: Artificial intelligence's impact on transformational nurse leadership. *Teaching and Learning in Nursing*, *19*(3), 298–300. DOI: 10.1016/j.teln.2024.04.017

Sutton, R. T., Pincock, D., Baumgart, D. C., Sadowski, D. C., Fedorak, R. N., & Kroeker, K. I. (2020). An overview of clinical decision support systems: Benefits, risks, and strategies for success. *NPJ Digital Medicine*, *3*(1), 17. DOI: 10.1038/s41746-020-0221-y

Thompson, C., & Dowding, D. (2009). *Essential decision making and clinical judgement for nurses*. Elsevier.

Topol, E. (2019). The Topol Review: preparing the healthcare workforce to deliver the digital future. NHS Health Education England., Available at https://topol.hee.nhs.uk, Retrieved January 2, 2026, from.

Trede, F., Macklin, R., & Bridges, D. (2012). Professional identity development: A review of the higher education literature. *Studies in Higher Education*, *37*(3), 365–384. DOI: 10.1080/03075079.2010.521237

Tung, T. (2025) 'Ethical and practical challenges of generative AI in healthcare', *Journal of Medical AI Ethics*, PMC [online]. Available at: https://pmc.ncbi.nlm.nih.gov/articles/PMC12665710 (Accessed: 2 January 2026).

UNESCO. (2023) *Guidance for generative AI in education and research*. Paris: UNESCO. Available at: https://www.unesco.org/en/articles/guidance-generative-ai-education-and-research (Accessed: 2 January 2026).

Wangpitipanit, S., Lininger, J., & Anderson, N. (2024). Exploring the deep learning of artificial intelligence in nursing: A concept analysis using Walker and Avant's approach. *BMC Nursing*, *23*(1), 529. DOI: 10.1186/s12912-024-02170-x

World Health Organization. (2021) *Ethics and governance of artificial intelligence for health*. Geneva: World Health Organization. Available at: https://www.who.int/publications/i/item/9789240029200 (Accessed: 2 January 2026).

Wu, Y., Wu, M., Wang, C., Lin, J., Liu, J., & Liu, S. (2024). Evaluating the prevalence of burnout among health care professionals related to electronic health record use: Systematic review and meta-analysis. *JMIR Medical Informatics*, *12*, e54811. DOI: 10.2196/54811

Zhang, J., & Zhang, Z. M. (2023). Ethics and governance of trustworthy medical artificial intelligence. *BMC Medical Informatics and Decision Making*, *23*(1), 7. DOI: 10.1186/s12911-023-02103-9

Chapter 13
Integrating Artificial Intelligence in Nursing Education and Leadership:
Opportunities, Challenges, and Future Directions

Areej Khalil Assayed
http://orcid.org/0009-0000-3315-8718
Westcliff University, USA

Shelley L. Spessard
http://orcid.org/0009-0003-1696-6213
Westcliff University, USA

Nura I. ALhababsah
Westcliff University, USA

Sana'a Khalil Alsayed
http://orcid.org/0009-0002-1419-219X
Philadelphia University, Jordan

ABSTRACT

This proposed chapter examines how (AI) is transforming the nursing education and leadership by changing the roles and responsibilities of nurses leaders and reshaping the way they design curricula .Effective nursing leadership plays a vital role in empowering and preparing the nurses for AI integration in nursing education

DOI: 10.4018/979-8-3373-8247-0.ch013

as this integration will dramatically change the traditional learning methodologies, enhance personalization, student involvement and administrative effectiveness. The chapter also highlights the opportunities of AI in nursing practice and how integrating AI tools can provide nursing students, nurses and clinicians with smarter solutions While AI offers opportunities to enhance nursing education, leadership effciency and instructional support, it also raises challenges related to privacy, equity, and ethical issues related to AI health technologies.

INTRODUCTION

Nowadays, artificial intelligence shapes the routines for learners and instructors alike. Not just tools on screens, these systems now can be adapted and simulated in a smart way. For example, classrooms are different now, more responsive and engaging. Yet plenty remain unsure if they know enough to include such tech well (Khlaif et al., 2025). As things change, schools find attention pulled toward firm plans: helping instructors learn AI use wisely, backing moral choices, shaping class time around care-focused thinking, good decisions, keeping patients safe.

Behind the scenes, hospital training crews adjust workflows using similar technology and more nursing teachers seem open to working with artificial intelligence. In Saudi Arabia, one snapshot survey found most nursing learners - 92.2 percent out of 322 - felt favorably about AI tools in healthcare and showed eagerness to try them while studying (Alanzi & Al-Shakihs, 2025). Earlier summaries of multiple studies agree: exposure to smart systems tends to lift student motivation, sharpen real-world skills, and boost confidence heading into jobs; yet worries linger around fairness questions and how courses are built moving forward (AlAli et al., 2025). When looked at as a whole, the evidence suggests updates to nurse education must balance tech fluency with strong values and sharp judgment on digital dilemmas.

This chapter explores the impact of artificial intelligence as a transformative force that reframes how nurses enhance their academic knowledge and leadership skills to provide high-quality medical care and it also focuses on how AI is developing nursing education and leadership by reshaping the roles of nurse leaders and the way curricula is designed by utilizing a variety of recommended AI tools leading to improvement in the standards of healthcare delivery.

AI AND THE FUTURE OF NURSING EDUCATION

Nursing education is changing rapidly as AI plays a significant role in reshaping health care systems, clinical practice and nursing curricula in addition to offering valuable opportunities to develop the nursing field and transform teaching and instructional methodologies which lead to enhance nurses' knowledge and care delivery practices. AI in nursing education employs intelligent, high- tech systems to support teaching, learning, and assessment, as well as clinical training through data-driven and adaptive tools.

Preparing nursing students to engage with AI-driven health technologies requires to modify Nursing curricula particularly at the undergraduate level, Such curricula should include content related to advanced technologies, including data analysis, machine learning, higher-order thinking skills, AI algorithms, and the ethical use of AI in nursing education and practice, as these technologies continue to reshape traditional approaches to nursing teaching and clinical practice (Buchanan et al., 2020).

El Arab et al. (2025) focused on the importance of integrating AI literacy into nursing education programs and highlighted that AI-powered educational technologies, including simulation platforms, virtual reality, and chatbot systems are greatly important for developing critical thinking, decision-making, and communication skills, as equipping students with these skills are necessary to for them to function effectively in high-technology health care environments. AI is also transforming traditional models of nursing education by shifting from teacher-centered to student-centered learning through adaptive systems and AI-powered tools that respond to individual learning needs and align naturally with competency-based education.

Although the use of AI in nursing education is vital to develop students 'learning experiences and improve efficiency, but it has to be implemented carefully and sensibly due to its potential risks, for example the use of AI chatbot systems including ChatGPT has raised concerns related to academic integrity, intellectual property, privacy, ethical considerations, data security, and resistance to pedagogical change, in addition to other concerns among nurse educators regarding the potential displacement of teaching roles which De Gagne (2023) addressed when he stated that AI technologies can support human interaction, critical thinking, and creativity by enabling personalized learning experiences and assisting nurse educators with administrative tasks, such as grading and attendance management rather than replace them or diminish their roles in teaching and learning.

Shift Toward Education 5.0

Universally, technological systems are moving from Industry 4.0 to Industry 5.0, which affecting different aspect of fields, including education (Assayed et al., 2023), Banking sector as well as in health services. Accordingly, Basulto-Ribeiro and Teixeira (2024) described Healthcare 5.0 as an era in which technology not only supports but also enhances the capabilities of healthcare professionals, increasing collaboration between doctors, patients, and technologies. Moreover, healthcare 5.0

puts emphasis on utilizing AI technology in order to enhance the quality of patient care, health care services, workforce experiences, and overall patient engagement, thereby increasing the targeted benefits across the sector of health care (Assayed et al., 2025).

As (Buchanan et al., 2020) stated that while Industry 4.0 was used to enhance health care efficiency and clinical processes, but its application often prioritized technical functionality over patient-centered needs as it focused on automation, data analytics, AI technology, and interconnected digital systems. In contrast, Industry 5.0 places nurses and patients at the center by using intelligent systems for patients and the professional expertise of nurses. This approach highlights the importance of balancing technological advancements with compassion and humanity (El Arab et al., 2025; World Health Organization, 2021). Ultimately, with nursing in Industry 5.0, nurses should use AI as a helping tool to decision making, patient care and training, whilst maintaining the caring and empathetic nature of the nursing profession.

The aim of Education 5.0 in nursing is enhancing the collaboration between humans and intelligent systems while creating flexible and adaptive learning environments that support personalized engagement and competency development (De Gagne, 2023). This perspective is supported within the domain of nursing education where digital competencies including critical thinking, creativity, collaborative and digital skills are increasingly essential. Such competencies are vital for the effective employment of AI tools by nurses while maintaining empathetic, patient-centered care (Judijanto, 2025). Furthermore, Education 5.0 promotes alignment between curricular outcomes and the evolving needs of the workplace and society, enabling nurses to continually develop their skills and contribute to health care advancement (Shahidi Hamedani et al., 2024).

The main objective of Education 5.0 in nursing is to create flexible and adaptive learning environments that support personalized engagement and competency development along with increasing collaboration between humans and intelligent systems. (De Gagne, 2023). Because education 5.0 is human-centered, it promotes alignment between curricular outcomes and the evolving needs of the workplace and society, enabling nurses to continually develop their skills and contribute to health care advancement (Shahidi Hamedani et al., 2024) which makes it one of paramount as digital competencies including critical thinking, creativity, collaborative problem-solving and digital skills are increasingly essential and they are vital for the effective employment of AI tools by nurses while maintaining empathetic, patient-centered care (Judijanto, 2025).

AI-Enhanced Learning Environments

Creating AI-enhanced learning environments in nursing education requires full integration with AI learning settings, including virtual classrooms, adaptive learning platforms, generative AI tools, and intelligent learning systems which support, personalize, and improve teaching, learning, and assessment processes. Such environment is positively influence multiple aspects of nursing education, including clinical competency development, student engagement, and the achievement of learning outcomes, similarly (Labrague et al., 2025; Marboah Kusi & Nono Wete, 2025) stated that AI-based learning systems provide individualized and interactive learning experiences that enable students to engage with real-life case studies and simulations, allowing them to develop practical competencies in authentic clinical contexts.

Integrating AI into nursing education has significantly reshaped teaching as it has become more engaging, interactive, and individualized, thereby the students' conceptual understanding and practical skills will be enhanced as well. As (Cucci et al., 2025) highlighted that there are many AI tools such as virtual patients (VPs) and AI chatbot systems like ChatGPT have been shown to increase student engagement and confidence while supporting the development of fundamental competencies, including communication and clinical decision-making skills.

AI-enhanced learning environments play a very important role in managing cognitive load and fostering resilience among nursing students particularly when they are in complex and high-pressure learning settings such as clinical simulations and skills-based training in addition to other settings where students need to develop their theoretical knowledge, technical skills, ethical judgment, and patient communication. Moreover, AI-enhanced environments create psychologically safe spaces for repeated practice, enabling students to learn from errors without fear of patient harm. AI-enhanced learning environments also support the development of students' academic and emotional capacities by shaping how they manage stress, adapt over time, and sustain performance in high-pressure clinical roles (De Gagne, 2023; El Arab et al., 2025).

AI and Nursing Leadership Transformation

Changing Roles of Nurse Leaders

AI plays a crucial role in reshaping how the medical sector is managed and how patients receive care which also requires a transformative change in nursing leadership as Sullivan et al. (2024) emphasized that future nurse leaders must champion the integration of AI as a tool for innovation while maintaining ethical practice. Therefore, nursing leadership during AI era has to be flexible and capable of addressing emerging challenges while strengthening patient-centered care.

The integration of AI within the nursing leadership has several challenges because it overlaps with health care providers, patients, organizational management, leadership structures, ethical considerations as well as other technological systems. These interdependencies create a "wicked problem," characterized mainly by complexity, dynamism, and networked relationships. Effective AI leadership therefore demands specialized skills and competencies to identify appropriate areas for AI integration, influence professional attitudes and behaviors, and manage complex relationships at the intersection of health care systems and AI technologies.

Nurse leaders have a major impact on developing comprehensive strategic plans that include ongoing professional development and soft skills-building to equip leadership teams with both technical and interpersonal qualifications that are needed for effective AI integration (Sriharan et al., 2024).

Human-Centered Leadership

The rapid innovation and integration of AI technologies have increased the demand for leadership approaches within different industries, including education, healthcare or others (Assayed & Assayed, 2026)

Human-centered leadership seeks to advance the development and application of AI in ways that sustain and reshape the roles of nurses, retain patient trust, and enhance clinical decision-making in addition to the focus on efficiency and automation. Similarly, Domfeh et al. (2022) conveyed that optimum performance is central to Human–Artificial Intelligence systems. Accordingly, AI system design and governance frameworks must integrate safety, trust, empathy, and reliability while being supported by regulatory standards established by governments to ensure appropriate functionality and accountability. By supporting nurses' resilience, confidence, and participation in AI-related initiatives, leaders foster a culture of trust and adaptability, so this approach not only improves workforce readiness but also ensures that the adoption of AI contributes to the building of sustainable practice environments in which nurses emotionally and professionally thrive in their practice, even in highly complex and demanding healthcare environments (De Gagne, 2023; El Arab et al., 2025).

In fact, nurse leaders must show an individual leadership skills so that they can overcome the traditional practices within care settings that preserving compassionate, patient-centered care remains a central responsibility of nurse leaders in AI-supported healthcare environments, as (Stuart-Pesevic & Talarico, 2024) highlighted that nurse leaders should build genuine relationships and foster authentic connections with stakeholders, so that they can influence change and contribute to be more responsive and patient-centered care models.

OPPORTUNITIES FOR AI IN NURSING PRACTICE AND LEADERSHIP

In the 21st century artificial intelligence is considered a formal force in the health care industry today and particularly in education sectors. Which urges the need to redefine nursing practices, leadership governance and reshape the services provided in alignment with the current market and customer needs acknowledging the speed and automation of AI systems. In nursing practice, integrating the AI trends is challenging but opening a wide opportunity to advance the nursing care and leadership modalities.

Refining Nursing Expertise Through Augmented Intelligence

In some cultures, the nursing field is seen as ordinary practice as well as routine tasks though it requires a synthesis of data, understanding the entire context of medical cases, logical understanding and ethical reasoning. With the existence of AI systems, it is escalating the demand to enhance the nursing workforce competencies to pace with evolving technology and redefining clinical expertise through synergizing AI with human intelligence. Davenport, T. and Kalakota, R. (2019), and Topol explains that expert systems, in conjunction with AI, have the potential to augment clinical judgments by extracting probabilistic insights from massive data sets.

These advancements drive the nurses to anticipate the patients' needs rather than responding to it, through predictive analysis to recognize early signs for deterioration, find the gaps in care, and proactively provide the care, which will end with a thoughtful, more integrative, more synthetic clinical judgment in which empirical evidence and patient values converge.

Through collaboration with human intelligence, nurses have the opportunity to augment, rather than erode, professional autonomy in nursing practice.

Redefining Nursing Education and Knowledge Development

Moreover, this technology has great potential for changing nursing practice, particularly in relation to developing knowledge and creating opportunities for learning. Conventional models of learning face difficulties in meeting diverse needs in a changing practice environment where complexity is escalating and knowledge development is accelerating. There are obvious advantages of using learning technology and more intelligent processes of tutoring that improve the learning experience (El Arab et al., 2025).

Additionally, computer-assisted documentation will allow nurses more time for more patient-centered practice and professional development, thus creating more positive job satisfaction and professional purpose through reducing administrative burdens.

From a leadership perspective, there is potential for using workforce tools that will allow leaders to balance sustainability of their organization with their moral obligation to their workforce through automation of tasks that do not add value to creating a more efficient workplace.

Expanding the Strategic Influence of Nursing Leadership

There is a significant opportunity for AI systems to increase the strategic influence of nursing leadership within healthcare organizations. The role of nurses has always had an impactful presence on the success of operations, but it may have been less significant in relation to other aspects of strategy within healthcare organizations. The way in which nursing leadership influences strategy within healthcare organizations is through the use of nursing expertise to interpret the data generated by AI systems and inform policy based on evidence derived from the data (Kotp et al., 2025).

Nursing leadership's involvement with AI systems provides a significant role in defining the use of data, the voices that are represented, and the outcomes that are desired within healthcare organizations, ultimately increasing the prominence of nursing leadership as a bridge between technology, patients, and strategy within healthcare organizations.

Additionally, involvement with AI systems ensures that complex value-based issues, such as those related to equity, transparency, and accountability, are addressed proactively as opposed to reactively (Morley et al., 2020).

Advancing Equity and Population Health Impact

Nurses have a significant chance to contribute more to population health equity and population health strategies through their involvement with AI systems, as they have the potential to address disparities and inequalities within population health by utilizing AI systems as a tool for population health data analysis to identify the disparities. Accordingly, nurses have the opportunity to be involved in an informed supported role, as their close association with social and structural determinants of health provides a significant opportunity to address disparities and inequalities within population health strategies (World Health Organization, 2021).

Nursing has an opportunity to increase their influence and go beyond bedside nursing and into a role of advocacy and leadership within population health strategies, as AI systems have the potential to address disparities and inequalities within population health strategies, and an ethics-based approach provides a significant opportunity to address preventive strategies, outreach, and resource allocation strategies related to social determinants of health.

Opportunities Come with Responsibility

Recognize that the opportunities of AI come with a high responsibility. Therefore, the same opportunities that can improve the situation can deteriorate it if we fail to manage them well. Therefore, the true opportunity for nursing practice and leadership is not AI, but how nursing manages AI and information to empower nurses.

A Holistic View

The opportunities of AI present a wide, complex, and multi-layered array of opportunities for nursing practice and leadership. AI has the potential to enhance clinical judgment, education, workforce, strategic planning, equity, and the identity of the profession. The challenge of these opportunities is to encourage leaders to go beyond embracing technology to lead a transformation driven by technology. When AI is integrated with the people-centered values that are at the core of the nursing profession, it has the potential to improve health care and advance the position of the nursing profession in the health system. Figure 1 illustrates an integrative perspective on the opportunities of AI to support nursing practice and leadership.

Figure 1. Opportunities of AI in Nursing Practice and Leadership

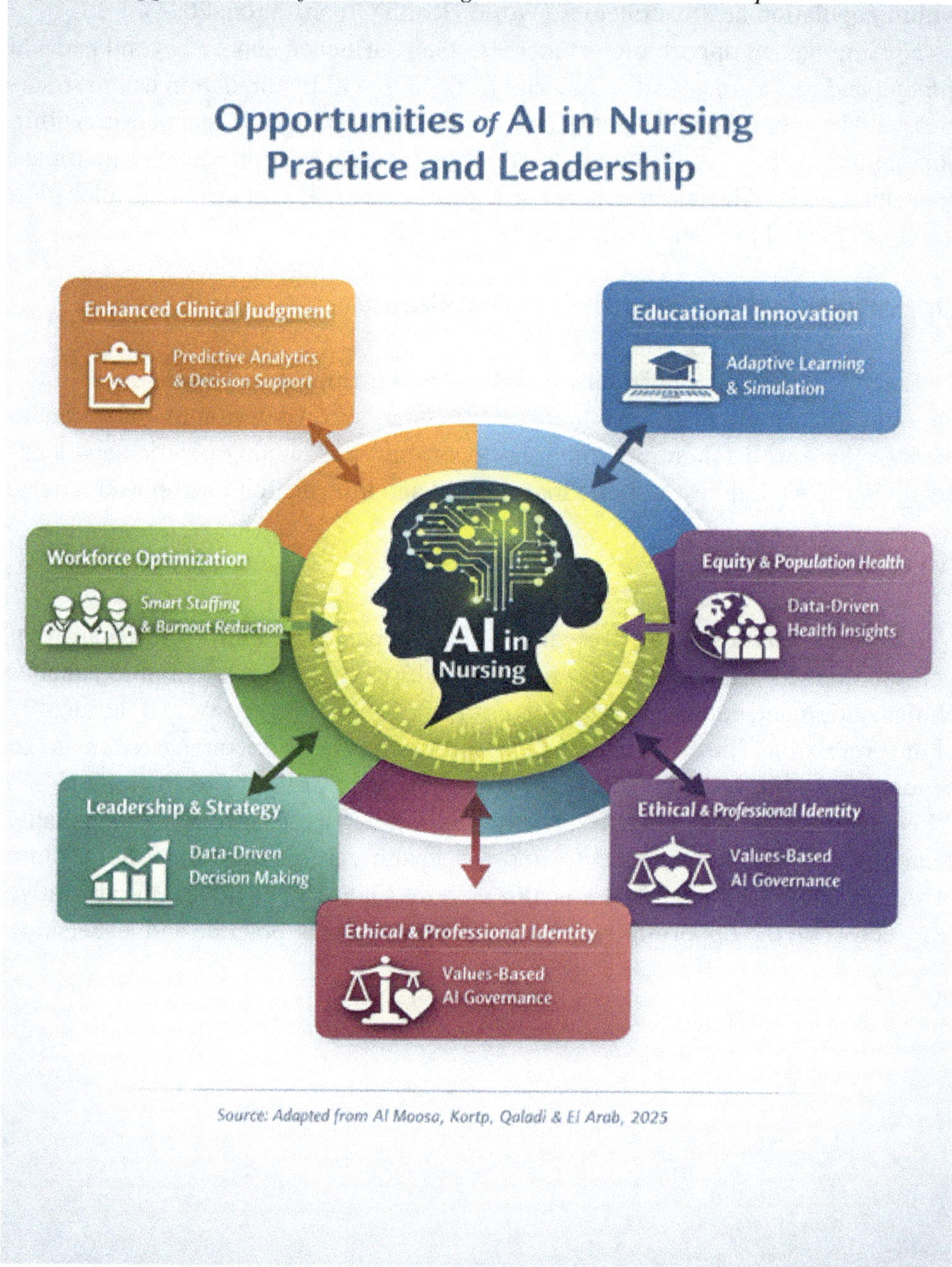

Note. This figure highlights the key opportunities that artificial intelligence can bring in nursing practice and leadership, which include enhanced judgment in practice, new approaches in education, workforce optimization, strategic leadership, equity and population health impact, and the development of an ethical and professional identity.

Strengthen Fair Rules and Shared Responsibility

A system watching right and wrong must keep asking questions - about fairness, about who owns information, about how choices are explained, about privacy, about blame when machines decide things. It has to do this over and over, adjusting as answers shift (Amann et al., 2020).

Using AI to enhance work without replacing human effort

When it comes to AI technology in medicine, worth appears only if humans lead. Not swapping out caregivers, clever tools help most when they stand alongside. Decisions, care, presence - those remain with people. Backed by Topol's 2019 findings, and it shows up again in Davenport and Kalakota's work from that year, they both focus on help comes from machines while direction comes from people.

Keep Evaluating and Improving

Trying out AI works best when treated like a loop that keeps refining itself. From a teaching standpoint, how well it works shows up in fairness and consequences, Organizations stay aligned with shifting demands by tweaking their AI systems over time - feedback helps them do that.

Trust and Professional Identity First

Trust matters most when bringing AI into health care, especially for nurses. Comfort comes through being able to question or adjust AI suggestions - without worrying about career fallout. When leaders act openly, listen closely, and value nursing knowledge, trust grows. This kind of setting supports a strong nurse role even as technology changes how care works (Booth et al., 2021).

CHALLENGES AND RISKS

Although the preceding nursing leadership tips can offer simple steps for ethical and conscientious ways to implement AI, it is also important to understand the risks involved with using AI. While AI can be leveraged to assist with nursing education and leadership, also there are risks involved with adopting AI that schools and healthcare companies should be aware of. These risks don't just affect the nuts and bolts of how we operate, they can affect students, faculty, nurse leaders, and the daily life of everyone who works in health care. Nursing is a profession rooted in creating safe environments and practicing with precision and care, so we must understand these risks involved before implementing and adopting technology.

Accuracy is the most immediate risk because nursing students are starting to notice that AI explanations can sound confident while still missing key clinical details. In one recent survey, students said the output was helpful, but also easy to misread as reliable when it was incomplete or subtly wrong, and they were unsure how to decide when to trust it (Han et al., 2025). That uncertainty matters in nursing education, where clinical judgment develops through repeated practice with an expert's reasoning, not just exposure to correct answers. If an AI tool omits a contraindication, skips a safety check, or compresses a clinical rationale, students may rehearse the wrong thinking pattern even when the wording sounds "right." As AI becomes more common in simulation and decision-support, fidelity will also include reasoning fidelity, meaning the system should model safe, realistic clinical logic that supports, rather than distorts, student development.

Equity is one of the ethical principles that continues to elevate concerns. AI models train on existing data, and those data are likely to contain patterns and biases related to race, gender, age, and socioeconomic status, among other factors. Nursing faculty shared specific concerns around what equity "look-for" would be, as well as worries automated feedback, learning pathway recommendations, or triggers for remediation could unfairly disadvantage students from marginalized backgrounds or widen gaps in opportunity and supports (Rony et al., 2025). These sentiments were echoed in scholarship from higher education which critiques AI-focused learning research for centering little to no inquiry into justice or fairness while relegating the responsibility for equity discussions to faculty after tools have been widely adopted (Zawacki-Richter et al., 2019). For nursing programs striving to create clinicians who provide culturally responsive care, injustice is not a theoretical concern. The ways in which biased feedback and unequal learning supports shape how learners perform clinical reasoning, construct professional identity, and advocate for patients can have material impacts.

Privacy is a relevant and important concern. AI-augmented learning environments may be required to collect and process large amounts of data about student performance and decision-making patterns. In simulation-based nursing education, AI tools may capture or record sensitive data in order to individualize learning experiences or automate debriefing processes. Simulation experts have raised alarms that without clear protections, this data may be misused or inadvertently exposed, creating risks of student privacy and diminished trust (Jung, 2023). Students may also feel surveilled by these systems, rather than supported, if data use is not transparent.

Opacity also complicates the use of AI. Many AI systems are "black boxes" in that it is difficult or impossible for faculty or students to see how a particular conclusion was reached. AI ethics scholars have argued that AI systems and technologies cannot be considered trustworthy if their outputs cannot be explained or questioned (Floridi & Cowls, 2019). In educational settings like nursing where critical thinking and evidence-based decisions should be taught, this is crucial. If students cannot see how AI came up with their recommendations and or scores, they are losing valuable teachable moments from the reasoning process.

The risks of AI adoption in nursing education exist in human and organizational fields as well. While nursing educators are naturally curious and excited about AI, they may also feel underprepared or anxious about the impact on their practice. When researchers surveyed nursing faculty on AI use, there was a clear faculty desire for more guidelines, defined policy, and professional development prior to implementing AI in their classrooms (Rony et al., 2025). Nurse leaders and executives experience these same challenges as well. One recent literature review on AI and the workforce showed that health and nursing organizations are likely to have insufficient infrastructure, resources, or governance to effectively and ethically adopt AI (Alenezi et al., 2024). If organizations aren't ready as a whole, AI adoption may feel siloed, unsupported, and/or contrary to teaching and learning goals.

Finally, there are academic integrity and responsible use concerns. Students and faculty have expressed confusion about when and how they should be using AI and citing it properly. They have expressed fear that AI could negatively impact their learning if overused. This has led to mixed messages and expectations for students between courses and faculty members. Some scholars have suggested that if institutions do not establish policies or communicate student expectations, AI will be used in ways that could inadvertently harm student learning or assessment (Ramírez-Baraldes et al., 2025).

When decisions about AI are grounded in ethics and pedagogical theory, risks can be minimized and the promise of AI embraced for nursing education.

ESSENTIAL PROFESSIONAL DEVELOPMENT FOR AI-READY LEADERSHIP

AI is currently being integrated into nursing education, clinical practice, and health system management. Because of this, professional development to prepare nurses for an AI-ready workforce is no longer optional or tangentially required nursing leadership competencies. Successful AI implementation in nursing will depend less on how complex AI tools are and more on whether nurses and nurse leaders know when and how to use these tools, how to think critically about their output, and how to ensure they are being leveraged to align with professional standards of care, ethical frameworks, and patient-centered care (Pawar & Shaha, 2025). Without intentional and sustained professional development, AI technologies risk being underused, misused, or implemented in ways that undermine trust, equity, and professional autonomy.

Evidence of an essential preparedness gap between current strategic interest and planned capacity is emerging in national and international scholarship. Although AI and related digital transformation activities are widely seen as strategic priorities in healthcare, many organizations have not yet established the leadership capacity or workforce readiness to bring that priority to practice (Aldrich et al., 2025). According to results from an American Organization for Nursing Leadership (AONL) Think Tank, nearly 90% of healthcare executives and nurse leaders surveyed name AI and digital transformation as top organizational priorities, but a majority say their organizations have not invested in the appropriate planning, resources, and professional development (Aldrich et al., 2025). These findings highlight the need for AI-ready nursing leaders who can connect digital strategy, education, and practice.

A foundational goal of professional development must be applied AI literacy for nurses and nurse leaders at all levels, not only informaticists or those at the leadership level. Applied AI literacy includes knowledge about how AI systems work (e.g., how algorithms are trained, data quality affects outputs, and how bias and lack of transparency affect the strength of recommendations) as well as basic scientific principles that inform AI decision-making. Umbrella and systematic reviews of nurses' and nurse educators' perspectives on AI in health care education and practice have found strong interest and positivity about AI potential but low confidence in their ability to interpret AI outputs or system limitations (El Arab et al., 2025; El-Banna et al., 2025). Professional development must go beyond demonstrations of tools and include foundational knowledge of data, algorithms, and the ability to question and evaluate AI-supported decisions critically.

An essential component of professional development is also hands-on learning applied in realistic clinical and educational contexts. Recommendations from the AONL Think Tank include embedding AI education into nursing curricula and professional development through case studies, simulation, and practice-based scenarios that allow learners to apply AI tools and outputs to realistic clinical decision-making, documentation support, staffing, and workload management while still being accountable for final decision-making (Aldrich et al., 2025). This approach reflects more general findings that AI is most helpful and accepted when it augments, rather than replaces, professional clinical reasoning and care delivery (Alenezi et al., 2024).

Ethical competence must also be a defining part of AI-ready professional development. AI technologies bring with them many ethical issues related to data privacy, surveillance, transparency, bias, and responsibility that have direct implications for patient safety, professional practice, and health equity. Although the broad ethical principles that AI implementation should respect are generally well established in scholarship on AI and health ethics (Floridi & Cowls, 2019), these are not always clear to nurses about how they are or should be realized in practice. Emerging research in AI-integrated simulation and education finds that bias and algorithmic discrimination, consent and data security, and appropriate versus overuse continue to be problems as AI is applied to health education, care delivery, and clinical decision-making (Jung, 2023; El Arab et al., 2025). In both research and application, ethical considerations around AI in health care are rapidly emerging and must be made an explicit part of AI-ready professional development.

For nurse leaders, professional development for AI-readiness also extends into organizational and pedagogical leadership. Leaders must be prepared to guide how AI and related data analytics are built into curricula, assessment, simulation, workforce, and staffing models, care delivery operations, and organizational digital transformation strategy. The AONL Guiding Principles for Digital Transformation, developed by an AONL Expert Panel of healthcare executives, chief nursing officers, and academic leaders, state that "digital strategy is also the responsibility of nurse leaders and their involvement is expected by their teams and key stakeholders" and that nurse leaders must "advocate for digital adoption and integration that align with organizational strategy, culture and values," "seek input and alignment across teams," and "should own up to and/or lead digital transformation activities" (Aldrich et al., 2025, 1–3). This requires nurse leaders who are able to understand and teach not only AI applications but also their educational impact on learning, as well as their operational impact on nursing practice, including nursing workflows, staffing models, and interdisciplinary communication.

Change leadership and communication skills are likely to be particularly important for nurses and nurse leaders in AI-enabled care and educational environments. AI adoption and use in nursing can generate fear or resistance about job displacement, decreased autonomy, and being monitored. A review of nurse leaders' responses to AI-readiness found significant variability in leaders' knowledge about and plans for AI readiness and implementation, indicating a need for more targeted professional development, including communication and change leadership skills (Ahmed et al., 2025). Essential professional development for AI-readiness in leadership should prepare nurses and nurse leaders to overcome resistance, foster trust, communicate transparently with nurses and other stakeholders, and directly engage nurses in AI design, implementation, and evaluation.

Importantly, professional development for AI-readiness must be longitudinal, embedded in organizational structures, and ongoing, not delivered as a single training event. Evidence from the fields of nursing education, healthcare leadership, and higher education's digital transformation consistently show that short, one-time professional development events are less impactful than longitudinal, applied learning models such as communities of practice, interdisciplinary partnerships, mentoring, and assessment (El Arab et al., 2025; Pawar & Shaha, 2025). The AONL Think Tank recommendations further call for standardized competencies and readiness assessments across stakeholder groups (students, faculty, and practicing nurses) to guide appropriate and tailored professional development for AI (Aldrich et al., 2025).

Finally, essential professional development for AI-readiness must also allow nurses to take active roles in AI's future and development as applied in healthcare. In order to understand how and where AI should be used and governed in nursing, nurse educators and leaders must be able to interpret and explain AI and be prepared to question and test AI-supported decisions, escalate concerns, and advocate for patients. Leadership that does not provide this essential and applied professional development risks sending a message that AI, not nurses and nursing values, will determine how nurses practice and care is delivered.

As artificial intelligence technologies advance and proliferate in nursing education and practice, leaders must keep forefront the idea that these technologies should never replace the humanistic elements of nursing. Studies related to workforce and leadership concerns in healthcare show artificial intelligence can best function when it enhances and extends empathy, professional identity, and relationship-based care instead of replacing them (Alenezi et al., 2024). As AI becomes more integrated into educational and clinical systems, nursing leaders have a responsibility to hold firmly to the nursing worldview and to reassert the value of human relationships and professional judgment amid technological and commercial pressures that seek to displace or redefine them.

The future of AI in nursing education and leadership will likely depend less on the speed of adoption and more on alignment. When guided by pedagogy, ethical leadership, and professional values, AI can strengthen nursing education, safeguard patient care, and support excellence in practice within an increasingly complex healthcare environment.

RECOMMENDED AI TOOLS FOR NURSING EDUCATION AND LEADERSHIP

Artificial intelligence shows up in nursing less like a gadget, more like layers of tools reshaping how insights form, decisions unfold, support grows, authority shifts. Much like simulators, digital charts, online course platforms did earlier, AI matters not because it's new, yet due to the principles built into it and how those guide real-world choices. What nurses face today isn't about proving AI strong enough - it's about weaving it through training and guidance so clinical wisdom deepens, ethics stay clear, healing stays central.

Open access research now highlights how AI in health training must balance tech capabilities with human choices - how people guide systems matters just as much as code. Nursing faces a task: pick smart tools that do more than speed things up - they must honor care built on trust and responsibility. These suggestions sort digital aids by role in teaching nurses and guiding teams, spotlighting roles where judgment, fairness, and focus on patients grow stronger.

Adaptive Learning Platforms: The challenge of precision without pedagogical simplification

Learning paths shift based on how students respond when artificial intelligence guides the way. Tailored lessons show up in tough subjects - pharmacology sits beside pathophysiology, both shaped around each learner's pace. Instead of everyone moving step by step together like old classroom models demand, these digital helpers notice who struggles and who doesn't. One student might loop back through concepts while another moves ahead without pause. Flexibility becomes real once instruction stops pretending every mind works the same. Complex ideas meet individual rhythms rather than fixed timetables set long before anyone walked in. The system watches, adjusts, reshapes - all quietly behind screens where growth gets measured differently now.

A fresh approach unfolded when nursing instructors tackled repeated mistakes in giving medicines by new learners. Rather than adding extra classroom hours, they turned to insights pulled from smart software that tracks where students stumble - especially with dose math and how drugs move through bodies. Once the patterns emerged from the system's reports, teachers guided conversations helping pupils link those digital findings to sharper reasoning skills. This blend of machine feedback and human reflection reshaped how lessons were shaped in training nurses (Integration of artificial intelligence in nursing education, 2025).

Still, experts warn putting too much weight on adaptive tests can narrow education down to just what shows up in scores. Because of this, lessons might skip over ethics, personal growth in the field, and understanding emotions - things nurses need most. When tools shape teaching too tightly, softer but vital skills start fading out. What gets measured often pushes aside what matters just as much. These human elements anchor real care work, even if they do not appear on exams. Williamson and Eynon pointed this out back in 2020.

Still, knowing what's fair matters a lot. When confusion exists, artificial intelligence might lead learners to act with less integrity. For this reason, nursing leaders must lay down straightforward guidelines - making it known that technology should only support caregiving, never taking over the role of personal connection.

FUTURE DIRECTIONS

As artificial intelligence continues to develop, the future of nursing education and leadership depends less on technological capabilities and more on vision. The literature suggests that regardless of which educational or practice application is under consideration, artificial intelligence is most often viewed not as a replacement for educators, nurse leaders, or clinical judgment, but rather as an enabling technology that may allow for an extension of human reasoning, deepened learning, and support of complex decision-making processes, when applied mindfully and with care. Thus, the next phase of AI integration in nursing must be marked by human-centered design, ethical stewardship, and a focus on long-term professional development.

One main area of focus in the future will be shifting from adoption that is reactionary or convenience-based to purposeful, pedagogically-aligned design. Studies about AI integration in higher education have shown that in the past, implementations were often done because the technology was available instead of because it was necessary from a teaching and learning perspective (Zawacki-Richter et al., 2019). This problem is likely to be amplified in nursing education, where use of AI tools can have outsized implications. AI should be selected for and molded according to clearly stated learning objectives, such as clinical reasoning, ethical judgment, and safe patient care, so that, when educators are leading the process, AI will function as a means of deepening rather than cheapening professional preparation.

Ethical governance will also shape future AI use in nursing education and practice. Although the general principles of ethical AI have been well established, including transparency, justice, and accountability (Floridi & Cowls, 2019), nursing education specifically needs frameworks that consider patient safety and equity in care, as well as professional responsibility and accountability. Recent literature in healthcare education has similarly focused on the need for anticipatory ethics, in which AI's risks are considered, such as bias, data use and storage, and system limitations, and ideally addressed by educational institutions before implementation rather than in response to harm (Artificial Intelligence in Healthcare Education, 2023). In the future, progress will be marked by values such as these being translated into clear institutional policies to guide both education and practice.

Preparation of AI-ready nurse leaders is another crucial area of future focus. Research on educators' and leaders' understanding of AI in healthcare systems shows a knowledge gap in which many stakeholders are aware of AI's potential in the future but not confident in their ability to evaluate, implement, or govern AI tools and resources (assayed et al., 2025). Leadership development, then, must go beyond technical training to include such skills as ethical reasoning, change management, and the ability to engage critically with AI-generated recommendations or data visualizations. Nurse leaders who are prepared to ask the right questions of AI systems will be best positioned to ensure that their use supports clinical and educational judgment, rather than supplanting it.

Simulation and other experiential learning environments are likely to grow in importance as well. AI-enhanced simulation could allow for greater personalization and adaptivity in learning experiences, supporting both reflective practice and clinical decision-making in safe spaces (Jung, 2023). However, important for the future of AI in simulation will be continuing to maintain and emphasize the educator's role as a facilitator and mentor. AI should not be used to replace or automate assessment or judgment. On the contrary, when AI is used to identify learning patterns or student behaviors and guided by expert faculty, AI-generated data may be used to support simulation debriefing and deepen student self-reflection.

Effective and sustainable AI integration in nursing education will increasingly rely on interdisciplinary collaboration. Nurse educators, educational technologists, ethicists, data scientists, and healthcare administrators will all need to work together to ensure AI's successful use. As noted in the literature, AI in education initiatives is most likely to be successful and sustainable when educators are active partners in development and evaluation, rather than passive end-users of externally developed systems (Ramírez-Baraldes et al., 2025). Interdisciplinary work will help to ensure alignment between innovation and professional standards and values.

Looking ahead, AI in nursing education will also need to remain grounded in the human elements of nursing. Research into workforce and leadership in the age of AI has emphasized that the technology is most likely to be a benefit to the field and individual learners when it does not erode empathy, professional identity, or relational care (Alenezi et al., 2024). Nursing leaders have a responsibility to continuously reiterate the nursing worldview when AI is becoming more integrated into educational and clinical systems, to ensure that technology is always being used to support nursing practice and not vice versa.

In the future, the integration of AI in nursing education and leadership will be characterized less by acceleration and more by alignment. AI integration that is driven by pedagogy, ethical leadership, and professional values is uniquely positioned to support and strengthen nursing education, to protect patient care, and to support excellence in a rapidly changing healthcare environment.

CONCLUSION

This chapter demonstrates that AI is not merely a technological advancement but a transformative force that reshapes how nurses learn, lead, and deliver care and it also explores how artificial intelligence is transforming nursing education and leadership by reshaping the roles and responsibilities of nurse leaders and the ways curricula are designed as AI-supported systems assist nurse leaders by improving clinical insight, predictive staffing, operational efficiency, and evidence-based decision-making, ultimately supporting patient safety and workforce wellbeing.

It is a fact that effective nursing leadership plays a vital role in empowering and preparing nurses for AI integration, as this integration is changing traditional learning methodologies while enhancing personalization, student engagement, and administrative effectiveness. Generally, AI is emerging as a significant influence on educational design and leadership practice, so nursing students are increasingly required to develop not only foundational clinical knowledge but also advanced academic skills such as critical thinking, clinical decision-making, and problem-solving.

The chapter also highlights the opportunities AI presents for nursing practice and AI-enhanced learning environments demonstrating how thoughtful integration of AI tools can provide nursing students, nurses, and clinicians with smarter solutions and richer learning experiences that they need to strengthen their academic engagement, clinical competence, and decision-making through personalization and interactivity. The chapter also focuses on human-centered leadership that emerges as an essential requirement in the AI era because it enables nurse leaders to balance innovation with professional responsibility.

While AI offers significant benefits for nursing education and leadership efficiency, it also raises important complexities related to privacy, equity, ethical governance, and the potential displacement of human roles within healthcare; consequently, nursing care should be grounded in compassion, ethical reasoning, and relational practice

This chapter emphasizes the need for structured training and professional development programs that prepare nurses to use AI tools effectively and provide them with AI literacy, critical evaluation skills, and professional confidence. Such programs should be embedded within the organizational frameworks and governance structures that proactively address data privacy, transparency, equity, and academic integrity prior to AI adoption. This chapter also provides insight into how nurses and nurse leaders can engage with recommended AI tools in ways that allow them to shape technological implementation rather than be shaped by it.

AI has the potential to strengthen nursing education, enhance leadership capacity, and improve the quality and sustainability of healthcare delivery. As a general rule, the future integration of AI in nursing depends on leaders who should lead with trust, and ethical clarity, ensuring that AI remains an asset to nursing and to patients rather than a force that reshapes the profession in unintended or inequitable ways.

REFERENCES

Ahmed, A. A.. (2025). Empowering nurse leaders: Readiness for AI integration and perceived benefits of predictive analytics. *BMC Nursing*, *24*(1), 56. DOI: 10.1186/s12912-024-02653-x PMID: 39819624

AlAli, M. F., Qtait, M., Al-Alwayssa, R. M., Alqaissi, N., & Jaradat, Y. (2025). The impact of artificial intelligence on nursing students: A systematic review. *South Eastern European Journal of Public Health*, 797–808. Advance online publication. DOI: 10.70135/seejph.vi.4633

Alanzi, T. M., & Al-Shakihs, A. H. (2025). Readiness and acceptance of nursing students regarding AI-based health care technology in training. *JMIR Nursing*, *8*, e71653. DOI: 10.2196/71653 PMID: 40737490

Aldrich, K., Chipps, E., & Mook, P. J. (2025). Driving innovations: Nursing leadership think tank explores AI solutions. *Nurse Leader*, *23*(3), 236–238. DOI: 10.1016/j.mnl.2025.04.001

Alenezi, A., Alshammari, M. H., & Ibrahim, I. A. (2024). Optimizing Nursing Productivity: Exploring the Role of Artificial Intelligence, Technology Integration, Competencies, and Leadership. Journal of Nursing Management, 2024(1). Portico. DOI: 10.1155/2024/8371068

Amann, J., Blasimme, A., Vayena, E., Frey, D., & Madai, V. I. (2020). Explainability for artificial intelligence in healthcare: A multidisciplinary perspective. *BMC Medical Informatics and Decision Making*, *20*(1), 1–9. DOI: 10.1186/s12911-020-01332-6 PMID: 33256715

Assayed, A. K., & Assayed, S. K. (2026). AI-Driven Educational Leadership: Empowering Leaders, Staff, and Students in the Digital Age. In *Enhancing Student Support and Learning Through Conversational AI* (pp. 1-18). IGI Global Scientific Publishing.

Assayed, S. K., Alkhatib, M., & Shaalan, K. (2023, June). Advising chatbot for high school in smart cities. In *2023 8th International Conference on Smart and Sustainable Technologies (SpliTech)* (pp. 1-6). IEEE. DOI: 10.23919/SpliTech58164.2023.10193065

Assayed, S. K., Shieh, C. S., & Gupta, S. K. (2025). Engineering intelligent healthcare systems: Understanding medical queries with AI and NLP. *Journal of Engineering and Applied Sciences (Asian Research Publishing Network)*, *72*(1), 212. DOI: 10.1186/s44147-025-00800-y

Basulo-Ribeiro, J., & Teixeira, L. (2024). The future of healthcare with Industry 5.0: Preliminary interview-based qualitative analysis. *Future Internet, 16*(3), 68. DOI: 10.3390/fi16030068

Booth, R. G.. (2021). Ethical challenges of AI in nursing and healthcare leadership. *Journal of Nursing Management, 29*(5), 1234–1243.

Buchanan, C., Howitt, M. L., Wilson, R., Booth, R. G., Risling, T., & Bamford, M. (2020). Predicted influences of artificial intelligence on nursing education: Scoping review (Preprint). https://doi.org/DOI: 10.2196/preprints.23933

Cucci, F., Marasciulo, D., Romani, M., Soldano, G., Cascio, D., De Nunzio, G., Caldararo, C., Rubbi, I., Vitale, E., Lupo, R., & Conte, L. (2025). The contribution of artificial intelligence in nursing education: A scoping review of the literature. *Nursing Reports, 15*(8), 283. DOI: 10.3390/nursrep15080283 PMID: 40863670

Davenport, T. H., & Kalakota, R. (2019). The potential for artificial intelligence in healthcare. *Future Healthcare Journal, 6*(2), 94–98. DOI: 10.7861/futurehosp.6-2-94 PMID: 31363513

De Gagne, J. C. (2023). The state of artificial intelligence in nursing education: Past, present, and future directions. *International Journal of Environmental Research and Public Health, 20*(6), 4884. DOI: 10.3390/ijerph20064884 PMID: 36981790

Domfeh, E. A., Weyori, B., Appiahene, P., Mensah, J., Awarayi, N., & Afrifa, S. (2022). Human-centered artificial intelligence: A review. https://doi.org/DOI: 10.22541/au.166013641.15972664/v1

El Arab, R. A., Al Moosa, O. A., Abuadas, F. H., & Somerville, J. (2025). The role of artificial intelligence in nursing education and practice: An umbrella review. *Journal of Medical Internet Research, 27*, e69881. DOI: 10.2196/69881 PMID: 40072926

El-Banna, M. M., Sajid, M. R., Rizvi, M. R., Sami, W., & McNelis, A. M. (2025). AI literacy and competency in nursing education: Preparing students and faculty members for an AI-enabled future. *Frontiers in Medicine, 12*, 1681784. DOI: 10.3389/fmed.2025.1681784 PMID: 41384110

Floridi, L., & Cowls, J. (2019). A unified framework of five principles for AI in society. *Harvard Data Science Review, 1*(1). Advance online publication. DOI: 10.1162/99608f92.8cd550d1

Han, S., Han, J., & Cho, M. (2025). Nursing students' perceptions, benefits, and challenges of using artificial intelligence in academic settings. *Nursing Reports, 15*(2), 283–298. DOI: 10.3390/nursrep15020068 PMID: 39997804

Judijanto, L., Ili, L., & Wardhana, M. G. (2025). Education 5.0: Collaboration and creativity in improving students' digital intelligence. *International Journal of Teaching and Learning*, *3*(4), 369–382.

Jung, S. (2023). Challenges and future directions for artificial intelligence integrated nursing simulation education. *Korean Journal of Women Health Nursing*, *29*(3), 239–242. DOI: 10.4069/kjwhn.2023.09.06.1 PMID: 37813667

Khlaif, Z. N., Salameh, N., Ajouz, M., & Alwawi, A. (2025). Using generative AI in nursing education: Students' perceptions. *BMC Medical Education*, *25*(1), 926. DOI: 10.1186/s12909-025-07416-z PMID: 40598139

Kotp, M. H., Ismail, H. A., Basyouny, H. A. A., & Elmoaty, A. E. (2025). Nurse leaders' readiness for AI integration: Implications for healthcare management. *BMC Nursing*, *24*, 56. DOI: 10.1186/s12912-024-02653-x PMID: 39819624

Labrague, L. J., Al Sabei, S., & Al Yahyaei, A. (2025). Artificial intelligence in nursing education: A review of AI-based teaching pedagogies. *Teaching and Learning in Nursing*, *20*(3), 210–221. DOI: 10.1016/j.teln.2025.01.019

Morley, J., Floridi, L., Kinsey, L., & Elhalal, A. (2020). From what to how: Ethical implementation of AI in healthcare. *AI & Society*, *35*(2), 457–468.

Pawar, P., & Shaha, S. R. (2025). Digital transformation in higher education: Innovations, strategies, and challenges. In *Higher Education 4.0: Strategies for digital success* (1st ed.). Dreambook Publishing House.

Ramírez-Baraldes, A., González, M. A., & Avendaño, C. (2025). Artificial intelligence in nursing: New opportunities and challenges. *European Journal of Education*, *60*(1), 123–140. DOI: 10.1111/ejed.70033

Rony, M. K. K., Ahmad, S., Tanha, S. M., Das, D. C., Akter, M. R., Khatun, M. A., Begum, M. H. B., Khalil, M. I., Peu, U. R., Parvin, M. R., Alrazeeni, D. M., & Akter, F. (2025). Nursing educators' perspectives on the integration of artificial intelligence into academic settings. *SAGE Open Nursing*, *11*, 23779608251342931. Advance online publication. DOI: 10.1177/23779608251342931 PMID: 40386172

Shahidi Hamedani, S., Aslam, S., Mundher Oraibi, B. A., Wah, Y. B., & Shahidi Hamedani, S. (2024). Transitioning towards tomorrow's workforce: Education 5.0 in the landscape of Society 5.0: A systematic literature review. *Education Sciences*, *14*(10), 1041. DOI: 10.3390/educsci14101041

Sriharan, A., Sekercioglu, N., Mitchell, C., Senkaiahliyan, S., Hertelendy, A., Porter, T., & Banaszak-Holl, J. (2024). Leadership for AI transformation in health care organization: Scoping review. *Journal of Medical Internet Research, 26*, e54556. DOI: 10.2196/54556 PMID: 39009038

Stuart-Pesevic, N., & Talarico, S. (2024). Nursing leadership. *Nurse Leader, 22*(5), 526–530. DOI: 10.1016/j.mnl.2024.07.001

Sullivan, D., Hall, V. P., & Morrison, J. (2024). Navigating the future: Artificial intelligence's impact on transformational nurse leadership. *Teaching and Learning in Nursing, 19*(3), 298–300. DOI: 10.1016/j.teln.2024.04.017

Topol, E. (2019). *Deep medicine: How artificial intelligence can make healthcare human again*. Basic Books.

Williamson, B., & Eynon, R. (2020). Historical threads, missing links, and future directions in AI in education. *Learning, Media and Technology, 45*(3), 223–235. DOI: 10.1080/17439884.2020.1798995

World Health Organization. (2021). *Ethics and governance of artificial intelligence for health*. WHO.

World Health Organization. (2024). *Ethics and governance of artificial intelligence for health: Large multi-modal models*. World Health Organization.

Zawacki-Richter, O., Marín, V. I., Bond, M., & Gouverneur, F. (2019). Systematic review of research on artificial intelligence applications in higher education: Where are the educators? *International Journal of Educational Technology in Higher Education, 16*(1), 39. DOI: 10.1186/s41239-019-0171-0

Compilation of References

Abernethy, A., Adams, L., Barrett, M., Bechtel, C., Brennan, P., Butte, A., Faulkner, J., Fontaine, E., Friedhoff, S., Halamka, J., Howell, M., Johnson, K., Long, P., McGraw, D., Miller, R., Lee, P., Perlin, J., Rucker, D., Sandy, L., & Valdes, K. (2022). (2022). The Promise of Digital Health: Then, Now, and the Future. *NAM Perspectives*, *6*(22). Advance online publication. DOI: 10.31478/202206e

Abualruz, H., Yasin, I., Sabra, M A A., & Abunab, H. Y. (2025). The role of artificial intelligence in enhancing triage decisions in healthcare settings: A systematic review. . *Applied Nursing Research*, *62*, 151576. DOI: 10.1016/j.apnr.2025.152024

Acharya, D. B., Kuppan, K., & Divya, B. (2025). Agentic AI: Autonomous intelligence for complex goals—A comprehensive survey. *IEEE Access : Practical Innovations, Open Solutions*, *13*, 18912–18936. DOI: 10.1109/ACCESS.2025.3532853

Adeniyi, A. O., Arowoogun, J. O., Chidi, R., Okolo, C. A., & Babawarun, O. (2024). The impact of electronic health records on patient care and outcomes: A comprehensive review. *World Journal of Advanced Research and Reviews*, *21*(2), 1446–1455. DOI: 10.30574/wjarr.2024.21.2.0592

Agrawal, A., Soni, R., Gupta, D., & Dubey, G. (2024). The role of robotics in medical science: Advancements, applications, and future directions. *Journal of Autonomous Intelligence*, *7*(3), 1–27. DOI: 10.32629/jai.v7i3.1008

Ahmed, A. A.. (2025). Empowering nurse leaders: Readiness for AI integration and perceived benefits of predictive analytics. *BMC Nursing*, *24*(1), 56. DOI: 10.1186/s12912-024-02653-x PMID: 39819624

Ahmed, S. F., Sharmin, S., Kuldeep, S. A., & Gandomi, A. H. (2025). Transformative impacts of the Internet of Medical Things on modern healthcare. [CoLab]. *Results in Engineering*, *25*, 103787. DOI: 10.1016/j.rineng.2024.103787

Ajegbile, M. D., Olaboye, J. A., Maha, C. C., Igwama, G. T., & Abdul, S. (2024). The role of data-driven initiatives in enhancing healthcare delivery and patient retention. *World Journal of Biology Pharmacy and Health Sciences*, *19*(1), 234–242. DOI: 10.30574/wjbphs.2024.19.1.0435

Ajjawi, R., Tai, J., Dollinger, M., Dawson, P., Boud, D., & Bearman, M. (2024). From authentic assessment to authenticity in assessment: Broadening perspectives. *Assessment & Evaluation in Higher Education*, *49*(4), 499–510. DOI: 10.1080/02602938.2023.2271193

Akhmedov, B. A. (2025). Integrating ICT and artificial intelligence in teaching philological disciplines: a focus on machine translation of textual data. *Экономика и социум*, (6-1 (133)), 115-122.

Al Khatib, I., Shamayleh, A., & Ndiaye, M. (2024). Healthcare and the Internet of Medical Things: Applications, trends, key challenges, and proposed resolutions. [MDPI]. *Informatics (MDPI)*, *11*(3), 47. DOI: 10.3390/informatics11030047

Al Sadi, K., & Balachandran, W. (2023). Prediction model of Type 2 diabetes mellitus for Oman prediabetes patients using artificial neural network and six machine learning classifiers. *Applied Sciences (Basel, Switzerland)*, *13*(4), 2344. DOI: 10.3390/app13042344

AlAli, M. F., Qtait, M., Al-Alwayssa, R. M., Alqaissi, N., & Jaradat, Y. (2025). The impact of artificial intelligence on nursing students: A systematic review. *South Eastern European Journal of Public Health*, 797–808. Advance online publication. DOI: 10.70135/seejph.vi.4633

Alanazi, A. (2025). Assessing Clinicians' Legal Concerns and the Need for a Regulatory Framework for AI in Healthcare: A Mixed-Methods Study. *Health Care*, *13*(13), 1487. DOI: 10.3390/healthcare13131487 PMID: 40648512

Alanazi, M. A., Shaban, M. M., Ramadan, O. M. E., Zaky, M. E., Mohammed, H. H., Amer, F. G. M., & Shaban, M. (2024). Navigating end-of-life decision-making in nursing: A systematic review of ethical challenges and palliative care practices. *BMC Nursing*, *23*(1), 467. DOI: 10.1186/s12912-024-02087-5

Alanzi, T. M., & Al-Shakihs, A. H. (2025). Readiness and acceptance of nursing students regarding AI-based health care technology in training. *JMIR Nursing*, *8*, e71653. DOI: 10.2196/71653 PMID: 40737490

Alder, S. (2026, January 2). Effects of Poor Communication in Healthcare—2026 Update. *The HIPAA Journal*. https://www.hipaajournal.com/effects-of-poor-communication-in-healthcare/

Alderman, J. E., Palmer, J., Laws, E., McCradden, M. D., Ordish, J., Ghassemi, M., Pfohl, S. R., Rostamzadeh, N., Cole-Lewis, H., Glocker, B., Calvert, M., Pollard, T. J., Gill, J., Gath, J., Adebajo, A., Beng, J., Leung, C. H., Kuku, S., Farmer, L.-A., & Liu, X. (2025). Tackling algorithmic bias and promoting transparency in health datasets: The STANDING Together consensus recommendations. *The Lancet. Digital Health*, *7*(1), e64–e88. DOI: 10.1016/S2589-7500(24)00224-3 PMID: 39701919

Aldrich, K., Chipps, E., & Mook, P. J. (2025). Driving innovations: Nursing leadership think tank explores AI solutions. *Nurse Leader*, *23*(3), 236–238. DOI: 10.1016/j.mnl.2025.04.001

Alenezi, A., Alshammari, M. H., & Ibrahim, I. A. (2024). Optimizing nursing Productivity: Exploring the role of Artificial Intelligence, Technology Integration, competencies, and Leadership. *Journal of Nursing Management*, *2024*(1), 8371068. DOI: 10.1155/2024/8371068

Alfakhry, G., Naeem, A., AboHajar, M. B., Alfakhry, A., Mohandes, A. F., Ali, I., Makhoul, E., Ahmed, N., Abla, M. M., Alhomsi, K., & Jamous, I. (2023, January 3). Revealing the significant shortcomings in the learning environment at the three largest medical schools in Syria: What's next? *BMC Medical Education*, *23*(1), 2. DOI: 10.1186/s12909-022-03978-4 PMID: 36597081

Alharbi, T. A. F., Rababa, M., Alsuwayl, H., Alsubail, A., & Alenizi, W. S. (2025). Diagnostic challenges and patient safety: the critical role of accuracy: a systematic review. *Journal of Multidisciplinary Healthcare*, *18*, 3051–3064. DOI: 10.2147/JMDH.S512254

Ali Mohamad, T., Bastone, A., Bernhard, F., & Schiavone, F. (2023). How artificial intelligence impacts the competitive position of healthcare organizations. *Journal of Organizational Change Management*, *36*(8), 49–70. DOI: 10.1108/JOCM-03-2023-0057

Ali, A. M., Abdelhafeez, A., Soliman, T. H., & ELMenshawy, K. (2024). A probabilistic hesitant fuzzy MCDM approach to selecting treatment policy for COVID-19. Decision making: applications in management and engineering, 7(1), 131-144. DOI: 10.31181/dmame712024917

Ali, H. (2022). Reinforcement learning in healthcare: Optimizing treatment strategies, dynamic resource allocation, and adaptive clinical decision-making. *Int J Comput Appl Technol Res*, *11*(3), 88–104.

Almagharbeh, W. T. (2025). The impact of AI-based decision support systems on nursing workflows in critical care units. *International Nursing Review*, *72*(2), e13011. DOI: 10.1111/inr.13011

Almagharbeh, W. T., Alfanash, H. A., Alnawafleh, K. A., Alasmari, A. A., Alsaraireh, F. A., Dreidi, M. M., & Nashwan, A. J. (2025). Application of artificial intelligence in nursing practice: A qualitative study of Jordanian nurses' perspectives. *BMC Nursing*, *24*(1), 92. DOI: 10.1186/s12912-024-02658-6 PMID: 39863852

Almotairi, M. A., Alotaibi, A. S. M., Alharbi, K. F. N., Alqarni, A. M. G., Alshammari, M. S. F., Alqasir, M. A., Alshammari, F. N. S., Alrowaily, S. A. T., Bellen, A. C., Alsoaib, A., Alraggas, T. M., Alojairi, A. A., Alessa, N. H., Alrabeeah, R. T., Alshehri, W. D., & Alqahtani, S. T. A. (2024). Nursing Documentation as a Foundation of Safe, Ethical, and Accountable Care: A Systematic Review. *Journal of Angiotherapy*, *8*(5), 1–13. DOI: 10.25163/angiotherapy.8510497

Alnawafleh, K. A. (2024). The Impact of AI on Nursing Workload and Stress Levels in Critical Care Settings. *Pakistan Journal of Life and Social Sciences*, *22*(2), 8529–8542. DOI: 10.57239/PJLSS-2024-22.2.00643

Alobayli, F., O'Connor, S., Holloway, A., & Cresswell, K. (2023). Electronic Health Record Stress and Burnout Among Clinicians in Hospital Settings: A Systematic Review. *Digital Health*, *9*, 20552076231220241. DOI: 10.1177/20552076231220241 PMID: 38130797

Alowais, S. A., Alghamdi, S. S., Alsuhebany, N., Alqahtani, T., Alshaya, A. I., Almohareb, S. N., Aldairem, A., Alrashed, M., Bin Saleh, K., Badreldin, H. A., Al Yami, M. S., Al Harbi, S., & Albekairy, A. M. (2023). Revolutionizing healthcare: The role of artificial intelligence in clinical practice. *BMC Medical Education*, *23*(1), 689. DOI: 10.1186/s12909-023-04698-z

Alruwaili, A. N., Alshammari, A. M., Alhaiti, A., Elsharkawy, N. B., Ali, S. I., & Elsayed Ramadan, O. M. (2025). 'Neonatal nurses' experiences with generative AI in clinical decision-making: A qualitative exploration in high-risk NICUs'. *BMC Nursing*, *24*(1), 1–20. DOI: 10.1186/s12912-025-03044-6

AlSaad, R., Abd-Alrazaq, A., Boughorbel, S., Ahmed, A., Renault, M. A., Damseh, R., & Sheikh, J. (2024). Multimodal large language models in health care: Applications, challenges, and future outlook. *Journal of Medical Internet Research*, *26*, e59505. DOI: 10.2196/59505 PMID: 39321458

Alsayed, S., Assayed, S. K., Alkhatib, M., & Shaalan, K. (2024). Impact of artificial intelligence chatbots on student well-being and mental health: A systematic review. *People and Behavior Analysis*, *2*(2), 1–3. DOI: 10.31098/pba.v2i2.2411

Alshalawi, M. A., Almuhlafi, J. M., Alsubiei, S. M., Al-Shamrani, S. E., Alotaibi, M. M., Alenzi, S. M., & Alotaibi, A. H. (2024). The Role Of Clinic Development Strategies In Enhancing Care Coordination And Clinical Workflow: A Systematic Evaluation Of Evidence. *The Review of Diabetic Studies; RDS*, •••, 182–190.

Al-Thani, N. A., Al-Ansari, T., & Haouari, M. (2022). Integrated TOPSIS-COV approach for selecting a sustainable PET waste management technology: A case study in Qatar. *Heliyon*, *8*(8), e10274. Advance online publication. DOI: 10.1016/j.heliyon.2022.e10274 PMID: 36061036

Alwashmi, M. F., Hawboldt, J., Davis, E., Marra, C., & Gamble, J. M. (2021). "The use of digital health technologies for remote monitoring in chronic disease management: An overview." Frontiers in Public Health, Volume 9. *Article*, *652456*, 1–10. DOI: 10.3389/fpubh.2021.652456

Alzghaibi, H. (2025). Nurses' perspectives on AI-Enabled wearable health technologies: Opportunities and challenges in clinical practice. *BMC Nursing*, *24*(1), 799. DOI: 10.1186/s12912-025-03343-y

Amann, J., Blasimme, A., Vayena, E., Frey, D., & Madai, V. I. (2020). Explainability for artificial intelligence in healthcare: A multidisciplinary perspective. *BMC Medical Informatics and Decision Making*, *20*(1), 310. Advance online publication. DOI: 10.1186/s12911-020-01332-6 PMID: 33256715

Amiot, F., & Potier, B. (2025). Artificial intelligence and emergency medicine: Balancing opportunities and challenges. *JMIR Medical Informatics*, *13*(1), e70903. DOI: 10.2196/70903

Amjad, A., Kordel, P., & Fernandes, G. (2023). A review on innovation in healthcare sector (telehealth) through artificial intelligence. *Sustainability (Basel)*, *15*(8), 6655. Advance online publication. DOI: 10.3390/su15086655

Andrade, A. N., Cabral, A. T., Bellini, B., Facco Rodrigues, V., da Rosa Righi, R., André da Costa, C., & Barbosa, J. L. V. (2024). IoT-based vital sign monitoring: A literature review. *Smart Health (Amsterdam, Netherlands)*, *32*, 100462. Advance online publication. DOI: 10.1016/j.smhl.2024.100462

Apathy, N. C., Rotenstein, L. S., Bates, D. W., & Holmgren, A. J. (2022). Documentation dynamics: Note composition, burden, and physician efficiency. *Journal of the American Medical Informatics Association : JAMIA*, *29*(3), 674–685.

Aquino, Y. S. J. (2023). Making decisions: Bias in artificial intelligence and data-driven diagnostic tools. *Australian Journal of General Practice*, *52*(7), 439–442. DOI: 10.31128/AJGP-12-22-6630 PMID: 37423238

Araouchi, Z., & Adda, M. (2025). A Comprehensive Literature Review on AI-Assisted Multimodal Triage Systems for Health Centers. . *Procedia Computer Science*, *250*, 311–318. DOI: 10.1016/j.procs.2025.03.029

Arinze, C. A., Izionworu, V. O., Isong, D., Daudu, C. D., & Adefemi, A. (2024). Integrating artificial intelligence into engineering processes for improved efficiency and safety in oil and gas operations. *Open Access Research Journal of Engineering and Technology*, *6*(1), 39–51. DOI: 10.53022/oarjet.2024.6.1.0012

Arslan, A. E., Arslan, O., & Kandemir, S. Y. (2021). AHP–TOPSIS hybrid decision-making analysis: Simav integrated system case study. *Journal of Thermal Analysis and Calorimetry*, *145*(3), 1191–1202. Advance online publication. DOI: 10.1007/s10973-020-10270-4

Asgari, E., Kaur, J., Nuredini, G., Balloch, J., Taylor, A. M., Sebire, N., Robinson, R., Peters, C., Sridharan, S., & Pimenta, D. (2024). Impact of Electronic Health Record Use on Cognitive Load and Burnout Among Clinicians: Narrative Review. *JMIR Medical Informatics*, *12*(1), e55499. DOI: 10.2196/55499 PMID: 38607672

Asha, R., Sangeetha, J., Adaikkammai, A., Thilagam, T., & Aparna, P. (2026). Machine Learning and Computational Intelligence for Smart Healthcare: Advancing Diagnosis and Treatment. In *Applied AI and Computational Intelligence in Diagnostics and Decision-Making* (pp. 87-110). IGI Global Scientific Publishing.

Ashburner, J. M., Chang, Y., Wang, X., Khurshid, S., Anderson, C. D., Dahal, K., Weisenfeld, D., Cai, T., Liao, K. P., Wagholikar, K. B., Murphy, S. N., Atlas, S. J., Lubitz, S. A., & Singer, D. E. (2022). Natural language processing to improve prediction of incident atrial fibrillation using electronic health records. . *Journal of the American Heart Association*, *11*(15), e023123. DOI: 10.1161/JAHA.122.026014

Assayed, A. K., & Assayed, S. K. (2026). AI-Driven Educational Leadership: Empowering Leaders, Staff, and Students in the Digital Age. In *Enhancing Student Support and Learning Through Conversational AI* (pp. 1-18). IGI Global Scientific Publishing.

Assayed, S. K., Alkhatib, M., & Shaalan, K. (2023, June). Advising chatbot for high school in smart cities. In *2023 8th International Conference on Smart and Sustainable Technologies (SpliTech)* (pp. 1-6). IEEE. DOI: 10.23919/SpliTech58164.2023.10193065

Assayed, S. K. (2025a). *Transforming healthcare through generative and agentic AI: A systematic review*. In *Proceedings of the 10th International Conference on Information Technology Trends (ITT)* (pp. 124–129). IEEE. https://doi.org/DOI: 10.1109/ITT69610.2025.11352935

Assayed, S. K. (Ed.). (2025a). *Educational Applications of Natural Language Processing, Chatbots, and AI*. IGI Global. DOI: 10.4018/979-8-3373-6791-0

Assayed, S. K. (Ed.). (2025b). *Enhancing Student Support and Learning Through Conversational AI*. IGI Global. DOI: 10.4018/979-8-3373-3316-8

Assayed, S. K., Alkhatib, M., & Shaalan, K. (2024). Transforming student advising in smart cities: A deep learning conversational AI chatbot. In *Proceedings of the 2024 Mediterranean Smart Cities Conference (MSCC)* (pp. 1–6). IEEE. https://doi.org/DOI: 10.1109/MSCC62288.2024.10696988

Assayed, S. K., Alkhatib, M., Shaalan, K. F., & Alsayed, S. (2025). HSGAdviser: AI speech assistant for enabling sustainable education solutions. In *Proceedings of the 2025 1st International Conference on Computational Intelligence Approaches and Applications (ICCIAA)* (pp. 1–6). IEEE. https://doi.org/DOI: 10.1109/ICCIAA65327.2025.11013058

Assayed, S. K., Shieh, C. S., & Gupta, S. K. (2025). Engineering intelligent healthcare systems: Understanding medical queries with AI and NLP. *Journal of Engineering and Applied Sciences (Asian Research Publishing Network)*, *72*(1), 212. DOI: 10.1186/s44147-025-00800-y

Assayed, S., & Maheshwari, P. (2023). Agent-based simulation for university students admission: Medical colleges in Jordan universities. *Computer Science & Engineering* [CSEIJ]. *International Journal (Toronto, Ont.)*, *13*(1).

Assayed, S., Shaalan, K., Al-Sayed, S., & Alkhatib, M. (2023). Psychological emotion recognition of students using machine learning based chatbot. [IJAIA]. *International Journal of Artificial Intelligence & Applications*, *14*(2), 29–39. DOI: 10.5121/ijaia.2023.14203

Astbury, H., Fortune, E., Dal Ponte, C., Lyons, K., & Shaw, L. (2025). Generative artificial intelligence for teaching and assessment in health professions education: A scoping review. *Nurse Education in Practice*, •••, 104697.

Ayan, E., & Ünver, H. M. (2019, April). Diagnosis of pneumonia from chest X-ray images using deep learning. In 2019 Scientific meeting on electrical-electronics & biomedical engineering and computer science (EBBT) (pp. 1-5). Ieee. DOI: 10.1109/EBBT.2019.8741582

Azari, A., Nabizadeh, R., Mahvi, A. H., & Nasseri, S. (2022). Integrated Fuzzy AHP-TOPSIS for selecting the best color removal process using carbon-based adsorbent materials: Multi-criteria decision making vs. systematic review approaches and modeling of textile wastewater treatment in real conditions. *International Journal of Environmental Analytical Chemistry*, *102*(18), 7329–7344. DOI: 10.1080/03067319.2020.1828395

Azeroual, O. (2024). Can generative AI transform data quality? A critical discussion of ChatGPT's capabilities. *Academia Engineering, 1*(4).

Babapour, A. R., Gahassab-Mozaffari, N., & Fathnezhad-Kazemi, A. (2022). Nurses' job stress and its impact on quality of life and caring behaviors: A cross-sectional study. *BMC Nursing*, *21*(1), 75. DOI: 10.1186/s12912-022-00852-y

Badawy, M., Ramadan, N., & Hefny, H. A. (2023). Healthcare predictive analytics using machine learning and deep learning techniques: A survey. *Journal of Electrical Systems and Information Technology*, *10*(1), 40. DOI: 10.1186/s43067-023-00108-y

Badola, A., Chauhan, R., Bhatt, C., Devliyal, S., Kumar, G., & Pillai, R. (2024). Deep learning–based frailty detection in conjunction with telemedicine. In *Proceedings of the 2024 IEEE 9th International Conference for Convergence in Technology (I2CT)* (pp. 1–7). IEEE. DOI: 10.1109/I2CT61223.2024.10544058

Badr, J., Motulsky, A., & Denis, J. (2024). Digital health technologies and inequalities: A scoping review of potential impacts and policy recommendations. *Health Policy (Amsterdam)*, *146*, 105122. DOI: 10.1016/j.healthpol.2024.105122 PMID: 38986333

Baidoo-Anu, D., & Ansah, L. O. (2023). Education in the era of generative artificial intelligence (AI): Understanding the potential benefits of ChatGPT in promoting teaching and learning. *Journal of Artificial Intelligence*, *7*(1), 52–62.

Baig, M. M., Hobson, C., GholamHosseini, H., Ullah, E., & Afifi, S. (2024). Generative AI in improving personalized patient care plans: Opportunities and barriers towards its wider adoption. . *Applied Sciences (Basel, Switzerland)*, *14*(23), 9876. DOI: 10.3390/app142310899

Bakker, C. J., Wyatt, T. H., Breth, M. C., Gao, G., Janeway, L. M., Lee, M. A., Martin, C. L., & Tiase, V. L. (2023). Nurses' roles in mHealth app development: Scoping review. *JMIR Nursing*, *6*, e46058. DOI: 10.2196/46058

Barak-Corren, Y., Wolf, R., Rozenblum, R., Creedon, J. K., Lipsett, S. C., Lyons, T. W., Michelson, K. A., Miller, K. A., Shapiro, D. J., Reis, B. Y., & Fine, A. M. (2024). Harnessing the power of generative AI for clinical summaries: Perspectives from emergency physicians. *Annals of Emergency Medicine*, *84*(2), 128–138. DOI: 10.1016/j.annemergmed.2024.01.039

Barnard, J. (2019). *Clinical decision-making by acute medicine advanced nurse practitioners*. Sheffield Hallam University.

Basu, D., Kashid, S., Pawar, S., & Datta, D. (2020, December). An integrated detection and treatment recommendation framework for breast cancer using convolutional neural networks and TOPSIS. In 2020 IEEE 17th India Council International Conference (INDICON) (pp. 1-7). IEEE. DOI: 10.1109/INDICON49873.2020.9342266

Basulo-Ribeiro, J., & Teixeira, L. (2024). The future of healthcare with Industry 5.0: Preliminary interview-based qualitative analysis. *Future Internet*, *16*(3), 68. DOI: 10.3390/fi16030068

Bates, D. W., Cheng, H. Y., Cheung, N. T., Jew, R., Mir, F., Tamblyn, R., & Li, Y.-C. (2022). 'Improving smart medication management': An online expert discussion. . *BMJ Health & Care Informatics*, *29*(1), e100345. Advance online publication. DOI: 10.1136/bmjhci-2021-100540

Batra, P., & Dave, D. M. (2024). Revolutionizing healthcare platforms: The impact of AI on patient engagement and treatment efficacy. [IJSR]. *International Journal of Scientific Research*, *13*, 613–624.

Bednorz, A., Mak, J. K., Jylhävä, J., & Religa, D. (2023). Use of electronic medical records (EMR) in gerontology: Benefits, considerations and a promising future. *Clinical Interventions in Aging*, *18*, 2171–2183. DOI: 10.2147/CIA.S400887

Benner, P. (1984). *From novice to expert: Excellence and power in clinical nursing practice*. Addison-Wesley. DOI: 10.1097/00000446-198412000-00027

Bharti, U., Bajaj, D., Batra, H., Lalit, S., Lalit, S., & Gangwani, A. Medbot: Conversational artificial intelligence powered chatbot for delivering tele-health after covid-19. In2020 5th international conference on communication and electronics systems (ICCES) 2020 Jun 10 (pp. 870-875). IEEE

Bhimavarapu, U. (2026). AI in Healthcare: Automating Hospital Operations for Better Patient Care. In *Evaluation and Assessment of AI-Driven Systems in Hospitals* (pp. 279-306). IGI Global Scientific Publishing.

Bhuyan, S. S., Sateesh, V., Mukul, N., Galvankar, A., Mahmood, A., Nauman, M., Rai, A., Bordoloi, K., Basu, U., & Samuel, J. (2025). Generative Artificial Intelligence Use in Healthcare: Opportunities for Clinical Excellence and Administrative Efficiency. *Journal of Medical Systems*, *49*(1), 10. DOI: 10.1007/s10916-024-02136-1 PMID: 39820845

Bibri, S. E. (2021). Artificial intelligence-driven smart sustainable healthcare. *Sustainable Cities and Society*, *72*, 103098. DOI: 10.1016/j.scs.2021.103098

Bickmore, T. W., Trinh, H., Olafsson, S., O'Leary, T. K., Asadi, R., Rickles, N. M., & Cruz, R. (2018). Patient and consumer safety risks when using conversational assistants for medical information. *Journal of Medical Internet Research*, *20*(9), e11510. DOI: 10.2196/11510 PMID: 30181110

Bienefeld, N., Keller, E., & Grote, G. (2024). Human-AI Teaming in Critical Care: A Comparative Analysis of Data Scientists' and Clinicians' Perspectives on AI Augmentation and Automation. *Journal of Medical Internet Research*, *26*, e50130. DOI: 10.2196/50130 PMID: 39038285

Biot, C., Tabbuso, T., & Marechal, Y. (2026). Artificial Intelligence for Hospital Scheduling: A Simple, Reproducible, and Effective Model. *Cureus*, *18*(1), e101412. DOI: 10.7759/cureus.101412 PMID: 41536626

Biswas, A., & Talukdar, W. (2024). Intelligent Clinical Documentation: Harnessing Generative AI for Patient-Centric Clinical Note Generation. *International Journal of Innovative Science and Research Technology (IJISRT)*, 994–1008. DOI: 10.38124/ijisrt/IJISRT24MAY1483

Blease, C. (2024). Open AI meets open notes: Surveillance capitalism, patient privacy and online record access. *Journal of Medical Ethics*, *50*(2), 84–89. DOI: 10.1136/jme-2023-109574 PMID: 38050159

Boddington, G. (2021). The Internet of Bodies—alive, connected and collective: The virtual physical future of our bodies and our senses. *AI & Society*, *38*(5), 1897–1913. DOI: 10.1007/s00146-020-01137-1 PMID: 33584018

Booth, R. G.. (2021). Ethical challenges of AI in nursing and healthcare leadership. *Journal of Nursing Management*, *29*(5), 1234–1243.

Booth, R. G., Strudwick, G., McBride, S., O'Connor, S., & López, A. L. (2023). How artificial intelligence can improve nursing practice. *Nursing Outlook*, *71*(2), 101912. DOI: 10.1016/j.outlook.2022.101912 PMID: 36690529

Borycki, E. M., & Kushniruk, A. W. (2023). Health technology, quality and safety in a learning health system. *Healthcare Management Forum, 36*(2), 79–85. DOI: 10.1177/08404704221139383

Botrugno, C. (2019). Information technologies in healthcare: Enhancing or dehumanising doctor–patient interaction? *Health, 25*(4), 475–493. DOI: 10.1177/1363459319891213

Boulesnane, A., Saidi, Y., Kamel, O., Bouhamed, M. M., & Mennour, R. (2022, October 12). Dzchatbot: A medical assistant chatbot in the Algerian Arabic dialect using seq2seq model. In *2022 4th International Conference on Pattern Analysis and Intelligent Systems (PAIS)* (pp. 1–8). IEEE. DOI: 10.1109/PAIS56586.2022.9946867

Bowles, T., Trentino, K. M., Lloyd, A., Trentino, L., Jones, G., Murray, K., Thompson, A., Halpin, S., & Waterer, G. (2024). Outcomes in patients receiving continuous monitoring of vital signs on general wards: A systematic review and meta-analysis of randomised controlled trials. *Digital Health, 10*, 20552076241288826. DOI: 10.1177/20552076241288826 PMID: 39398891

Bragazzi, N. L., & Garbarino, S. (2024). Toward Clinical Generative AI: Conceptual framework. *JMIR AI, 3*, e55957. DOI: 10.2196/55957

Braun, E. J., Singh, S., Penlesky, A. C., Strong, E. A., Holt, J. M., Fletcher, K. E., Stadler, M. E., Nattinger, A. B., & Crotty, B. H. (2022). Nursing implications of an early warning system implemented to reduce adverse events: A qualitative study. *BMJ Quality & Safety, 31*(10), 716–724. DOI: 10.1136/bmjqs-2021-014498

Bruggen, S., & Sah, V. (2025). AI-driven virtual health systems integrating federated learning for decentralized telemedicine. Journal of Nano Molecular Intelligence and Virtual Health Systems. DOI: 10.70023/nmivhs.251101

Buchanan, C., Howitt, M. L., Wilson, R., Booth, R. G., Risling, T., & Bamford, M. (2020). Predicted influences of artificial intelligence on nursing education: Scoping review (Preprint). https://doi.org/DOI: 10.2196/preprints.23933

Buchanan, C., Howitt, M. L., Wilson, R., Booth, R. G., Risling, T., & Bamford, M. (2020). Predicted influences of artificial intelligence on the domains of nursing: Scoping review. *JMIR Nursing, 3*(1), e23939. DOI: 10.2196/23939

Bugaj, M., Kliestik, T., & Lăzăroiu, G. (2023). Generative artificial intelligence-based diagnostic algorithms in disease risk detection and personalized healthcare procedures. *Contemporary Readings in Law and Social Justice, 15*(1), 9–26. DOI: 10.22381/CRLSJ15120231

Campanozzi, L. L., Gibelli, F., Bailo, P., Nittari, G., Sirignano, A., & Ricci, G. (2023). The role of digital literacy in achieving health equity in the third millennium society: A literature review. *Frontiers in Public Health, 11*, 1109323. DOI: 10.3389/fpubh.2023.1109323

Cant, R. P., & Cooper, S. J. (2017). Use of simulation-based learning in undergraduate nurse education: An umbrella systematic review. *Nurse Education Today, 49*, 63–71. DOI: 10.1016/j.nedt.2016.11.015

Carayon, P., Hoonakker, P., Hundt, A. S., & Salwei, M. E. (2020). Work system design for patient safety. *Applied Ergonomics, 82*, 102914. DOI: 10.1016/j.apergo.2019.102914

Car, J., Sheikh, A., Wicks, P., & Williams, M. S. (2019). Beyond the hype of big data and artificial intelligence: Building foundations for knowledge and wisdom. *BMC Medicine, 17*(1), 143. DOI: 10.1186/s12916-019-1382-x

Cascella, M., Scarpati, G., Bignami, E., Cuomo, A., Vittori, A., Di Gennaro, P., Crispo, A., & Coluccia, S. (2023). Utilizing an artificial intelligence framework (conditional generative adversarial network) to enhance telemedicine strategies for cancer pain management. *Journal of Anesthesia, Analgesia and Critical Care, 3*(1), 104. Advance online publication. DOI: 10.1186/s44158-023-00104-8 PMID: 37386680

Chahal, A., & Gulia, P. (2019). Machine learning and deep learning. *International Journal of Innovative Technology and Exploring Engineering, 8*(12), 4910–4914. DOI: 10.35940/ijitee.L3550.1081219

Chandrakar, M. (2024). Telehealth and digital tools enhancing healthcare access in rural systems. *Discover Public Health, 21*(1), 144. DOI: 10.1186/s12982-024-00271-1

Chatterjee, B., Mohseni, P., & Sen, S. (2022). Bioelectronic sensor nodes for Internet of Bodies. arXiv. https://arxiv.org/abs/2212.11370

Chaturvedi, U., Chauhan, S. B., & Singh, I. (2025). The impact of artificial intelligence on remote healthcare: Enhancing patient engagement, connectivity, and overcoming challenges. *Intelligent Pharmacy, 3*(5), 323–329. DOI: 10.1016/j.ipha.2024.12.003

Chen, A., Liu, L., & Zhu, T. (2024). Advancing the democratization of generative artificial intelligence in healthcare: A narrative review. *Journal of Hospital Management and Health Policy, 8*, 8. DOI: 10.21037/jhmhp-24-54

Chen, K. K., & Banerjee, A. (2021). *The digital transformation of medical education* (Vol. 14). SAGE Publications Sage UK.

Cheungpasitporn, W., Thongprayoon, C., & Kashani, K. (2025). Artificial intelligence in critical care nephrology: Current applications, emerging techniques, and challenges. *Kidney360.*

Chin, M. H., Afsar-Manesh, N., Bierman, A. S., Chang, C., Colón-Rodríguez, C. J., Dullabh, P., & Hightower, M. (2023). Guiding principles to address the impact of algorithm bias on racial and ethnic disparities in health and health care. *JAMA Network Open, 6*(12), e2345050–e2345050. DOI: 10.1001/jamanetworkopen.2023.45050 PMID: 38100101

Chinta, S. V., Wang, Z., Palikhe, A., Zhang, X., Kashif, A., Smith, M. A., Liu, J., & Zhang, W. (2025). AI-driven healthcare: A review on ensuring fairness and mitigating bias. *PLOS Digital Health, 4*(5), e0000864. DOI: 10.1371/journal.pdig.0000864 PMID: 40392801

Cho, A., Min, I. K., Hong, S., Chung, H. S., Lee, H. S., & Kim, J. H. (2022). Effect of applying a real-time medical record input assistance system with voice artificial intelligence on triage task performance in the emergency department: Prospective interventional study. *JMIR Medical Informatics, 10*(8), e39892. DOI: 10.2196/39892

Choi, J., Woo, S., & Ferrell, A. (2023). Artificial intelligence–assisted telehealth for nursing: A scoping review. *Journal of Telemedicine and Telecare, 31*(1), 140–149. DOI: 10.1177/1357633X231167613 PMID: 37071572

Choudhury, A., & Asan, O. (2020). Role of artificial intelligence in patient safety outcomes: Systematic literature review. *JMIR Medical Informatics, 8*(7), e18599. DOI: 10.2196/18599 PMID: 32706688

Christopherjames, J. E., Saravanan, M., Thiyam, D. B., Sahib, M. Y., Ganapathi, M. V., & Milton, A. (2021, August 4). Natural language processing based human assistive health conversational agent for multi-users. In *2021 Second International Conference on Electronics and Sustainable Communication Systems (ICESC)* (pp. 1414–1420). IEEE. DOI: 10.1109/ICESC51422.2021.9532913

Christopoulou, S. (2024). Machine learning models and technologies for evidence-based telehealth and smart care: A review. *BioMedInformatics, 4*(1), 42. Advance online publication. DOI: 10.3390/biomedinformatics4010042

Cohran, A. (2025). *Impact of integrating generative artificial intelligence into organizational processes on individual performance*. Benedictine University.

Colacci, M.. (2025). Sociodemographic bias in clinical machine learning models: A scoping review. *Journal of Clinical Machine Learning, 12*(4), 1–15.

Colasacco, C. J., & Born, H. L. (2024). A Case of Artificial Intelligence Chatbot Hallucination. *JAMA Otolaryngology-Head & Neck Surgery, 150*(6), 457–458. DOI: 10.1001/jamaoto.2024.0428 PMID: 38635259

Comito, C., Falcone, D., & Forestiero, A. (2022). AI-driven clinical decision support: Enhancing disease diagnosis exploiting patients similarity. . *IEEE Access : Practical Innovations, Open Solutions, 10*, 123456–123469. DOI: 10.1109/ACCESS.2022.3142100

Connolly, F., Byrne, D., Lydon, S., Walsh, C., & O'Connor, P. (2017). Barriers and facilitators related to the implementation of a physiological track and trigger system: A systematic review of the qualitative evidence. *International Journal for Quality in Health Care : Journal of the International Society for Quality in Health Care, 29*(8), 973–980. DOI: 10.1093/intqhc/mzx148 PMID: 29177409

Coutu, F.-A., Iorio, O. C., & Ross, B. A. (2023). Remote patient monitoring strategies and wearable technology in chronic obstructive pulmonary disease. *Frontiers in Medicine, 10*, 1236598. DOI: 10.3389/fmed.2023.1236598 PMID: 37663662

Cresswell, K., Papoutsi, C., Simon, G. E., Bates, D. W., & Sheikh, A. (2025). Advancing learning health systems: Leveraging routine data for improvement and research. *NPJ Digital Medicine, 8*, 12. DOI: 10.1038/s41746-024-01045-4

Cucci, F., Marasciulo, D., Romani, M., Soldano, G., Cascio, D., De Nunzio, G., Caldararo, C., Rubbi, I., Vitale, E., Lupo, R., & Conte, L. (2025). The contribution of artificial intelligence in nursing education: A scoping review of the literature. *Nursing Reports, 15*(8), 283. DOI: 10.3390/nursrep15080283 PMID: 40863670

da Silva Tiago, R., & Mitchell, A. (2024) 'Integrating digital transformation in nursing education: best practices and challenges in curriculum development', in *Digital transformation in higher education*, Part B. Bingley: Emerald Publishing Limited, pp. 57–101.

Dai, T., & Swaminathan, J. M. (2025). Artificial intelligence and operations: A foundational framework of emerging research and practice. *Production and Operations Management*, 10591478251412943. DOI: 10.1177/10591478251412943

Dall'Ora, C., Ball, J., Reinius, M., & Griffiths, P. (2020). Burnout in nursing. *Journal of Advanced Nursing, 76*(12), 3364–3376. DOI: 10.1111/jan.14539 PMID: 32503559

Das, T. K., & Mohapatro, A. (2025). Text summarization: An application of generative AI. In Vajjhala, N. R., Roy, S. S., Taşcı, B., & Hoque Chowdhury, M. E. (Eds.), *Generative artificial intelligence (AI) approaches for industrial applications* (Vol. 24, pp. xx–xx). Springer., DOI: 10.1007/978-3-031-76710-4_16

Datta, A., & Sen, S. (2023). Invited: IoB: The vision of the Internet of Bodies. *Proceedings of the IEEE Midwest Symposium on Circuits and Systems (MWSCAS)*, 444–448. DBLPDOI: 10.1109/MWSCAS57524.2023.10405903

Davenport, T. H., & Kalakota, R. (2019). The potential for artificial intelligence in healthcare. *Future Healthcare Journal*, *6*(2), 94–98. DOI: 10.7861/futurehosp.6-2-94 PMID: 31363513

De Gagne, J. C. (2023). The state of artificial intelligence in nursing education: Past, present, and future directions. *International Journal of Environmental Research and Public Health*, *20*(6), 4884. DOI: 10.3390/ijerph20064884 PMID: 36981790

De Lathauwer, I. L. J., Nieuwenhuys, W. W., Hafkamp, F., Regis, M., Brouwers, R. W. M., Funk, M., & Kemps, H. M. C. (2025). Remote patient monitoring in heart failure: A comprehensive meta-analysis of effective programme components for hospitalization and mortality reduction. *European Journal of Heart Failure*, *27*(9), 1670–1685. Advance online publication. DOI: 10.1002/ejhf.3568 PMID: 39834044

de Paula, P. A. B., Severino, J. V. B., Berger, M. N., Veiga, M. H., Ribeiro, K. D. P., & Loures, F. S.. (2025). Improving documentation quality and patient interaction with AI. *Journal of Medical Artificial Intelligence*, •••, 8.

de Waal, C.. (2025). Accuracy of vital sign monitoring using a photoplethysmography upper arm wearable in hospitalised patients. *Journal of Clinical Monitoring and Computing*. Advance online publication. DOI: 10.1007/s10877-025-01358-z

Delardes, B., McLeod, L., Chakraborty, S., & Bowles, K.-A. (2020). What is the effect of electronic clinical handovers on patient outcomes? A systematic review. *Health Informatics Journal*, *26*(4), 2422–2434. DOI: 10.1177/1460458220905162 PMID: 32114869

Dinesh, & Kumar, S. (2024). Integrated VIKOR-TOPSIS strategy based on picture fuzzy knowledge and accuracy measures with application in waste-water treatment. Evolutionary Intelligence, 17(5), 3891-3920. DOI: 10.1007/s12065-024-00963-2

Domfeh, E. A., Weyori, B., Appiahene, P., Mensah, J., Awarayi, N., & Afrifa, S. (2022). Human-centered artificial intelligence: A review. https://doi.org/DOI: 10.22541/au.166013641.15972664/v1

Dorsey, E. R., & Topol, E. J. (2016). State of telehealth. *The New England Journal of Medicine*, *375*(2), 154–161. DOI: 10.1056/NEJMra1601705 PMID: 27410924

Dubey, R., & Tiwari, A. (2023). Artificial intelligence and remote patient monitoring in US healthcare market: A literature review. *Journal of Market Access & Health Policy*, *11*(1), 2205618. DOI: 10.1080/20016689.2023.2205618 PMID: 37151736

Edelson, D. P., Churpek, M. M., Carey, K. A., Lin, Z., Huang, C., Siner, J. M., Johnson, J., Krumholz, H. M., & Rhodes, D. J. (2024). Early warning scores with and without artificial intelligence. *JAMA Network Open*, *7*(10), e2438986. DOI: 10.1001/jamanetworkopen.2024.38986 PMID: 39405061

Eggins, S., & Slade, D. (2015). Communication in Clinical Handover: Improving the Safety and Quality of the Patient Experience. *Journal of Public Health Research*, *4*(3), 666. DOI: 10.4081/jphr.2015.666 PMID: 26753165

Eggins, S., & Slade, D. (2015). Communication in clinical handover: Improving the safety of patients. *Journal of Health Services Research & Policy.*

El Arab, R. A., & Al Moosa, O. A. (2025). Systematic review of cost effectiveness and budget impact of artificial intelligence in healthcare. *NPJ Digital Medicine*, *8*(1), 172. Advance online publication. DOI: 10.1038/s41746-025-01722-y PMID: 40858882

El Arab, R. A., Al Moosa, O. A., Abuadas, F. H., & Somerville, J. (2025). The role of artificial intelligence in nursing education and practice: An umbrella review. *Journal of Medical Internet Research*, *27*, e69881. DOI: 10.2196/69881 PMID: 40072926

El-Banna, M. M., Sajid, M. R., Rizvi, M. R., Sami, W., & McNelis, A. M. (2025). AI literacy and competency in nursing education: Preparing students and faculty members for an AI-enabled future. *Frontiers in Medicine*, *12*, 1681784. DOI: 10.3389/fmed.2025.1681784 PMID: 41384110

El-deep, S. E., Abohany, A. A., Sallam, K. M., & Abd El-Mageed, A. A. (2025). A comprehensive survey on impact of applying various technologies on the Internet of Medical Things. [SpringerLink]. *Artificial Intelligence Review*, *58*(3), 86. DOI: 10.1007/s10462-024-11063-z

Elhaddad, M., & Hamam, S. (2024). AI-driven clinical decision support systems: An ongoing pursuit of potential. . *Cureus*, *16*, e12345. DOI: 10.7759/cureus.57728

El-Khoury, M., & Arikan, C. L. (2021). From the Internet of Things toward the Internet of Bodies: Ethical and legal considerations. Journal of Strategic Contracting and Negotiation, 7(2), 307–314. RSD Journal Ewoh, P., & Vartiainen, T. (2024). Vulnerability to cyberattacks and sociotechnical solutions for health care systems: Systematic review. Journal of Medical Internet Research, 26, e46904. https://doi .org/DOI: 10.1002/jsc.2411

Ergin, E., Karaarslan, D., Şahan, S., & Çınar Yücel, Ş. (2022). Artificial intelligence and robot nurses: from nurse managers' perspective: a descriptive cross-sectional study. *Journal of Nursing Management*, *30*(8), 3853–3862. DOI: 10.1111/jonm.13646

Esteva, A., Robicquet, A., Ramsundar, B., Kuleshov, V., DePristo, M., Chou, K., Cui, C., Corrado, G., Thrun, S., & Dean, J. (2021). A guide to deep learning in healthcare. *Nature Medicine*, *27*(7), 1129–1145. DOI: 10.1038/s41591-021-01312-x

European Commission. (2021) *Proposal for a regulation laying down harmonised rules on artificial intelligence (Artificial Intelligence Act).* Brussels: European Commission. Available at: https://eur-lex.europa.eu/legal-content/EN/TXT/?uri=CELEX%3A52021PC0206 (Accessed: 2 January 2026).

Fahim, Y. A., Hasani, I. W., Kabba, S., & Ragab, W. M. (2025). Artificial intelligence in healthcare and medicine. *European Journal of Medical Research*, *30*(1), 848. DOI: 10.1186/s40001-025-03196-w PMID: 40988064

Falco, G., Shneiderman, B., Badger, J., Carrier, R., Dahbura, A., Danks, D., Eling, M., Goodloe, A., Gupta, J., Hart, C., Jirotka, M., Johnson, H., LaPointe, C., Llorens, A. J., Mackworth, A. K., Maple, C., Pálsson, S. E., Pasquale, F., Winfield, A., & Yeong, Z. K. (2021). Governing AI safety through independent audits. *Nature Machine Intelligence*, *3*(7), 566–571. DOI: 10.1038/s42256-021-00370-7

Farrokhi, M., Fallahian, A. H., Rahmani, E., Aghajan, A., Alipour, M., Khouzani, P. J., Hezarani, H. B., Sabzehie, H., Pirouzan, M., Pirouzan, Z., & Dalvandi, B. (2025). Current applications, challenges, and future directions of artificial intelligence in emergency medicine: A narrative review. *Archives of Academic Emergency Medicine*, *13*(1), e45.

Fatai, A., Sattayarom, C., Laochai, W., & Faksook, E. (2025). Effectiveness of AI-assisted ESI triage on accuracy and selected outcomes in emergency nursing: A systematic review.. *Journal of Emergency Nursing: JEN*, *51*, 45–54. DOI: 10.1016/j.jen.2024.10.003

Felix, F. A. S., & Martins, L. E. G. (2024). IoT devices in use in healthcare applications: A systematic literature review. [SpringerLink]. *Research on Biomedical Engineering*, *40*(3-4), 547–561. DOI: 10.1007/s42600-024-00356-5

Floridi, L., & Cowls, J. (2019). A unified framework of five principles for AI in society. *Harvard Data Science Review*, *1*(1). Advance online publication. DOI: 10.1162/99608f92.8cd550d1

Floridi, L., Cowls, J., Beltrametti, M., Chatila, R., Chazerand, P., Dignum, V., Luetge, C., Madelin, R., Pagallo, U., Rossi, F., Schafer, B., Valcke, P., & Vayena, E. (2018). AI4People—An ethical framework. *Minds and Machines*, *28*(4), 689–707. DOI: 10.1007/s11023-018-9482-5 PMID: 30930541

Foad, N. C., Lippert, J., & Lippert, W. C. (2026, January 1). (n.d.). Bridging Inpatient and Outpatient Care: A Scoping Review on Discharge Summary Documentation Timeliness and Quality. *Journal of Brown Hospital Medicine*, *5*(1), 151812. DOI: 10.56305/001c.151812 PMID: 41488445

Frasca, M., La Torre, D., Pravettoni, G., & Cutica, I. (2024). Explainable and interpretable artificial intelligence in medicine: A systematic bibliometric review. *Discover Artificial Intelligence*, *4*(1), 15. DOI: 10.1007/s44163-024-00114-7

Gaffney, A., Woolhandler, S., Cai, C., Bor, D., Himmelstein, J., McCormick, D., & Himmelstein, D. U. (2022a). Medical Documentation Burden Among US Office-Based Physicians in 2019: A National Study. *JAMA Internal Medicine*, *182*(5), 564–566. DOI: 10.1001/jamainternmed.2022.0372 PMID: 35344006

Galanis, P., Moisoglou, I., Katsiroumpa, A., Vraka, I., Siskou, O., Konstantakopoulou, O., Meimeti, E., & Kaitelidou, D. (2023). Increased Job Burnout and Reduced Job Satisfaction for Nurses Compared to Other Healthcare Workers after the COVID-19 Pandemic. *Nursing Reports*, *13*(3), 1090–1100. DOI: 10.3390/nursrep13030095

Ganapathy, K., Haranath, S. P., Baez, A. A., & Scott, B. K. (2022). Telemedicine to expand access to critical care around the world. *Critical Care Clinics*, *38*(4), 809–826. DOI: 10.1016/j.ccc.2022.06.007 PMID: 36162912

Garg, L., Basterrech, S., Banerjee, C., & Sharma, T. K. (2021). *Artificial intelligence in healthcare*. Springer.

Garg, S. (2025). The role of generative AI in personalized medicine and treatment recommendations. *Clinical Medicine and Health Research Journal*, *5*(2), 1214–1227. DOI: 10.18535/cmhrj.v5i02.463

Geetha, S., Srinidhii, P., & Madhusudanan, J. (2026). Assessment of AI's Impact on Precision Medicine and Personalized Healthcare in Clinical Environments. In *Evaluation and Assessment of AI-Driven Systems in Hospitals* (pp. 139–168). IGI Global Scientific Publishing.

Genes, N., Simon, G., Koziatek, C., Kim, J. G., Woo, K., Dahn, C., Chan, L., & Wiesenfeld, B. (2025). Generative Artificial Intelligence Summaries to Facilitate Emergency Department Handoff. *Applied Clinical Informatics*, *16*(04), 1185–1191. DOI: 10.1055/a-2681-5008 PMID: 40795949

Genovese, A., Borna, S., Gomez-Cabello, C. A., Haider, S. A., Prabha, S., Forte, A. J., & Veenstra, B. R. (2024). Artificial intelligence in clinical settings: A systematic review of its role in language translation and interpretation. *Annals of Translational Medicine*, *12*(6), 117. DOI: 10.21037/atm-24-162

Gerlach, M., Renggli, F. J., Bieri, J. S., Sariyar, M., & Golz, C. (2025). Exploring nurse perspectives on AI-based shift scheduling for fairness, transparency, and work-life balance. *BMC Nursing, 24*(1), 1161. DOI: 10.1186/s12912-025-03808-0

Gesner, E., Dykes, P. C., Zhang, L., & Gazarian, P. (2022). Documentation Burden in Nursing and Its Role in Clinician Burnout Syndrome. *Applied Clinical Informatics, 13*(05), 983–990. DOI: 10.1055/s-0042-1757157 PMID: 36261113

Ghassemi, M., Oakden-Rayner, L., & Beam, A. L. (2021). The false hope of current AI in healthcare. *The Lancet. Digital Health, 3*(11), e745–e750. DOI: 10.1016/S2589-7500(21)00208-9 PMID: 34711379

Goddard, K., Roudsari, A., & Wyatt, J. C. (2012). Automation bias: A systematic review of frequency, effect mediators, and mitigators. *Journal of the American Medical Informatics Association : JAMIA, 19*(1), 121–127. DOI: 10.1136/amiajnl-2011-000089

Göktepe, N., & Sarıköse, S. (2025). Perspectives and Experiences of Nurse Managers on the Impact of Artificial Intelligence on Nursing Work Environments and Managerial Processes: A Qualitative Study. *International Nursing Review, 72*(2), e70043. DOI: 10.1111/inr.70043

Gopal, G., Suter-Crazzolara, C., Toldo, L., & Eberhardt, W. (2019). Digital transformation in healthcare–architectures of present and future information technologies. [CCLM]. *Clinical Chemistry and Laboratory Medicine, 57*(3), 328–335. DOI: 10.1515/cclm-2018-0658

Gosmar, D., & Dahl, D. A. Hallucination mitigation using agentic ai natural language-based frameworks (2025). *arXiv preprint arXiv:2501.13946*. https://doi.org//arXiv.2501.13946DOI: 10.48550

Gottesman, O., Futoma, J., Liu, Y., Parbhoo, S., Celi, L., Brunskill, E., & Doshi-Velez, F. (2020). *Interpretable off-policy evaluation in reinforcement learning by highlighting influential transitions.* Paper presented at the International Conference on Machine Learning.

Greenhalgh, T., Wherton, J., Papoutsi, C., Lynch, J., Hughes, G., Hinder, S., Fahy, N., Procter, R., & Shaw, S. (2017). Beyond adoption: A new framework for theorizing and evaluating nonadoption, abandonment, and challenges to the scale-up, spread, and sustainability of health and care technologies. *Journal of Medical Internet Research, 19*(11), e8775. DOI: 10.2196/jmir.8775

Gregoriou, P. L., Charalambous, A., Rousou, E., Papastavrou, E., & Merkouris, A. (2025). Attitudes of Physicians and Nurses Toward Interprofessional Collaboration: A Systematic Literature Review. *Materia Socio-Medica, 37*(1), 64–73. DOI: 10.5455/msm.2025.37.64-73 PMID: 40098756

Hallaj, S., Heinke, A., Kalaw, F. G. P., Gim, N., Blazes, M., Owen, J., Dysinger, E., Benton, E. S., Cordier, B. A., Evans, N. G., Li-Pook-Than, J., Snyder, M. P., Nebeker, C., Zangwill, L. M., Baxter, S. L., McWeeney, S., Lee, C. S., Lee, A. Y., & Patel, B. (2025). Navigating open data sharing and privacy in the age of clinical AI research: From reidentification to pseudo-reidentification. *EClinicalMedicine, 91*, 103729. DOI: 10.1016/j.eclinm.2025.103729 PMID: 41542222

Hameed, K., Naha, R., & Hameed, F. (2024). Digital transformation for sustainable health and well-being: A review and future research directions. *Discover Sustainability, 5*(1), 104. DOI: 10.1007/s43621-024-00273-8

Han, J., Park, J., Huh, J., Oh, U., Do, J., & Kim, D. (2024). AscleAI: A LLM-based Clinical Note Management System for Enhancing Clinician Productivity. *Extended Abstracts of the CHI Conference on Human Factors in Computing Systems, CHI EA '24*, 1–7. DOI: 10.1145/3613905.3650784

Han, R., Acosta, J. N., Shakeri, Z., Ioannidis, J. P. A., Topol, E. J., & Rajpurkar, P. (2024). Randomised controlled trials evaluating artificial intelligence in clinical practice: A scoping review. *The Lancet. Digital Health, 6*(5), e367–e373. DOI: 10.1016/S2589-7500(24)00047-5 PMID: 38670745

Han, S., Han, J., & Cho, M. (2025). Nursing students' perceptions, benefits, and challenges of using artificial intelligence in academic settings. *Nursing Reports, 15*(2), 283–298. DOI: 10.3390/nursrep15020068 PMID: 39997804

Harder, N. (2025). Comparing artificial intelligence-enhanced virtual reality and traditional simulated patient learning: Perceptions of realism and educational impact. *Journal of Nursing Simulation, 19*(1), 1–10.

Hasanzadeh, F., Josephson, C. B., Waters, G., Adedinsewo, D., Azizi, Z., & White, J. A. (2025). Bias recognition and mitigation strategies in artificial intelligence healthcare applications. *NPJ Digital Medicine, 8*(1), 154. DOI: 10.1038/s41746-025-01503-7 PMID: 40069303

Haviana, E., Putriani, N. D., Novika, P. W., Pujadi, A., & Asfo, N. S. (2025). The Effect of Company Policy on Employee Compliance with the Implementation of AI to Maintain Company Data Security. [IJHESS]. *International Journal of Health, Economics, and Social Sciences, 7*(1), 468–473.

He, P., Huang, D., Wu, D., He, H., Wei, Y., Cui, Y., Wang, R., & Peng, L. (2024). A survey of Internet of Medical Things: Technology, application and future directions. Digital Communications and Networks. Advance online publication. sciencedirect. comDOI: 10.1016/j.dcan.2024.11.013

Hicks, M. H., Tore, M., Michard, F., & Khanna, A. K. (2025). Portable wireless monitoring of vital signs in hospital wards. *BJA Education*, *25*(7), 265–272. DOI: 10.1016/j.bjae.2025.04.004 PMID: 40575591

Ho, L. H., Lin, Y. L., & Chen, T. Y. (2020). A Pearson-like correlation-based TOPSIS method with interval-valued Pythagorean fuzzy uncertainty and its application to multiple criteria decision analysis of stroke rehabilitation treatments. *Neural Computing & Applications*, *32*(12), 8265–8295. DOI: 10.1007/s00521-019-04304-8

Hosseinzadegan, F., Salamatbakhsh, M., Salehzadeh, M., Nournezhad, H., & Mohammadpour, Y. (2025). Hospital errors and their consequences among healthcare professionals a: Descriptive correlational investigation. *Annals of Medicine and Surgery (London)*, *87*(7), 4026–4033. DOI: 10.1097/MS9.0000000000003280 PMID: 40852022

Howcroft, A., Bennett-Weston, A., Khan, A., Griffiths, J., Gay, S., & Howick, J. (2025). AI chatbots versus human healthcare professionals: A systematic review and meta-analysis of empathy in patient care. *British Medical Bulletin*, *156*(1), ldaf017. Advance online publication. DOI: 10.1093/bmb/ldaf017

Huang, J., Neill, L., Wittbrodt, M., Melnick, D., Klug, M., Thompson, M., Bailitz, J., Loftus, T., Malik, S., Phull, A., Weston, V., Heller, J. A., & Etemadi, M. (2023). Generative artificial intelligence for chest radiograph interpretation in the emergency department. . *JAMA Network Open*, *6*(10), e2312345. DOI: 10.1001/jamanetworkopen.2023.36100

Huang, Y., Wang, J., Wang, S., & Zhang, Y. (2023). Internet of medical things: A systematic review. *Neurocomputing*, *557*, 126719. Advance online publication. DOI: 10.1016/j.neucom.2023.126719

Hudson, T. J., Albrecht, M., Smith, T. R., Ator, G. A., Thompson, J. A., Shah, T., & Shanks, D. (2025). Impact of Ambient Artificial Intelligence Documentation on Cognitive Load. *Mayo Clinic Proceedings. Digital Health*, *3*(1), 100193. DOI: 10.1016/j.mcpdig.2024.100193 PMID: 40206994

Indu, V. T., Elumalai, M., & Gracious, L. A. (2026). Optimization Algorithms for Machine Learning Model Enhancement in Healthcare. In *AI Model Design and Data Managementfor Disease Prediction* (pp. 159–192). IGI Global Scientific Publishing.

International Council of Nurses. (2021) *The ICN code of ethics for nurses*. Geneva: International Council of Nurses. Available at: https://www.icn.ch/sites/default/files/inline-files/ICN_Code-of-Ethics_EN_Web.pdf (Accessed: 2 January 2026).

Ip, W., Xenochristou, M., Sui, E., Ruan, E., Ribeira, R., Dash, D., Srinivasan, M., Artandi, M., Omiye, J. A., Scoulios, N., & Hofmann, H. L. (2024). 'Hospitalization prediction from the emergency department using computer vision AI with short patient video clips', *npj. Digital Medicine*, *7*(1), 371.

Islam, M. M., Maddison, R., Talukder, A., & Kamal, A. H. M. (2023). "Artificial intelligence in remote patient monitoring: A systematic review." Sensors, Volume 23, Issue 3. *Article*, *1234*, 1–20. DOI: 10.3390/s23031234

Ivers, N., Jamtvedt, G., Flottorp, S., Young, J. M., Odgaard-Jensen, J., French, S. D., O'Brien, M. A., Johansen, M., Grimshaw, J., & Oxman, A. D. (2012). Audit and feedback: Effects on professional practice and healthcare outcomes. *The Cochrane Library*, *2012*(7), 6. DOI: 10.1002/14651858.CD000259.pub3

Jain, N. (2024). Revolutionizing patient care: The impact of ChatGPT and generative AI in healthcare. *International Journal of Scientific and Research Publications*, *14*(11), 24–38. DOI: 10.29322/IJSRP.14.11.2024.p15506

Jha, D., Durak, G., Sharma, V., Keles, E., Cicek, V., Zhang, Z., Srivastava, A., Rauniyar, A., Hagos, D. H., Tomar, N. K., Miller, F. H., Topcu, A., Yazidi, A., Håkegård, J. E., & Bagci, U. (2025). A Conceptual Framework for Applying Ethical Principles of AI to Medical Practice. *Bioengineering (Basel, Switzerland)*, *12*(2), 180. DOI: 10.3390/bioengineering12020180 PMID: 40001699

Jiang, F., Jiang, Y., Zhi, H., Dong, Y., Li, H., Ma, S., Wang, Y., Dong, Q., Shen, H., & Wang, Y. (2017). Artificial intelligence in healthcare: Past, present and future. *Stroke and Vascular Neurology*, *2*(4), 230–243. DOI: 10.1136/svn-2017-000101

Jiang, F., Jiang, Y., Zhi, H., Dong, Y., Li, H., Ma, S., Wang, Y., Dong, Q., Shen, H., & Wang, Y. (2021). Artificial intelligence in healthcare: Past, present and future. *Stroke and Vascular Neurology*, *6*(3), 230–243. DOI: 10.1136/svn-2020-000101

Jones, M. C.. (2023). Navigating data governance associated with real-world health data: Legal and information governance structures in the UK. *BMJ Open*, *13*(10), e069925. DOI: 10.1136/bmjopen-2022-069925

Joshi, M., Iqbal, F. M., Sharabiani, M., Ashrafian, H., Arora, S., McAndrew, K., Khan, S., Cooke, G., & Darzi, A. (2025). Performance of continuous digital monitoring of vital signs with a wearable sensor in acute hospital settings. *Sensors (Basel)*, *25*(9), 2644. DOI: 10.3390/s25092644 PMID: 40363083

Joshi, M., Pezzotti, N., & Browne, J. T. (2023). Human–AI relationship in healthcare. In *Explainable AI in Healthcare* (pp. 1–22). Chapman and Hall/CRC. DOI: 10.1201/9781003333425-1

Judijanto, L., Ili, L., & Wardhana, M. G. (2025). Education 5.0: Collaboration and creativity in improving students' digital intelligence. *International Journal of Teaching and Learning*, *3*(4), 369–382.

Jukanti, M. (2025). Ai in healthcare: Revolutionizing medical diagnosis. *Journal Of Engineering And Computer Sciences*, *4*(7), 1087–1093.

Jung, S. (2023). Challenges and future directions for artificial intelligence integrated nursing simulation education. *Korean Journal of Women Health Nursing*, *29*(3), 239–242. DOI: 10.4069/kjwhn.2023.09.06.1 PMID: 37813667

Kabir, M. R., Shishir, F. S., Shomaji, S., & Ray, S. (2025). Digital twins in healthcare IoT: A systematic review. *High-Confidence Computing*, *5*(3), 100340. DOI: 10.1016/j.hcc.2025.100340

Kakhi, K., Jagatheesaperumal, S. K., Khosravi, A., Alizadehsani, R., & Acharya, U. R. (2025). Fatigue monitoring using wearables and AI: Trends, challenges, and future opportunities. *Computers in Biology and Medicine*, *195*, 110461. DOI: 10.1016/j.compbiomed.2025.110461 PMID: 40580618

Karunanayake, N. (2025). Next-generation agentic AI for transforming healthcare. *Informatics and Health*, *2*(2), 73–83. DOI: 10.1016/j.infoh.2025.03.001

Kaur, H., Selvakumar, P., Haashni, S., Anute, N., Sharma, M., & Manjunath, T. C. (2025). Representations in developing thinking regarding probabilities in higher education. In Anastasiadou, S., & Seremeti, L. (Eds.), *Modes of representation in developing statistical thinking in education* (pp. 89–118). IGI Global Scientific Publishing. , DOI: 10.4018/979-8-3693-9934-7.ch006

Kazerouni, A., Aghdam, E. K., Heidari, M., Azad, R., Fayyaz, M., Hacihaliloglu, I., & Merhof, D. (2022). Diffusion models for medical image analysis. *arXiv preprint arXiv:2211.07804.*

Kelly, C. J., Karthikesalingam, A., Suleyman, M., Corrado, G., & King, D. (2019). Key challenges for delivering clinical impact with artificial intelligence. *BMC Medicine*, *17*(1), 195. DOI: 10.1186/s12916-019-1426-2

Kelly, S., Pryor, C., Stephens, M., & Heaslip, V. (2025). Exploring the presence and impact of advanced nursing roles in care homes and charitable organisations: An international systematic scoping review. *Journal of Advanced Nursing*, jan.70212. DOI: 10.1111/jan.70212

Khan, F. A. (2025). AI in clinical diagnostics: Is overreliance eroding clinical expertise? *PLOS Digital Health*, *4*(8), e0000959. DOI: 10.1371/journal.pdig.0000959 PMID: 40758655

Khanna, A., Selvaraj, P., Gupta, D., Sheikh, T. H., Pareek, P. K., & Shankar, V. (2023). Internet of things and deep learning enabled healthcare disease diagnosis using biomedical electrocardiogram signals. *Expert Systems: International Journal of Knowledge Engineering and Neural Networks*, *40*(4), e12864. DOI: 10.1111/exsy.12864

Khan, S., & Alam, M. (2021). Wearable Internet of Things for personalized healthcare: Study of trends and latent research. In Das, H. (Eds.), *Health informatics: A computational perspective in healthcare* (pp. 43–60). Springer., DOI: 10.1007/978-981-15-9735-0_3

Khlaif, Z. N., Salameh, N., Ajouz, M., & Alwawi, A. (2025). Using generative AI in nursing education: Students' perceptions. *BMC Medical Education*, *25*(1), 926. DOI: 10.1186/s12909-025-07416-z PMID: 40598139

Khude, H., & Shende, P. (2025). AI-driven clinical decision support systems: Revolutionizing medication selection and personalized drug therapy. *Advances in Integrative Medicine*, *12*(4), 100529. DOI: 10.1016/j.aimed.2025.100529

Khullar, D., Casalino, L. P., Qian, Y., Lu, Y., Chang, E., & Aneja, S. (2021). Public vs physician views of liability for artificial intelligence in health care. *Journal of the American Medical Informatics Association : JAMIA*, *28*(7), 1574–1577. DOI: 10.1093/jamia/ocab055 PMID: 33871009

Khurram Shahzad Warraich, M., Usman, H., Zakir, S., & Mehboob, M. (2025). Ethical Governance of artificial intelligence Hallucinations in legal practice. *Social Sciences Spectrum*, *4*(2), 603–615. DOI: 10.71085/sss.04.02.297

Kim, S. K., & Huh, J. H. (2020). Artificial neural network blockchain techniques for healthcare system: Focusing on the personal health records. *Electronics (Basel)*, *9*(5), 763. DOI: 10.3390/electronics9050763

Kirubakaran, D. (2025). Review on emerging frontiers in medical sensing: Innovations shaping the future of healthcare. *Biomedical Materials & Devices*, *3*, 385. DOI: 10.1007/s44174-025-00385-3

Kline, A., Wang, H., Li, Y., Dennis, S., Hutch, M., Xu, Z., Wang, F., Cheng, F., & Luo, Y. (2022). Multimodal machine learning in precision health: A scoping review. *NPJ Digital Medicine*, *5*(1), 171. DOI: 10.1038/s41746-022-00712-8 PMID: 36344814

Knevel, R., & Liao, K. P. (2023). From real-world electronic health record data to real-world results using artificial intelligence. *Annals of the Rheumatic Diseases*, *82*(3), 306–311. DOI: 10.1136/ard-2022-222626

Kothinti, R. R.Rishi Reddy Kothinti. (2024). Deep learning in healthcare: Transforming disease diagnosis, personalized treatment, and clinical decision-making through AI-driven innovations. *World Journal of Advanced Research and Reviews*, *24*(2), 2841–2856. DOI: 10.30574/wjarr.2024.24.2.3435

Kreimeyer, K., Foster, M., & Pandey, A.. (2017). Natural language processing systems for clinical text. *Journal of Biomedical Informatics*, *65*, 14–29. DOI: 10.1016/j.jbi.2017.07.012 PMID: 28729030

Kruse, C. S., Krowski, N., Rodriguez, B., Tran, L., Vela, J., & Brooks, M. (2017). Telehealth and patient satisfaction: A systematic review and narrative analysis. *BMJ Open*, *7*(8), e016242. DOI: 10.1136/bmjopen-2017-016242 PMID: 28775188

Kumar, A., U, P. R., & Maben, M. (2025). Heart disease prediction using machine learning algorithms. In *Proceedings of the 2025 Third International Conference on Networks, Multimedia and Information Technology (NMITCON)* (pp. 1–6). IEEE. https://doi.org/DOI: 10.1109/NMITCON65824.2025.11187908

Kumar, M. S., & Ganesh, D. (2024). Improving telemedicine through IoT and cloud computing. *Advances in Engineering and Intelligence Systems*, *3*(3), 123–135.

Kumar, V., & Garg, M. L. (2017, November). Deep learning in predictive analytics: A survey. In *2017 International Conference on Emerging Trends in Computing and Communication Technologies (ICETCCT)* (pp. 1-6). IEEE. DOI: 10.1109/ICETCCT.2017.8280331

Kutney-Lee, A., & Kelly, D. (2011). The effect of hospital EHR adoption. *Health Services Research*, *46*(3), 884–905. DOI: 10.1111/j.1475-6773.2010.01231.x

Kwan, H. Y. (2024). User-focused telehealth powered by LLMs: Bridging the gap between technology and human-centric care delivery. In *Proceedings of the International Conference on Cognitive Computing and Artificial Intelligence* (pp. 187–191). IEEE. DOI: 10.1109/CCAI61966.2024.10603150

Labrague, L. J., Al Sabei, S., & Al Yahyaei, A. (2025). Artificial intelligence in nursing education: A review of AI-based teaching pedagogies. *Teaching and Learning in Nursing*, *20*(3), 210–221. DOI: 10.1016/j.teln.2025.01.019

Lang, O., Yaya-Stupp, D., Traynis, I., & Cole-Lewis, H. (2024). Using generative AI to investigate medical imagery models and datasets.. *The Lancet. Digital Health*, *6*, e354–e366. DOI: 10.1016/S2589-7500(24)00017-9

Laranjo, L., Dunn, A. G., Tong, H. L., Kocaballi, A. B., Chen, J., Bashir, R., Surian, D., Gallego, B., Magrabi, F., Lau, A. Y. S., & Coiera, E. (2018). Conversational agents in healthcare a systematic review. *Journal of the American Medical Informatics Association : JAMIA*, *25*(9), 1248–1258. DOI: 10.1093/jamia/ocy072 PMID: 30010941

Lee, C., Vogt, K. A., & Kumar, S. (2024). Prospects for AI clinical summarization to reduce the burden of patient chart review. *Frontiers in Digital Health*, *6*, 1475092. Advance online publication. DOI: 10.3389/fdgth.2024.1475092 PMID: 39575412

Lee, D., & Yoon, S. N. (2021). Application of artificial intelligence-based technologies in the healthcare industry: Opportunities and challenges. *International Journal of Environmental Research and Public Health*, *18*(1), 271. Advance online publication. DOI: 10.3390/ijerph18010271 PMID: 33401373

Lee, J. O., Zhou, H. Y., Berzin, T. M., Sodickson, D. K., & Rajpurkar, P. (2025). Multimodal generative AI for interpreting 3D medical images and videos. . *NPJ Digital Medicine*, *8*(1), 45–57. DOI: 10.1038/s41746-025-01649-4

Lee, K., Liu, Z., Mai, Y., Jun, T., Ma, M., Wang, T., Ai, L., Calay, E., Oh, W., Stolovitzky, G., Schadt, E., & Wang, X. (2024). Optimizing clinical trial eligibility design using natural language processing models and real-world data: Algorithm development and validation. . *JMIR AI*, *5*, e34567. DOI: 10.2196/50800

Leiserowitz, G., Mansfield, J., MacDonald, S., & Jost, M. (2025). Patient Attitudes Toward Ambient Voice Technology: Preimplementation Patient Survey in an Academic Medical Center. *JMIR Medical Informatics*, *13*(1), e77901. DOI: 10.2196/77901 PMID: 41308194

Liao, L., Yang, G. H., & Shah, C. (2023, February 27). Proactive conversational agents. In *Proceedings of the Sixteenth ACM International Conference on Web Search and Data Mining* (pp. 1244–1247). ACM. https://doi.org/DOI: 10.1145/3539597.3572724

Li, H., Yazdi, M., Huang, C. G., & Peng, W. (2022). A reliable probabilistic risk-based decision-making method: Bayesian Technique for Order of Preference by Similarity to Ideal Solution (B-TOPSIS). *Soft Computing*, *26*(22), 12137–12153. DOI: 10.1007/s00500-022-07462-5

Lin, C., & Kuo, C. F. (2025). Roles and potential of large language models in healthcare. *Biomedical Journal*, *48*(5), 100868. DOI: 10.1016/j.bj.2025.100868 PMID: 40311872

Liu, J., & Liu, H. (2025). Research on flexible sensors for wearable devices: A review. *Nanomaterials (Basel, Switzerland)*, *15*(7), 520. DOI: 10.3390/nano15070520 PMID: 40214565

Liu, X., Faes, L., & Kale, A. U.. (2019). Deep learning in healthcare. *The Lancet. Digital Health*, *1*(6), e271–e297. DOI: 10.1016/S2589-7500(19)30123-2 PMID: 33323251

Liu, X., Gao, K., Liu, B., Pan, C., Liang, K., Yan, L., & Pan, S. (2021). Advances in deep learning-based medical image analysis. *Health Data Science*, *2021*, 8786793. DOI: 10.34133/2021/8786793 PMID: 38487506

Liu, X., Peng, Y., Yang, Q., Wang, X., & Cui, N. (2021). Determining optimal deficit irrigation and fertilization to increase mango yield, quality, and WUE in a dry hot environment based on TOPSIS. *Agricultural Water Management*, *245*, 106650. DOI: 10.1016/j.agwat.2020.106650

Li, Y., Wen, G., Hu, Y., Luo, M., Fan, B., Wang, C., & Yang, P. (2021). Multi-source Seq2seq guided by knowledge for Chinese healthcare consultation. *Journal of Biomedical Informatics*, *117*, 103727. DOI: 10.1016/j.jbi.2021.103727 PMID: 33713854

Longoni, C., Bonezzi, A., & Morewedge, C. K. (2019). Resistance to medical artificial intelligence. *The Journal of Consumer Research*, *46*(4), 629–650. DOI: 10.1093/jcr/ucz013

Lukac, P. J., Turner, W., Vangala, S., Chin, A. T., Khalili, J., Shih, Y.-C. T., Sarkisian, C., Cheng, E. M., & Mafi, J. N. (2025). Ambient AI Scribes in Clinical Practice: A Randomized Trial. *NEJM AI*, *2*(12), AIoa2501000. DOI: 10.1056/AIoa2501000

Lukkien, D. R., Stolwijk, N. E., Askari, S. I., Hofstede, B. M., Nap, H. H., Boon, W. P., & Minkman, M. M. (2024). AI-assisted decision-making in long-term care: Qualitative study on prerequisites for responsible innovation. *JMIR Nursing*, *7*(1), e55962. DOI: 10.2196/55962 PMID: 39052315

Maithili, K., Ponmalar, A., Yamini, B., Karthikeyan, M., Anish, T. P., Maheswari, B., & Subramanian, R. S. (2024). Advances in AI and Machine Learning for Healthcare Informatics. In *Machine Learning and Generative AI in Smart Healthcare* (pp. 1–22). IGI Global. DOI: 10.4018/979-8-3693-3719-6.ch001

Malekpoor, H., Mishra, N., & Kumar, S. (2022). A novel TOPSIS–CBR goal programming approach to sustainable healthcare treatment. *Annals of Operations Research*, *312*(2), 1403–1425. DOI: 10.1007/s10479-018-2992-y

Malekpoor, H., Mishra, N., Sumalya, S., & Kumari, S. (2017). An efficient approach to radiotherapy dose planning problem: A TOPSIS case-based reasoning approach. *International Journal of Systems Science: Operations & Logistics*, *4*(1), 4–12. DOI: 10.1080/23302674.2015.1135354

Mann, K. D., Good, N. M., Fatehi, F., Khanna, S., Campbell, V., Conway, R., Sullivan, C., Staib, A., Joyce, C., & Cook, D. (2021). Predicting patient deterioration: A review of tools in the digital hospital setting. . *Journal of Medical Internet Research*, *23*(9), e23456. DOI: 10.2196/28209

Marinescu, M.-R., Ionescu, O. N., Pachiu, C. I., Dinescu, M. A., Muller, R., & uchea, M. P. (2025). Next-gen healthcare devices: Evolution of MEMS and BioMEMS in the era of the Internet of Bodies for personalized medicine. *Micromachines*, *16*(10), 1182. DOI: 10.3390/mi16101182 PMID: 41156428

Márquez Fosser, S., Mahmoud, N., Habib, B., & Weir, D. L. (2021). Smart about medications (SAM): A digital solution to enhance medication management following hospital discharge. . *Journal of the American Medical Informatics Association : JAMIA*, *28*, 2105–2112. DOI: 10.1093/jamia/ocab095

Marshall, N., Carsey, E., Chen, P., Bain, A., Bernard, P., & Patton, L. (2025). 'Pediatric nurses' perceptions of the quality and usefulness of clinical summaries: Surgeons versus generative AI'. *Journal of Pediatric Surgical Nursing*, *14*(4), 126–131. DOI: 10.1177/23320249251362849

Martinez, V. A., Betts, R. K., Scruth, E. A., Buckley, J. D., Cadiz, V. R., Bertrand, L. D., Paulson, S. S., Dummett, B. A., Abhyankar, S. S., Reyes, V. M., Hatton, J. R., Sulit, R., & Liu, V. X. (2022). The Kaiser Permanente Northern California Advance Alert Monitor Program: An automated early warning system for adults at risk for in-hospital clinical deterioration. . *Joint Commission Journal on Quality and Patient Safety*, *48*(8), 61–69. DOI: 10.1016/j.jcjq.2022.05.005

Matlhaba, K. (2024). Telehealth and Remote Monitoring. In *Enhancing Clinical Competence of Graduate Nurses*. Springer., DOI: 10.1007/978-3-031-81407-5_13

Matthew, A. J., Dhanalakshmi, R., & Vimal, S. (2025). A systematic review of Internet of Medical Things (IoMT) in healthcare. *Sci*, *7*(2), 36. DOI: 10.3390/sci7020036

Mazzeo, A. E. P., & dos Santos, L. W. (2025). Integration of biomedical devices and the internet of bodies revolution. Research. *Social Development*, *14*(5), e48921. DOI: 10.33448/rsd-v14i5.48921

Mbunge, E., Muchemwa, B., & Batani, J. (2021). Sensors and Healthcare 5.0: Transformative shift in virtual care through emerging digital health technologies. *Global Health Journal (Amsterdam, Netherlands)*, *5*(4), 169–177. DOI: 10.1016/j.glohj.2021.11.008

McGonigle, D., & Mastrian, K. (2021). *Nursing informatics and the foundation of knowledge* (5th ed.). Jones & Bartlett., DOI: 10.21019/9781284231542

Men, L., Ilk, N., Tang, X., & Liu, Y. (2021). Multi-disease prediction using LSTM recurrent neural networks. *Expert Systems with Applications*, *177*, 114905. DOI: 10.1016/j.eswa.2021.114905

Michalowski, M., Topaz, M., & Peltonen, L. M. (2025). An AI-Enabled Nursing Future With No Documentation Burden: A Vision for a New Reality. *Journal of Advanced Nursing*. PMID: 40129115

Michard, F., & Saugel, B. (2025). New sensors for the early detection of clinical deterioration on general wards and beyond – A clinician's perspective. *Journal of Clinical Monitoring and Computing*, *39*(2), 435–442. DOI: 10.1007/s10877-024-01235-1 PMID: 39546216

Miller, J. (n.d.). *MedQuAD* [Dataset]. Kaggle. https://www.kaggle.com/datasets/jpmiller/layoutlm

Mishra, A., Majumder, A., Kommineni, D., & Joseph, C. A. (2025). Role of generative artificial intelligence in personalized medicine: A systematic review. . *Cureus*, *17*, e14567. DOI: 10.7759/cureus.82310

Mittelstadt, B. D., Allo, P., Taddeo, M., Wachter, S., & Floridi, L. (2016). Ethics of algorithms. *Big Data & Society*, *3*(2), 2053951716679679. Advance online publication. DOI: 10.1177/2053951716679679

Mohammed, A. S., & Neravetla, A. R. (2024). "Understanding the impact of AI-driven clinical decision support systems." *15th IEEE International Conference on Healthcare Informatics*, pages 456-462. DOI: .DOI: 10.1109/ICCCNT61001.2024.10726136

Montejo, L., Fenton, A., & Davis, G. (2024). Artificial intelligence (AI) applications in healthcare and considerations for nursing education. *Nurse Education in Practice*, *80*, 104158. DOI: 10.1016/j.nepr.2024.104158

Moore, S. J., Garnett, A., Mason, K., Onigbinde, E., & Yurkiv, H. (2025). Nurses' Perceptions on the Usability of Electronic Health Records: A Scoping Review. *Science of Nursing and Health Practices = Science Infirmière et Pratiques en Santé*, *8*(1), 57–86. DOI: 10.62212/snahp.130

Moor, M., Rieck, B., Horn, M., Jutzeler, C. R., & Borgwardt, K. (2021). Early prediction of sepsis in the ICU using machine learning: A systematic review. *Frontiers in Medicine*, *8*, 607952. DOI: 10.3389/fmed.2021.607952 PMID: 34124082

Moran, S., Bailey, M. E., & Doody, O. (2024). Role and contribution of the nurse in caring for patients with palliative care needs: A scoping review. *PLoS One*, *19*(8), e0307188. DOI: 10.1371/journal.pone.0307188

Morley, J., Floridi, L., Kinsey, L., & Elhalal, A. (2019). From what to how: An initial review of publicly available AI ethics tools, methods and research to translate principles into practices. SSRN *Electronic Journal*. DOI: 10.2139/ssrn.3830348

Morley, J., Floridi, L., Kinsey, L., & Elhalal, A. (2020). From what to how: Ethical implementation of AI in healthcare. *AI & Society*, *35*(2), 457–468.

Morrish, D., Zayat, N., & Hoskins, I. A. (2024). Use of telehealth as an adjunct to conventional mental health care. *Obstetrics and Gynecology Clinics of North America*, *52*(1), 67–79. DOI: 10.1016/j.ogc.2024.09.006 PMID: 39880567

Morrow, E., Zidaru, T., Ross, F., Mason, C., Patel, K. D., Ream, M., & Stockley, R. (2023). Artificial intelligence technologies and compassion in healthcare. *Frontiers in Psychology*, *13*, 971044. DOI: 10.3389/fpsyg.2022.971044 PMID: 36733854

Nagendran, M., Chen, Y., Lovejoy, C. A., Gordon, A. C., Komorowski, M., Harvey, H., Topol, E. J., Ioannidis, J. P., Collins, G. S., & Maruthappu, M. (2020). Artificial intelligence versus clinicians: Systematic review of design, reporting standards, and claims of deep learning studies. *BMJ (Clinical Research Ed.)*, •••, 368. DOI: 10.1136/bmj.m689

Naghib, M., Chalechale, A., & Gharehchopogh, F. S. (2025). A comprehensive and systematic literature review on intrusion detection systems in the Internet of Medical Things: Current status, challenges, and opportunities. *Artificial Intelligence Review*, *58*(4), 114. Advance online publication. DOI: 10.1007/s10462-024-11101-w

Nahavandi, S. (2019). Industry 5.0—A human-centric solution. *Sustainability (Basel)*, *11*(16), 4371. Advance online publication. DOI: 10.3390/su11164371

Nasir, S., Khan, R. A., & Bai, S. (2024). Ethical framework for harnessing the power of AI in healthcare and beyond. *IEEE Access : Practical Innovations, Open Solutions*, *12*, 31014–31035. DOI: 10.1109/ACCESS.2024.3369912

Nazi, Z. A., & Peng, W. (2024). Large language models in healthcare and medical domain: A review. *Informatics (MDPI)*, *11*(3), 57. DOI: 10.3390/informatics11030057

Ndirangu-Mugo, E., Barros, L. M., Mutwiri, B. D., Shumba, C. S., Waweru, B., & Siika, W. W. (2022). Current state of critical care nursing worldwide. *Critical Care Clinics*, *38*(4), 657–693. DOI: 10.1016/j.ccc.2022.06.014 PMID: 36162904

Negro-Calduch, E., Azzopardi-Muscat, N., Krishnamurthy, R. S., & Novillo-Ortiz, D. (2021). Technological progress in electronic health record system optimization: Systematic review of systematic literature reviews.. *International Journal ofMedical Informatics*, *151*, 104467. DOI: 10.1016/j.ijmedinf.2021.104507

Nemati, M., Ansary, J., & Nemati, N. (2020). Machine-learning approaches in COVID-19 survival analysis and discharge-time likelihood prediction using clinical data. *Patterns (New York, N.Y.)*, *1*(5), 100074. DOI: 10.1016/j.patter.2020.100074 PMID: 32835314

Nematollahi Maleki, R., Shahbazi, S., Hosseinzadeh, M., Ghafourifard, M., Gholizad Gougjehyaran, H., & Faravan, A. (2025). Artificial intelligence-assisted nursing care: A concept analysis using Walker and Avant approach. *BMC Nursing*, *24*(1), 1175. DOI: 10.1186/s12912-025-03818-y PMID: 40993699

NHS England. (2025a) *The NHS long term plan*. London: NHS England. Available at: https://www.gov.uk/government/publications/10-year-health-plan-for-england-fit-for-the-future (Accessed: 2 January 2026).

NHS England. (2025b) *Data saves lives: reshaping health and social care with data*. London: NHS England. Available at: https://www.england.nhs.uk/digitaltechnology/data-saves-lives/ (Accessed: 2 January 2026).

NHS England. (2025c) *Multi-professional framework for advanced practice in England*. London: NHS England. Available at: https://advanced-practice.hee.nhs.uk/multi-professional-framework-for-advanced-practice/ (Accessed: 2 January 2026).

NHS England. (2025d) *Transformation Directorate: artificial intelligence – information governance guidance*. Available at: https://transform.england.nhs.uk/information-governance/guidance/artificial-intelligence/ (Accessed: 2 January 2026).

Nibbelink, C. W., & Brewer, B. B. (2018). Decision-making in nursing practice: An integrative literature review. *Journal of Clinical Nursing*, *27*(5–6), 917–928. DOI: 10.1111/jocn.14151

Nikolic, S., Ros, M., Al-Abdeli, Y. M., & Fairweather, H. (2025). Beyond assessment security: A critical policy analysis of four alternative strategies to uphold academic integrity and adopt the GenAI transformation of teaching and learning for an accredited engineering degree. *STEM Education*, *5*(4), 564–586. DOI: 10.3934/steme.2025027

Nkrumah, I. P., Engmann, F., & Adu-Manu, K. S. (2025). Ethical AI in healthcare: A comprehensive review addressing privacy, security, and fairness.

Noble, S. M., Mende, M., Grewal, D., & Parasuraman, A. (2022). The fifth industrial revolution: How harmonious human–machine collaboration is triggering a retail and service (r)evolution. *Journal of Retailing*, *98*(2), 199–208. DOI: 10.1016/j.jretai.2022.04.003

Norful, A. A., Brewer, K. C., Cahir, K. M., & Dierkes, A. M. (2024). Individual and organizational factors influencing well-being and burnout amongst healthcare assistants: A systematic review. *International Journal of Nursing Studies Advances*, *6*, 100187. DOI: 10.1016/j.ijnsa.2024.100187

Nouis, S. C., Uren, V., & Jariwala, S. (2025). Evaluating accountability, transparency, and bias in AI-assisted healthcare decision- making: A qualitative study of healthcare professionals' perspectives in the UK. *BMC Medical Ethics*, *26*(1), 89. DOI: 10.1186/s12910-025-01243-z PMID: 40629303

Nursing and Midwifery Council. (2018) *The Code: professional standards of practice and behaviour for nurses, midwives and nursing associates*. London: Nursing and Midwifery Council. Available at: https://www.nmc.org.uk/standards/code/ (Accessed: 2 January 2026).

Nutbeam, D. (2023). Artificial intelligence and health literacy—Proceed with caution. *Health Literacy and Communication Open*, *1*(1), 2263355. DOI: 10.1080/28355245.2023.2263355

Obermeyer, Z., Powers, B., Vogeli, C., & Mullainathan, S. (2019). Dissecting racial bias in an algorithm used to manage the health of populations. *Science*, *366*(6464), 447–453. DOI: 10.1126/science.aax2342

Oei, S. P., Bakkes, T. H. G. F., Mischi, M., Bouwman, R. A., van Sloun, R. J. G., & Turco, S. (2025). Artificial intelligence in clinical decision support and the prediction of adverse events. *Frontiers in Digital Health*, *7*, 1403047. DOI: 10.3389/fdgth.2025.1403047 PMID: 40520218

Okonji, O. R., Yunusov, K., & Gordon, B. (2024). Applications of generative AI in healthcare. *arXiv preprint arXiv:2406.10632*.

Olakotan, O., Samuriwo, R., Ismaila, H., & Atiku, S. (2025). Usability Challenges in Electronic Health Records: Impact on Documentation Burden and Clinical Workflow: A Scoping Review. *Journal of Evaluation in Clinical Practice*, *31*(4), e70189. DOI: 10.1111/jep.70189 PMID: 40581989

Olson, K. D., Meeker, D., Troup, M., Barker, T. D., Nguyen, V. H., Manders, J. B., Stults, C. D., Jones, V. G., Shah, S. D., Shah, T., & Schwamm, L. H. (2025). Use of Ambient AI Scribes to Reduce Administrative Burden and Professional Burnout. *JAMA Network Open*, *8*(10), e2534976. DOI: 10.1001/jamanetworkopen.2025.34976 PMID: 41037268

Omar, M., Sorin, V., Collins, J. D., Reich, D., Freeman, R., Gavin, N., Charney, A., Stump, L., Bragazzi, N. L., Nadkarni, G. N., & Klang, E. (2025). Multi-model assurance analysis showing large language models are highly vulnerable to adversarial hallucination attacks during clinical decision support. *Communications Medicine*, *5*(1), 330. DOI: 10.1038/s43856-025-01021-3 PMID: 40753316

Omrani, H., Alizadeh, A., & Emrouznejad, A. (2018). Finding the optimal combination of power plants alternatives: A multi response Taguchi-neural network using TOPSIS and fuzzy best-worst method. *Journal of Cleaner Production*, *203*, 210–223. DOI: 10.1016/j.jclepro.2018.08.238

Orenstein, E. W., Ferro, D. F., Bonafide, C. P., Landrigan, C. P., Gillespie, S., & Muthu, N. (2019). Hidden health IT hazards: A qualitative analysis of clinically meaningful documentation discrepancies at transfer out of the pediatric intensive care unit. *JAMIA Open*, *2*(3), 392–398. DOI: 10.1093/jamiaopen/ooz026 PMID: 31984372

Organisation for Economic Co-operation and Development. (2023). *Health at a Glance 2023: OECD Indicators*. OECD Publishing., DOI: 10.1787/7a7afb35-

Ouanes, K., & Farhah, N. (2024). Effectiveness of artificial intelligence (AI) in clinical decision support systems and care delivery. . *Journal of Medical Systems*, *48*(1), 56. Advance online publication. DOI: 10.1007/s10916-024-02098-4

Oyeniran, C. O., Adewusi, A. O., Adeleke, A. G., Akwawa, L. A., & Azubuko, C. F.Oyekunle Claudius OyeniranAdebunmi Okechukwu AdewusiAdams Gbolahan AdelekeLucy Anthony AkwawaChidimma Francisca Azubuko. (2022). Ethical AI: Addressing bias in machine learning models and software applications. *Computer Science & IT Research Journal*, *3*(3), 115–126. DOI: 10.51594/csitrj.v3i3.1559

Oyewole, A. T., Adeoye, O. B., Addy, W. A., Okoye, C. C., Ofodile, O. C., & Ugochukwu, C. E.Adedoyin Tolulope OyewoleOmotayo Bukola AdeoyeWilhelmina Afua AddyChinwe Chinazo OkoyeOnyeka Chrisanctus OfodileChinonye Esther Ugochukwu. (2024). Promoting sustainability in finance with AI: A review of current practices and future potential. *World Journal of Advanced Research and Reviews*, *21*(3), 590–607. DOI: 10.30574/wjarr.2024.21.3.0691

Özyurt, S. (2024). AI-assisted English language learning for cross-cultural medical education. *Experimental and Applied Medical Science*, *5*(2), 83–92. DOI: 10.46871/eams.1464830

Paarima, Y., Kisinna, A. A., & Ofei, A. M. A. (2024). Perceived organizational politics: Implications for nurses' stress and job satisfaction. *International Journal of Africa Nursing Sciences*, *20*, 100686. DOI: 10.1016/j.ijans.2024.100686

Pang, K., Li, L., Ouyang, W., Liu, X., & Tang, Y. (2022). Establishment of ICU mortality risk prediction models with machine learning algorithm using MIMIC-IV database. *Diagnostics (Basel)*, *12*(5), 1068. DOI: 10.3390/diagnostics12051068 PMID: 35626224

Pan, W. J., & Wang, S. F. (2025). Understanding patients' emotional needs to strengthen therapeutic relationships: A deep insight into narrative nursing. *World Journal of Psychiatry*, *15*(3), 103093. DOI: 10.5498/wjp.v15.i3.103093

Parihar, A., Prajapati, J. B., Prajapati, B. G., Trambadiya, B., Thakkar, A., & Engineer, P. (2024). Role of IoT in healthcare: Applications, security & privacy concerns. *Intelligent Pharmacy*, *2*(5), 707–714. DOI: 10.1016/j.ipha.2024.01.003

Pati, A. K. (2025). *Agentic AI: A Comprehensive Survey of Technologies, Applications, and Societal Implications*. IEEE., DOI: 10.1109/ACCESS.2025.3585609

Paul, M. M., Khera, N., Elugunti, P. R., Ruff, K. C., Hommos, M. S., Thomas, L. F., Nagaraja, V., Garrett, A. L., Pantoja-Smith, M., Delafield, N. L., Lizaola-Mayo, B. C., Kresin, M. M., Seetharam, M., Nagarakanti, S. R., & Kaur, M. (2025). The state of remote patient monitoring for chronic disease management in the United States. *Journal of Medical Internet Research*, *27*, e70422. DOI: 10.2196/70422 PMID: 40570326

Pavuluri, S., Sangal, R., Sather, J., & Taylor, R. A. (2024). Balancing act: The complex role of artificial intelligence in addressing burnout and healthcare workforce dynamics. *BMJ Health & Care Informatics*, *31*(1), e101120. DOI: 10.1136/bmjhci-2024-101120 PMID: 39181545

Pawar, U., O'shea, D., Rea, S., & O'reilly, R. (2020). *Explainable AI in healthcare*. Paper presented at the 2020 international conference on cyber situational awareness, data analytics and assessment (CyberSA). DOI: 10.1109/CyberSA49311.2020.9139655

Pawar, P., Anute, N., Tripathi, S., Ahluwalia, G. K., & Kalshetti, P. (2026). AI and its importance in the development of luxury consumption. In Vale, V. (Ed.), *Multidisciplinary approach to luxury consumption and AI* (pp. 1–34). IGI Global Scientific Publishing. , DOI: 10.4018/979-8-3693-8422-0.ch001

Pawar, P., & Shaha, S. R. (2025). Digital transformation in higher education: Innovations, strategies, and challenges. In *Higher Education 4.0: Strategies for digital success* (1st ed.). Dreambook Publishing House.

Peddisetti, V., Kandregula, P. K., & John, J. A. (2024). Smart medication management: Enhancing medication adherence with an IoT-based pill dispenser and smart cup. . *IEEE Journal of Biomedical and Health Informatics*, *28*, 2950–2958. DOI: 10.1109/JBHI.2024.3456789

Pelletier, J. H., Watson, K., Michel, J., McGregor, R., & Rush, S. Z. (2025). Effect of a generative artificial intelligence digital scribe on pediatric provider documentation time, cognitive burden, and burnout. *JAMIA Open*, *8*(4), ooaf068. DOI: 10.1093/jamiaopen/ooaf068

Perez, A. M. M. M., & Poletti, M. E. (2022). Characterization of digital systems used in medical X-ray imaging. *Radiation Physics and Chemistry*, *200*, 110307. DOI: 10.1016/j.radphyschem.2022.110307

Perkins, S. W., Muste, J. C., Alam, T., & Singh, R. P. (2024). Improving Clinical Documentation with Artificial Intelligence: A Systematic Review. *Perspectives in Health Information Management*, *21*(2), 1d. PMID: 40134899

Poalelungi, D. G., Musat, C. L., Fulga, A., Neagu, M., Neagu, A. I., Piraianu, A. I., & Fulga, I. (2023). Advancing patient care: How artificial intelligence is transforming healthcare. *Journal of Personalized Medicine*, *13*(8), 1214. DOI: 10.3390/jpm13081214

Pong, C., Tseng, R. M. W. W., Tham, Y. C., & Lum, E. (2024). Current implementation of digital health in chronic disease management: A scoping review. *Journal of Medical Internet Research*, *26*, e53576. DOI: 10.2196/53576

Poon, E. G., Lemak, C. H., Rojas, J. C., Guptill, J., & Classen, D. (2025). Adoption of artificial intelligence in healthcare: Survey of health system priorities, successes, and challenges. *Journal of the American Medical Informatics Association : JAMIA*, *32*(7), 1093–1100. DOI: 10.1093/jamia/ocaf065 PMID: 40323320

Prabhu, D., Tejasri, M. V. S. L., Saratha, B., & Anish, T. P. (2025, April). Future Horizons: Key Trends Shaping the Evolution of Machine Learning. In *2025 8th International Conference on Trends in Electronics and Informatics (ICOEI)* (pp. 1091-1099). IEEE.

Pramanik, B., Ghosh, D., Ghosh, D., & Paul, K. (2025). Beyond prediction: How generative AI is creating new healthcare realities. In *Revolutionizing Healthcare 5.0* (pp. 219–233). Springer.

Pramanik, R., Dey, S., Malakar, S., Mirjalili, S., & Sarkar, R. (2022). TOPSIS aided ensemble of CNN models for screening COVID-19 in chest X-ray images. *Scientific Reports*, *12*(1), 15409. DOI: 10.1038/s41598-022-18463-7 PMID: 36104401

Preiksaitis, C., & Rose, C. (2023). Opportunities, challenges, and future directions of generative artificial intelligence in medical education: A scoping review. *JMIR Medical Education*, *9*, e48785. DOI: 10.2196/48785

Pruski, M. (2024). Ethical challenges to the adoption of AI in healthcare: A review. *The New Bioethics : a Multidisciplinary Journal of Biotechnology and the Body*, *30*(4), 251–267. DOI: 10.1080/20502877.2025.2541438 PMID: 40779305

Rabbani, S. A., El-Tanani, M., Sharma, S., Rabbani, S. S., El-Tanani, Y., Kumar, R., & Saini, M. (2025). Generative artificial intelligence in healthcare. *BioMedInformatics*, *5*(3), 37. DOI: 10.3390/biomedinformatics5030037

Raghavan, S. (2025). Global advancements in international nursing science and healthcare innovation: Trends, challenges, and future directions. *Journal of Comprehensive Nursing Research*, *1*(2).

Rajkomar, A., Dean, J., & Kohane, I. (2019). Machine learning in medicine. *The New England Journal of Medicine*, *380*(14), 1347–1358. DOI: 10.1056/NEJMra1814259 PMID: 30943338

Rajput, K., Darzi, A., & Ghafur, S. (2025). Overlooked and under-reported: The impact of cyberattacks on primary care in the UK National Health Service. *The Lancet. Digital Health*, *7*(7), 100879. Advance online publication. DOI: 10.1016/j.landig.2025.100879

Ramadan, O. M. E., Alruwaili, M. M., Alruwaili, A. N., Elsehrawy, M. G., & Alanazi, S. (2024). Facilitators and barriers to AI adoption in nursing practice: A qualitative study of registered nurses' perspectives. *BMC Nursing*, *23*(1), 891. DOI: 10.1186/s12912-024-02571-y

Ramírez-Baraldes, A., González, M. A., & Avendaño, C. (2025). Artificial intelligence in nursing: New opportunities and challenges. *European Journal of Education*, *60*(1), 123–140. DOI: 10.1111/ejed.70033

Ramkumar, P., Kunze, K., Haeberle, H., Karnuta, J., Luu, B., Nwachukwu, B., & Williams, R. (2020). Clinical and research medical applications of artificial intelligence. *Arthroscopy*. Advance online publication. DOI: 10.1016/j.arthro.2020.08.009 PMID: 32828936

Rani, K., Vishnoi, H., & Mishra, M. (2023). *A mental health chatbot delivering cognitive behavior therapy and remote health monitoring using NLP and AI.* Paper presented at the 2023 International Conference on Disruptive Technologies (ICDT). DOI: 10.1109/ICDT57929.2023.10150665

Rao, V. M., Hla, M., Moor, M., Adithan, S., Kwak, S., Topol, E. J., & Rajpurkar, P. (2025). Multimodal generative AI for medical image interpretation. . *Nature*, *610*(8056), 62–70. DOI: 10.1038/s41586-025-08675-y

Rashid, S., & Nemati, A. (2024). Human-centered IoT-based health monitoring in the Healthcare 5.0 era: Literature descriptive analysis and future research guidelines. *Discover Internet of Things*, *4*(1), 26. DOI: 10.1007/s43926-024-00082-5

Ratwani, R. M., Savage, E., & Will, A.. (2018). Identifying EHR usability problems. *Journal of the American Medical Informatics Association : JAMIA*, *25*(7), 834–844. DOI: 10.1093/jamia/ocy024

Rejeb, A., Rejeb, K., Treiblmaier, H., Appolloni, A., Alghamdi, S., Alhasawi, Y., & Iranmanesh, M. (2023). The Internet of Things (IoT) in healthcare: Taking stock and moving forward. *Internet of Things : Engineering Cyber Physical Human Systems*, *22*, 100721. DOI: 10.1016/j.iot.2023.100721

Renggli, F. J., Gerlach, M., Bieri, J. S., Golz, C., & Sariyar, M. (2025). Integrating Nurse Preferences Into AI-Based Scheduling Systems: Qualitative Study. *JMIR Formative Research*, *9*(1), e67747. DOI: 10.2196/67747

Rezaei Bezanjani, B., Ghafouri, S. H., & Gholamrezaei, R. (2025). Privacy-preserving healthcare data in IoT: A synergistic approach with deep learning and blockchain. *The Journal of Supercomputing*, *81*(4), 533. DOI: 10.1007/s11227-025-06980-x

Rintyarna, B., Insantuan, O., Widiawati, I., & Purwoko, R. (2023). Telehealth in remote areas: A new artificial intelligence–based model. *The International Journal of Science in Society*, *5*(4), 243–254. Advance online publication. DOI: 10.54783/ijsoc.v5i4.782

Rodman, A., & Topol, E. J. (2025). Is generative artificial intelligence capable of clinical reasoning? *Lancet*, *405*(10480), 689. DOI: 10.1016/S0140-6736(25)00348-4 PMID: 40023638

Ronquillo, Y., Meyers, A., & Korvek, S. J. (2023, May 1). Digital health. In *StatPearls* [Internet]. StatPearls Publishing., Retrieved from https://www.ncbi.nlm.nih.gov/books/NBK470260/

Rony, M. K. K., Ahmad, S., Tanha, S. M., Das, D. C., Akter, M. R., Khatun, M. A., Begum, M. H. B., Khalil, M. I., Peu, U. R., Parvin, M. R., Alrazeeni, D. M., & Akter, F. (2025). Nursing educators' perspectives on the integration of artificial intelligence into academic settings. *SAGE Open Nursing*, *11*, 23779608251342931. Advance online publication. DOI: 10.1177/23779608251342931 PMID: 40386172

Rony, M. K. K., Alrazeeni, D. M., Akter, F., Nesa, L., Das, D. C., Uddin, M. J., & Parvin, M. R. (2024). The role of artificial intelligence in enhancing nurses' work-life balance. *Journal of Medicine, Surgery, and Public Health*, *3*, 100135. DOI: 10.1016/j.glmedi.2024.100135

Rossi, M., & Rehman, S. (2025). Integrating artificial intelligence into telemedicine: Evidence, challenges, and future directions. *Cureus*, *17*, e90829. Advance online publication. DOI: 10.7759/cureus.90829 PMID: 40988810

Rotenstein, L., Melnick, E. R., Iannaccone, C., Zhang, J., Mugal, A., Lipsitz, S. R., Healey, M. J., Holland, C., Snyder, R., Sinsky, C. A., Ting, D., & Bates, D. W. (2024). Virtual Scribes and Physician Time Spent on Electronic Health Records. *JAMA Network Open*, *7*(5), e2413140. DOI: 10.1001/jamanetworkopen.2024.13140 PMID: 38787556

Rowland, B., Saha, A., Motamedi, V., Bundy, R., Winsor, S., McNavish, D., Lippert, W., & Khanna, A. K. (2025). Impact on patient outcomes of continuous vital sign monitoring on medical wards: Propensity-matched analysis. *Journal of Medical Internet Research*, *27*, e66347. DOI: 10.2196/66347 PMID: 40068153

Ruiz, V. M., Goldsmith, M. P., Shi, L., Simpao, A. F., Gálvez, J. A., Naim, M. Y., Nadkarni, V., Gaynor, J. W., & Tsui, F. R. (2022). Early prediction of clinical deterioration using data-driven machine-learning modeling of electronic health records. . *The Journal of Thoracic and Cardiovascular Surgery*, *164*(1), 1083–1091. DOI: 10.1016/j.jtcvs.2021.10.060

Rutledge, C., & Gustin, T. (2021). Preparing nurses for roles in telehealth: Now is the time! *Online Journal of Issues in Nursing*, *26*(1). Advance online publication. DOI: 10.3912/OJIN.Vol26No01Man03

Saba, D., & Hadidi, A. (2025). Opportunities, challenges, and future directions of generative AI in healthcare. In *Generative Artificial Intelligence in Healthcare* (pp. 276–298).

Sabaghi, M., Mascle, C., & Baptiste, P. (2015). Application of DOE-TOPSIS technique in decision-making problems. *IFAC-PapersOnLine*, *48*(3), 773–777. DOI: 10.1016/j.ifacol.2015.06.176

Sai, S., Gaur, A., Sai, R., Chamola, V., Guizani, M., & Rodrigues, J. J. (2024). Generative AI for transformative healthcare. *IEEE Access : Practical Innovations, Open Solutions, 12*, 31078–31106. DOI: 10.1109/ACCESS.2024.3367715

Sameh, A., Rostami, M., Oussalah, M., Korpelainen, R., & Farrahi, V. (2025). Digital phenotypes and digital biomarkers for health and diseases: A systematic review of machine learning approaches utilizing passive non-invasive signals collected via wearable devices and smartphones. *Artificial Intelligence Review, 58*(2), 66. DOI: 10.1007/s10462-024-11009-5

Sam-Oyerinde, O. A., Idowu, O. O., & Idowu, O. P. (2025). The future of AI in healthcare. *Modern Technologies in Healthcare*, 290–320.

Schultz, C. (2023). Telehealth and remote patient monitoring innovations in nursing practice: State of the science. Online Journal of Issues in Nursing, 28(2). *Online Journal of Issues in Nursing, 1*(2). Advance online publication. DOI: 10.3912/OJIN.Vol28No02ST01

Scott-Marshall, H. K. (2024). Safe limits on work hours for the nursing profession: A rapid evidence review. *Frontiers in Global Women's Health, 5*, 1455422. DOI: 10.3389/fgwh.2024.1455422

Seenu, A., & Rani, P. S. (2024). From reactive to proactive: Redesigning patient care pathways. *European Data Science Journal, 2*(1).

Seibert, K., Domhoff, D., Bruch, D., Schulte-Althoff, M., Fürstenau, D., Biessmann, F., & Wolf-Ostermann, K. (2021). Application scenarios for artificial intelligence in nursing care: Rapid review. *Journal of Medical Internet Research, 23*(11), e26522. DOI: 10.2196/26522

Šekrst, K. (2025). Hallucinations. In *The Illusion Engine: The Quest for Machine Consciousness*. Springer., DOI: 10.1007/978-3-032-05562-0_12

Selvakumar, P., & Haashni, S. SudhaAnanthi G, Manjunath T C, (2026). "Cybernetic systems thinking: Foundations for organizational adaptability." In L. Tsvasman (Ed.), Cybernetic leadership for sustainable innovation, IGI Global Scientific Publishing, 99-124. DOI: .DOI: 10.4018/979-8-3373-2484-5.ch004

Selvaraj, S. (2024). Empowering patients with AI-driven personalized care. *International Journal of Scientific Research, 13*(7), 337–343.

Sendak, M. P., D'Arcy, J., Kashyap, S., Gao, M., Nichols, M., Corey, K., Ratliff, W., & Balu, S. (2020). A path for translation of machine learning products into healthcare delivery. *EMJ Innov, 10*, 19–00172.

Sendak, M. P., Gao, M., Brajer, N., & Balu, S. (2020). Presenting machine learning model information to clinical end users with model facts labels. *NPJ Digital Medicine, 3*(41), 41. Advance online publication. DOI: 10.1038/s41746-020-0253-3 PMID: 32219182

Shahidi Hamedani, S., Aslam, S., Mundher Oraibi, B. A., Wah, Y. B., & Shahidi Hamedani, S. (2024). Transitioning towards tomorrow's workforce: Education 5.0 in the landscape of Society 5.0: A systematic literature review. *Education Sciences, 14*(10), 1041. DOI: 10.3390/educsci14101041

Shajari, M., Kuruvinashetti, K., Komeili, A., & Sundararaj, U. (2023). The emergence of AI-based wearable sensors for digital health technology: A review. *Sensors (Basel), 23*(23), 9498. DOI: 10.3390/s23239498 PMID: 38067871

Shen, S., Qi, W., Zeng, J., Li, S., Liu, X., Zhu, X., & Lou, X. (2025). Passive sensing for mental health monitoring using machine learning with wearables and smartphones: Scoping review. *Journal of Medical Internet Research, 27*, e77066. DOI: 10.2196/77066 PMID: 40811794

Shoghli, A., Darvish, M., & Sadeghian, Y. (2024). Balancing innovation and privacy: Ethical challenges in AI-driven healthcare. *Journal of Research in Medical Sciences : the Official Journal of Isfahan University of Medical Sciences, 4*(1), 1–11.

Shortliffe, E. H., & Sepúlveda, M. J. (2018). Clinical decision support in the era of AI. *Journal of the American Medical Association, 320*(21), 2199–2200. DOI: 10.1001/jama.2018.17163 PMID: 30398550

Shortliffe, E. H., Sepùlveda, M.-J., & Patel, V. L. (2022). Framework for the evaluation of clinical AI systems. In *Intelligent systems in medicine and health: the role of AI* (pp. 479–503). Springer. DOI: 10.1007/978-3-031-09108-7_17

Siira, E., Johansson, H., & Nygren, J. (2025). Mapping and summarizing the research on AI systems for automating medical history taking and triage: A scoping review. *Journal of Medical Internet Research, 27*, e53741. DOI: 10.2196/53741

Singhal, K., Azizi, S., Tu, T., Mahdavi, S. S., Wei, J., Chung, H. W., Scales, N., Tanwani, A., Cole-Lewis, H., Pfohl, S., Payne, P., Seneviratne, M., Gamble, P., Kelly, C., Babiker, A., Schärli, N., Chowdhery, A., Mansfield, P., Demner-Fushman, D., & Natarajan, V. (2023). Large language models encode clinical knowledge. *Nature, 620*(7972), 172–180. Advance online publication. DOI: 10.1038/s41586-023-06291-2 PMID: 37438534

Singh, B., Lopez, D., & Ramadan, R. (2023). Internet of things in healthcare: A conventional literature review. *Health and Technology*, *13*(5), 699–719. Advance online publication. DOI: 10.1007/s12553-023-00771-1

Sinsky, C., Colligan, L., & Li, L.. (2016). Allocation of clinician time. *Annals of Internal Medicine*, *165*(11), 753–760. DOI: 10.7326/M16-0961 PMID: 27595430

Sittig, D. F., & Singh, H. (2010). A new sociotechnical model for studying health information technology in complex adaptive healthcare systems. *Quality & Safety in Health Care*, *19*(Suppl 3), i68–i74. DOI: 10.1136/qshc.2010.042085

Smokovski, I., Steinle, N., Behnke, A., Bhaskar, S. M. M., Grech, G., Richter, K., Niklewski, G., Birkenbihl, C., Parini, P., Andrews, R. J., Bauchner, H., & Golubnitschaja, O. (2024). Digital biomarkers: 3PM approach revolutionizing chronic disease management—EPMA 2024 position. *The EPMA Journal*, *15*(2), 149–162. DOI: 10.1007/s13167-024-00364-6 PMID: 38841615

Sriharan, A., Sekercioglu, N., Mitchell, C., Senkaiahliyan, S., Hertelendy, A., Porter, T., & Banaszak-Holl, J. (2024). Leadership for AI transformation in health care organization: Scoping review. *Journal of Medical Internet Research*, *26*, e54556. DOI: 10.2196/54556 PMID: 39009038

Stallinga, H. A., Ten Napel, H., Jansen, G. J., Geertzen, J. H., De Vries Robbé, P. F., & Roodbol, P. F. (2015). Does language ambiguity in clinical practice justify the introduction of standard terminology? An integrative review. *Journal of Clinical Nursing*, *24*(3–4), 344–352. DOI: 10.1111/jocn.12624 PMID: 24813851

Stanford, M., & Sorensen, Z. (2025). *Integrating generative AI in medical practice*. NuovoNova Ltd.

Stanford, M., & Sorensen, Z. (2025). *Integrating generative AI in medical practice: enhancing patient care and diagnostics with agentic AI systems*. NuovoNova Ltd.

Štirbanović, Z., Gardić, V., Stanujkić, D., Marković, R., Sokolović, J., & Stevanović, Z. (2021). Comparative MCDM analysis for AMD treatment method selection. *Water Resources Management*, *35*(11), 3737–3753. DOI: 10.1007/s11269-021-02914-3

Stirbu, V., Granlund, T., & Mikkonen, T. (2023). Continuous design control for machine learning in certified medical systems. *Software Quality Journal*, *31*(2), 307–333. DOI: 10.1007/s11219-022-09601-5

Stuart-Pesevic, N., & Talarico, S. (2024). Nursing leadership. *Nurse Leader*, *22*(5), 526–530. DOI: 10.1016/j.mnl.2024.07.001

Subasri, V., Baghbanzadeh, N., Celi, L. A., & Seyyed-Kalantari, L. (2025). Potential for near-term AI risks to evolve into existential threats in healthcare. *BMJ Health & Care Informatics*, *32*(1), e101130. DOI: 10.1136/bmjhci-2024-101130

Subramanian, R. S., Swetha, M., Krishnaveni, K., Thilagam, T., Saranya, K., Gracious, L. A., & Sudha, K. (2026). Transforming Education with NLP and Machine Learning: Innovations, Applications, and Future Prospects. In *Educational Applications of Natural Language Processing, Chatbots, and AI* (pp. 269-292). IGI Global Scientific Publishing.

Subramanyam, S. V. (2022). AI-powered process automation: Unlocking cost efficiency and operational excellence in healthcare systems. [IJARET]. *International Journal of Advanced Research in Engineering and Technology*, *13*(1), 86–102. DOI: 10.34218/IJARET_13_01_008

Sugapriya, S., Garg, S., Mahalle, A., Yewale, A. U., & Manjunath, T. C. (2026). Medical imaging and radiology: AI-powered diagnostics. In Ather, D., Mun, N., Jain, S., Jain, V., & Kukreja, V. (Eds.), *Applied AI and computational intelligence in diagnostics and decision-making* (pp. 191–218). IGI Global Scientific Publishing. , DOI: 10.4018/979-8-3373-3311-3.ch008

Sujan, M. A., Spurgeon, P., Inada-Kim, M., Rudd, M., Fitton, L., Horniblow, S., Cross, S., Chessum, P., & Cooke, M. (2014). Clinical handover within the emergency care pathway and the potential risks of clinical handover failure (ECHO): Primary research. *Health Services and Delivery Research*, *2*(5), 1–144. DOI: 10.3310/hsdr02050

Sullivan, B. A., & Keim-Malpass, J. (2021). BARRIERS to early detection of deterioration in hospitalized infants using predictive analytics. . *Hospital Pediatrics*, *11*(9), 897–903. DOI: 10.1542/hpeds.2020-004382

Sullivan, D., Hall, V. P., & Morrison, J. (2024). Navigating the future: Artificial intelligence's impact on transformational nurse leadership. *Teaching and Learning in Nursing*, *19*(3), 298–300. DOI: 10.1016/j.teln.2024.04.017

Sung, S.-F., Hu, Y.-H., & Chen, C.-Y. (2024). Disambiguating Clinical Abbreviations by One-to-All Classification: Algorithm Development and Validation Study. *JMIR Medical Informatics*, *12*(1), e56955. DOI: 10.2196/56955 PMID: 39352715

Sun, S., Simonsson, O., McGarvey, S., Torous, J., & Goldberg, S. B. (2024). Mobile phone interventions to improve health outcomes among patients with chronic diseases: An umbrella review and evidence synthesis from 34 meta-analyses. *The Lancet. Digital Health*, *6*(11), e857–e870. DOI: 10.1016/S2589-7500(24)00119-5 PMID: 39332937

Sun, X., Douiri, A., & Gulliford, M. (2022). Applying machine learning algorithms to electronic health records to predict pneumonia after respiratory tract infection. *Journal of Clinical Epidemiology, 145*, 154–163. DOI: 10.1016/j.jclinepi.2022.01.009 PMID: 35045315

Sutton, R. T., Pincock, D., Baumgart, D. C., Sadowski, D. C., Fedorak, R. N., & Kroeker, K. I. (2020). An overview of clinical decision support systems: Benefits, risks, and strategies for success. *NPJ Digital Medicine, 3*(1), 17. DOI: 10.1038/s41746-020-0221-y PMID: 32047862

Tabaie, Z., & Omidvar, A. (2023). Human body heat-driven thermoelectric generators as a sustainable power supply for wearable electronic devices: Recent advances, challenges, and future perspectives. *Heliyon, 9*(4), e14707. DOI: 10.1016/j.heliyon.2023.e14707 PMID: 37025803

Taherdoost, H. (2024). Wearable healthcare and continuous vital sign monitoring with IoT integration. *Computers, Materials & Continua, 81*(1), 79–104. DOI: 10.32604/cmc.2024.054378

Tamli, N., & Sain, M. (2023). Exploring innovative strategies for patient-centered care in nursing. *South Asian Journal of Research & Innovation, 10*(1), 19–30. DOI: 10.3126/jori.v10i1.66025

Tataei, A., Rahimi, B., Afshar, H. L., Alinejad, V., Jafarizadeh, H., & Parizad, N. (2023). The effects of electronic nursing handover on patient safety in the general (non-COVID-19) and COVID-19 intensive care units: A quasi-experimental study. *BMC Health Services Research, 23*(1), 527. DOI: 10.1186/s12913-023-09502-8 PMID: 37221502

Templin, T., Perez, M. W., Sylvia, S., Leek, J., & Sinnott-Armstrong, N. (2024). Addressing 6 challenges in generative AI for digital health: A scoping review. *PLOS Digital Health, 3*(5), e0000503. DOI: 10.1371/journal.pdig.0000503 PMID: 38781686

Teo, Z. L., Jin, L., Liu, N., Li, S., Miao, D., Zhang, X., Ng, W. Y., Tan, T. F., Lee, D. M., Chua, K. J., Heng, J., Liu, Y., Goh, R. S. M., & Ting, D. S. W. (2024). Federated machine learning in healthcare: A systematic review on clinical applications and technical architecture. *Cell Reports Medicine, 5*(2), 101419. DOI: 10.1016/j.xcrm.2024.101419 PMID: 38340728

Thatoi, P., Choudhary, R., & Shiwlani, A. (2023). Natural language processing (NLP) in the extraction of clinical information from electronic health records (EHRs) for cancer prognosis. . *International Journal of Medical Informatics, 169*, 104957. DOI: 10.1016/j.ijmedinf.2022.104957

Thirunavukarasu, A. J., Ting, D. S. J., Elangovan, K., Gutierrez, L., Tan, T. F., & Ting, D. S. W. (2023). Large language models in medicine. *Nature Medicine*, *29*(8), 1930–1940. DOI: 10.1038/s41591-023-02448-8 PMID: 37460753

Thompson, C., & Dowding, D. (2009). *Essential decision making and clinical judgement for nurses*. Elsevier.

Thottempudi, P., & Kumar, V. (2024). The Role of IoT in Modern Healthcare: Innovations and Challenges in Pandemic Era. In *Technologies for Sustainable Healthcare Development* (pp. 57–80). IGI Global. DOI: 10.4018/979-8-3693-2901-6.ch004

Thrall, J. H. (2024). Challenges of implementing artificial intelligence–enabled programs in the clinical practice of radiology. *Radiology. Artificial Intelligence*, *6*(5), e240411. DOI: 10.1148/ryai.240411 PMID: 39259022

Tischendorf, T., Hinsche, L., Hasseler, M., & Schaal, T. (2025). GenAI in nursing and clinical practice. *Journal of Public Health (Berlin)*. Advance online publication. DOI: 10.1007/s10389-025-02523-z

Topaz, M., Peltonen, L. M., & Zhang, Z. (2025). Beyond human ears: Navigating the uncharted risks of AI scribes in clinical practice. *NPJ Digital Medicine*, *8*(1), 569. DOI: 10.1038/s41746-025-01895-6 PMID: 40993221

Topaz, M., & Pruinelli, L. (2017). Big data and nursing. *Nursing Outlook*, *65*(1), 104–112. DOI: 10.1016/j.outlook.2016.10.003 PMID: 28106594

Topol, E. (2019). The Topol Review: preparing the healthcare workforce to deliver the digital future. NHS Health Education England., Available at https://topol.hee.nhs.uk, Retrieved January 2, 2026, from.

Topol, E. (2019). *Deep medicine: How artificial intelligence can make healthcare human again*. Basic Books.

Topol, E. J. (2019). High-performance medicine: The convergence of human and artificial intelligence. *Nature Medicine*, *25*(1), 44–56. DOI: 10.1038/s41591-018-0300-7 PMID: 30617339

Totten, A. M., Womack, D. M., Eden, K., McDonagh, M., Griffin, J., Grusing, S., & Hersh, W. (2016). Telehealth: Mapping the evidence for patient outcomes from systematic reviews. Europe PMC (PubMed Central). https://europepmc.org/article/MED/27536752

Trede, F., Macklin, R., & Bridges, D. (2012). Professional identity development: A review of the higher education literature. *Studies in Higher Education*, *37*(3), 365–384. DOI: 10.1080/03075079.2010.521237

Tripathy, S., Singh, R., & Ray, M. (2023). Natural language processing for COVID-19 consulting system. *Procedia Computer Science*, *218*, 1335–1341. DOI: 10.1016/j.procs.2023.01.112 PMID: 36743786

Tsvetanov, F. (2024). "Integrating AI technologies into remote monitoring patient systems." Engineering Proceedings, Volume 45, pages not available. DOI: .DOI: 10.3390/engproc2024070054

Tung, T. (2025) 'Ethical and practical challenges of generative AI in healthcare', *Journal of Medical AI Ethics*, PMC [online]. Available at: https://pmc.ncbi.nlm.nih.gov/articles/PMC12665710 (Accessed: 2 January 2026).

Tun, H. M., Rahman, H. A., Naing, L., & Malik, O. A. (2025). Trust in Artificial Intelligence–Based Clinical Decision Support Systems Among Health Care Workers: Systematic Review. *Journal of Medical Internet Research*, *27*(1), e69678. DOI: 10.2196/69678 PMID: 40772775

Tu, T., Schaekermann, M., Palepu, A., Saab, K., Freyberg, J., Tanno, R., Wang, A., Li, B., Amin, M., Cheng, Y., Vedadi, E., Tomasev, N., Azizi, S., Singhal, K., Hou, L., Webson, A., Kulkarni, K., Mahdavi, S. S., Semturs, C., & Natarajan, V. (2025). Towards conversational diagnostic artificial intelligence. *Nature*, *642*(8067), 442–450. DOI: 10.1038/s41586-025-08866-7 PMID: 40205050

U.S. Department of Health and Human Services. (2013). *HIPAA privacy rule*.

Umamaheswari, S., & Valarmathi, A. (2023, April 21). Role of artificial intelligence in the banking sector. *Journal of Survey in Fisheries Sciences.*, *10*(4S), 2841–2849.

Umberfield, E., Ghaferi, A. A., Krein, S. L., & Manojlovich, M. (2019). Using Incident Reports to Assess Communication Failures and Patient Outcomes. *Joint Commission Journal on Quality and Patient Safety*, *45*(6), 406–413. DOI: 10.1016/j.jcjq.2019.02.006 PMID: 30935883

Unanah, O. V., & Aidoo, E. M. (2025). AI technologies to reduce disparities in healthcare. *World Journal of Advanced Research and Reviews*, *25*(2), 2643–2664.

UNESCO. (2023) *Guidance for generative AI in education and research*. Paris: UNESCO. Available at: https://www.unesco.org/en/articles/guidance-generative-ai-education-and-research (Accessed: 2 January 2026).

Vaccari, I., Orani, V., Paglialonga, A., Cambiaso, E., & Giusto, D. D. (2021). A generative adversarial network (GAN) technique for internet of medical things data. . *Sensors (Basel)*, *21*(11), 3456. DOI: 10.3390/s21113726

Van der Laak, J., Litjens, G., & Ciompi, F. (2021). Deep learning in histopathology: The path to the clinic. *Nature Medicine, 27*(5), 775–784. DOI: 10.1038/s41591-021-01343-4

Van Veen, D., Van Uden, C., Blankemeier, L., Delbrouck, J.-B., Aali, A., Bluethgen, C., Pareek, A., Polacin, M., Reis, E. P., Seehofnerová, A., Rohatgi, N., Hosamani, P., Collins, W., Ahuja, N., Langlotz, C. P., Hom, J., Gatidis, S., Pauly, J., & Chaudhari, A. S. (2024). Adapted large language models can outperform medical experts in clinical text summarization. *Nature Medicine, 30*(4), 1134–1142. DOI: 10.1038/s41591-024-02855-5 PMID: 38413730

Veldhuis, L. I., Woittiez, N. J., Nanayakkara, P. W., & Ludikhuize, J. (2022). Artificial intelligence for the prediction of in-hospital clinical deterioration: A systematic review. *Critical Care Explorations, 4*(9), e0744. DOI: 10.1097/CCE.0000000000000744 PMID: 36046062

Villanueva-Miranda, I., Xiao, G., & Xie, Y. (2025). Artificial Intelligence in Early Warning Systems for Infectious Disease Surveillance: A Systematic Review. *Frontiers in Public Health, 13*, 1609615. DOI: 10.3389/fpubh.2025.1609615 PMID: 40626156

Wang, B., Shi, X., Han, X., & Xiao, G. (2024). The digital transformation of nursing practice. *Frontiers in Medicine, 11*, 1471527. DOI: 10.3389/fmed.2024.1471527 PMID: 39678028

Wangpitipanit, S., Lininger, J., & Anderson, N. (2024). Exploring the deep learning of artificial intelligence in nursing: A concept analysis using Walker and Avant's approach. *BMC Nursing, 23*(1), 529. DOI: 10.1186/s12912-024-02170-x

Wang, Y., Liu, Z. L., Yang, H., Li, R., Liao, S. J., Huang, Y., Peng, M.-H., Liu, X., Si, G.-Y., He, Q.-Z., & Zhang, Y. (2024). Prediction of viral pneumonia based on machine learning models analyzing pulmonary inflammation index scores. *Computers in Biology and Medicine, 169*, 107905. DOI: 10.1016/j.compbiomed.2023.107905 PMID: 38159398

Watson, A. L., Bond, C., Aveyard, H., Smith, G. D., & Jackson, D. (n.d.). Generative AI at the Bedside: An Integrative Review of Applications and Implications in Clinical Nursing Practice. *Journal of Clinical Nursing, n/a*(n/a). DOI: 10.1111/jocn.70151

Watson, B. M., & Wu, X. I. (2023). Sentinel Events and Miscommunication What do we know in 2021: A Language and Social Psychology Framework. *Health Communication, 38*(9), 1770–1779. DOI: 10.1080/10410236.2022.2031451 PMID: 35209746

Watson, J. (2008). *Nursing: The philosophy and science of caring* (Rev. ed.). University Press of Colorado.

Webb, C. A., & Fisher, H. (2025). Tracking psychopathology dimensions through passive smartphone sensing—Promises, pitfalls, and pathways to clinical integration. *JAMA Network Open*, *8*(7), e2519054. DOI: 10.1001/jamanetworkopen.2025.19054 PMID: 40608343

Weiner, E. B., Dankwa-Mullan, I., Nelson, W. A., & Hassanpour, S. (2025). Ethical challenges and evolving strategies in the integration of artificial intelligence into clinical practice. *PLOS Digital Health*, *4*(4), e0000810. DOI: 10.1371/journal.pdig.0000810 PMID: 40198594

Wilcox, L., Brewer, R., & Diaz, F. (2023). AI Consent Futures: A Case Study on Voice Data Collection with Clinicians. *Proc. ACM Hum.-Comput. Interact.*, *7*(CSCW2), 316:1-316:30. DOI: 10.1145/3610107

Williamson, B., & Eynon, R. (2020). Historical threads, missing links, and future directions in AI in education. *Learning, Media and Technology*, *45*(3), 223–235. DOI: 10.1080/17439884.2020.1798995

Witkowska-Zimny, M. (2025). Telemedicine/telehealth in smart hospital care. In *Smart hospital technologies* (pp. 251–264). DOI: 10.1016/B978-0-443-34226-4.00013-7

Woo, T., Ho, R., Tang, A., & Tam, W. (2020). Global prevalence of burnout symptoms among nurses: A systematic review and meta-analysis. *Journal of Psychiatric Research*, *123*, 9–20. DOI: 10.1016/j.jpsychires.2019.12.015 PMID: 32007680

World Health Organization. (2021) *Ethics and governance of artificial intelligence for health*. Geneva: World Health Organization. Available at: https://www.who.int/publications/i/item/9789240029200 (Accessed: 2 January 2026).

World Health Organization. (2021). *Ethics and governance of artificial intelligence for health*. WHO.

World Health Organization. (2021). *Global strategy on digital health 2020–2025*. World Health Organization.

World Health Organization. (2022). *Regional strategy for fostering digital health in the Eastern Mediterranean Region (2023–2027)* (EM/RC69/8). Cairo: World Health Organization, Regional Office for the Eastern Mediterranean. https://apps.who.int/iris/handle/10665/359945

World Health Organization. (2024). *Ethics and governance of artificial intelligence for health: Large multi-modal models*. World Health Organization.

World Health Organization. (n.d.). *Health equity*. World Health Organization. https://www.who.int/health-topics/health-equity#tab=tab_1

Wu, Y., Wu, M., Wang, C., Lin, J., Liu, J., & Liu, S. (2024). Evaluating the prevalence of burnout among health care professionals related to electronic health record use: Systematic review and meta-analysis. *JMIR Medical Informatics*, *12*, e54811. DOI: 10.2196/54811

Xiao, Z., & Han, X. (2023). Evaluation of the effectiveness of telehealth chronic disease management system: Systematic review and meta-analysis. *Journal of Medical Internet Research*, *25*, e44256. DOI: 10.2196/44256 PMID: 37103993

Yadav, A., Dandu, H., Parchani, G., Chokalingam, K., Kadambi, P., Mishra, R., Jahan, A., Teboul, J.-L., & Latour, J. M. (2024). Early detection of deteriorating patients in general wards through continuous contactless vital signs monitoring. *Frontiers in Medical Technology*, *6*, 1436034. DOI: 10.3389/fmedt.2024.1436034 PMID: 39328308

Yadav, N., Pandey, S., Gupta, A., Dudani, P., Gupta, S., & Rangarajan, K. (2023). Data Privacy in Healthcare: In the Era of Artificial Intelligence. *Indian Dermatology Online Journal*, *14*(6), 788–792. DOI: 10.4103/idoj.idoj_543_23 PMID: 38099022

Yun, S., Comín-Colet, J., Calero-Molina, E., Hidalgo, E., José-Bazán, N., Cobo Marcos, M., Soria, T., Llàcer, P., Fernández, C., García-Pinilla, J. M., Cruzado, C., González-Franco, Á., García-Marina, E. M., Morales-Rull, J. L., Solé, C., García-Romero, E., Núñez, J., Civera, J., Fernández, C., & Fernández, C. (2025). Evaluation of mobile health technology combining telemonitoring and teleintervention versus usual care in vulnerable-phase heart failure management (HERMeS): A multicentre, randomised controlled trial. *The Lancet. Digital Health*, *7*(5), 100866. DOI: 10.1016/j.landig.2025.02.006 PMID: 40374486

Zawacki-Richter, O., Marín, V. I., Bond, M., & Gouverneur, F. (2019). Systematic review of research on artificial intelligence applications in higher education: Where are the educators? *International Journal of Educational Technology in Higher Education*, *16*(1), 39. DOI: 10.1186/s41239-019-0171-0

Zhang, B., Chen, C., Lee, I., Lee, K., & Ong, K.-L. (2025). A survey on security and privacy issues in wearable health monitoring devices. *Computers & Security*, *155*, 104453. DOI: 10.1016/j.cose.2025.104453

Zhang, J., Zeng, Y., & Starly, B. (2021). Recurrent neural networks with long term temporal dependencies in machine tool wear diagnosis and prognosis. *SN Applied Sciences*, *3*(4), 442. DOI: 10.1007/s42452-021-04427-5 PMID: 33855273

Zhang, J., & Zhang, Z. M. (2023). Ethics and governance of trustworthy medical artificial intelligence. *BMC Medical Informatics and Decision Making*, *23*(1), 7. DOI: 10.1186/s12911-023-02103-9

Zhang, K., Jiang, Y., Xi, K., & Sun, N. (2025). Application of persuasive system design in mobile health interventions for chronic disease management: A mini review. *Frontiers in Public Health*, *13*, 1718371. DOI: 10.3389/fpubh.2025.1718371 PMID: 41358248

Zhang, Y., Li, X., Wang, H., & Chen, J. (2025). Advanced applications in chronic disease monitoring using IoT mobile sensing devices. *Frontiers in Public Health*, *13*, 1510456. DOI: 10.3389/fpubh.2025.1510456

Zhao, Y., Du, Y., Liu, Y., Deng, C., & Li, X. (2025). Artificial intelligence in chronic disease self-management: Current applications and future directions. *Frontiers in Public Health*, *13*, 1689911. DOI: 10.3389/fpubh.2025.1689911 PMID: 41358250

Zhi, W., Appling, A. P., Golden, H. E., Podgorski, J., & Li, L. (2024). Deep learning for water quality. *Nature Water*, *2*(3), 228–241. DOI: 10.1038/s44221-024-00202-z PMID: 38846520

Zhu, Z., & Zhu, M. (2023). The usage of Internet of Things in healthcare: A review of mechanisms, platforms, and opportunities from a new perspective. *Journal of Intelligent & Fuzzy Systems*, *45*(1), 1–18. DOI: 10.3233/JIFS-224166

Ziatdinov, R., Atteraya, M. S., & Nabiyev, R. (2024). The fifth industrial revolution as a transformative step towards Society 5.0. *Societies (Basel, Switzerland)*, *14*(2), 19. Advance online publication. DOI: 10.3390/soc14020019

About The Contributors

Suha Khalil Assayed holds a Ph.D. in Computer Science with a specialization in Artificial Intelligence. She is currently advancing her research as a Postdoctoral Researcher at the National Kaohsiung University of Science and Technology (NKUST), where she leads projects applying Natural Language Processing to healthcare, including disease prediction and AI-driven virtual health assistants. Dr. Assayed's research focuses on developing AI-driven chatbots and NLP-based systems to enhance both education and healthcare. She also serves as a keynote speaker on AI in healthcare, sharing insights on the role of intelligent systems in transforming medical practice and learning. With over 30 publications in reputable journals and international conferences, Dr. Assayed has made significant contributions to advancing the integration of deep learning, speech–text interaction, and language modeling across the health and education sectors.

Maha Mohammed Wahbi Atout is an Associate Professor of Pediatric Nursing at Philadelphia University, Jordan. She currently serves as Head of the International Projects Office, where she leads international collaborations, Erasmus+ projects, and institutional partnerships. Dr. Atout is also actively involved in quality assurance and academic accreditation processes, with extensive experience in curriculum development, research supervision, and international mobility programs. Her academic and professional interests focus on pediatric nursing, health education, and strengthening global academic cooperation.

Chin-Shiuh Shieh (Member, IEEE) received the M.S. degree in electrical engineering from National Taiwan University, Taipei, Taiwan, in 1991, and the Ph.D. degree from the Department of Computer Science and Engineering, National Sun Yat-sen University, Kaohsiung, Taiwan, in 2009. He joined as a Faculty Member of the Department of Electronic Engineering, National Kaohsiung University of Science and Technology, Kaohsiung, in August 1991, where he is currently a

Professor. His research interests include wireless networks and handover techniques. (Based on document published on 12 April 2024).

***

Abinaya M. is an Assistant Professor at Erode Sengunthar Engineering College with seven years of teaching experience. She holds an M.E. in Embedded System and Technologies from Mahendra Institute of Engineering and Technology and a B.E. in Electronics and Communication Engineering from Paavai College of Engineering. Her research interests include AI,Internet of Things (IoT), Embedded Systems, Wireless Sensor Networks, Signal Processing, and Computer Networks. She has published a patent in the field of IoT and presented papers at national and international conferences.

Syed Muqthadar Ali received B.Tech degree in CSE from Anwarul Uloom College of Engineering & Technology, Vikarabad, affiliated to Jawaharlal Nehru Technological University, Hyderabad, A.P. in 2003. He received his M.Tech Degree in CSE from CVR College of Engineering, Ibrahimpatnam, affiliated to Jawaharlal Nehru Technological University Hyderabad, Hyderabad, Telangana in 2013. He is currently working as a Senior Assistant Professor, Department of Computer Science & Engineering, CVR College of Engineering, Rangareddy, Telangana, India.

Sana Alsayed is an Assistant Professor of Psychological Counseling at Philadelphia University, Jordan. She has published several articles exploring the intersections of artificial intelligence, psychology, and emotions. Her research reflects an interdisciplinary approach to understanding human behavior and emotional well-being. Alongside her academic role, she serves as Library Director and Information Resources Manager at the university. Through her dual positions, she contributes to both educational development and applied research.

Muaath Ismail Alsufi is a medical researcher and senior medical scholar with a strong interest in the fields of clinical research, and bioinformatics. Enthusiastic to contribute development of the medical field in the connection of artificial intelligence and medicine.

Muthafar Alsufi is a training physician with a solid background in clinical research. More interests in applying the data science and AI in medical practice, with the goal of improving the diagnostic and minimizing errors as well as supporting the physician precision and the decision making.

Areej Khalil Assayed is an educator, academic leader, and trainer with over 25 years of experience in the field of education. She is the Head of the English Department and Humanities at Jordan International Schools (JIS) and a PhD candidate in Educational Leadership and Curriculum at Westcliff University, California, USA. Holding an MA in Linguistics and a BA in English Language and Literature, she has extensive expertise in curriculum development, instructional innovation, and teacher professional development. Her work integrates modern pedagogical approaches such as cooperative learning, multiple intelligences, and critical thinking, and she has conducted inspections for private schools in Jordan in collaboration with Accreditation International (AI). Her career reflects a strong commitment to advancing educational quality, fostering professional growth, and promoting the holistic development of learners.

Kathirvel Ayyaswamy, acquired, B.E.(CSE), M.E. (CSE) from Crescent Engineering College affiliated to University of Madras and Ph. D (CSE.) from Anna University. He is currently working as Professor, Dept of Computer Science and Engineering, Saveetha Engineering College, Chennai. In-charge for CSE Cyber Forensics Research Group. He is a studious researcher by himself, completed 18 sponsored research projects worth of Rs 103 lakhs and published more than 110 articles in journals and conferences. 6 research scholars have completed Ph. D and 7 under progress under his guidance. He is working as scientific and editorial board member of many journals. He has reviewed dozens of papers in many journals. He has author of 13 books. His research interests are protocol development for wireless ad hoc networks, security in ad hoc network, data communication and networks, mobile computing, wireless networks, WSN and DTN. He is a Life member of the ISTE (India), IACSIT (Singapore), Life Member IAENG (Hong Kong), Member ICST (Europe), IAES, etc. He has given a number of guest lecturers/expert talks and seminars, workshops and symposiums.

Naresh K K is an accomplished academic and data analytics professional with 3.8 years of combined teaching and industry experience. He currently serves as an Assistant Professor at Padmashree Institute of Management and Science, Bengaluru. Holding an MCA from KGiSL Institute of Information Management, he specializes in Data Analytics, Business Analytics, Machine Learning, and Artificial Intelligence. His expertise in Python, SQL, Power BI, and Tableau enables him to mentor students in data-driven problem-solving. He has presented papers at international conferences and is passionate about integrating analytical research and technology into management education.

Sagar Kukkamudi is a distinguished technology leader specializing in Enterprise Data Engineering, Cloud Analytics, and Real-time Data Processing for financial services, healthcare, and pharmaceuticals. With over 12 years of experience, he has architected scalable, high-performance platforms handling millions of daily transactions for organizations including Deloitte, Cardinal Health, Ameriprise Financial, Global Atlantic Financial and AstraZeneca. He holds a B.Tech in Information Technology from Jawaharlal Nehru Technological University and advanced cloud certifications including AWS Solutions Architect – Professional and Google Associate Cloud Engineer. Recognized as a thought leader, he has published research, contributed to industry standards, and spoken at major technology conferences. His work integrates AI-driven analytics, automated workflows, and cloud-native architectures, driving operational excellence and national-level impact in technology innovation.

M. Sadhasivam is an Assistant Professor in the Department of Artificial Intelligence and Data Science at Panimalar Engineering College. He is engaged in teaching and mentoring students in AI, data science, and related emerging technologies. His academic interests focus on applying intelligent systems and data-driven methods to real-world problems.

Dinesh M. G. is a faculty member at Easa College of Engineering and Technology, Coimbatore, Tamil Nadu. He specializes in engineering education and contributes to academic research, teaching, and student development. With a commitment to innovative learning, he actively engages in institutional growth and professional advancement.

A. Maheshwari is an Associate Professor in the Department of CINTEL at SRM Institute of Science and Technology (SRMIST), Kattankulathur, Tamil Nadu, India.He is actively engaged in teaching, research, and academic development in intelligent and interdisciplinary technologies. His research interests include emerging computing paradigms and their applications in engineering and technology.

T.C. Manjunath was born on 6th February 1967. He did his B.E. from RV College of Engg. in 1989 (B'lore Univ), M.E. in Robotics & Automation from Govt.'s LD College of Engg., (Gujarat Univ., Ahmedabad) in 1992 with FCD-First Rank & PhD in Systems & Control Engg. from IIT Bombay in the year 2007, got best research scholar award for the entire IITB. He is currently working as the Dean Research (R & D) and as Professor in Dept. of Computer Science & Engg. with specialization in IoT, Cyber Security, Blockchain Technology in Rajarajeswari College of Engineering, Bengaluru, Karnataka. He has got a teaching (academic), research & administrative experience of more than 35+ years (10 years as Principal

& 8 years as HoD, 1 year as Dean Research & rest as faculty) and has published more than 1500+ research papers in various national & international journals & conferences, with 175+ patents, 100+ book-chapters, 25 awards, 100s of Keynote talks and also published 25 text books in various field of science, engineering & technology, completed projects worth Rs. 9 Crores till date & guided 10 PhD scholars in VTU. He is a member of 30 Professional Society Chapters and is a fellow of IE, IETE, AMIEE, Sr. Member of IEEE and a chartered engineer.

Swati Mirlekar is an Assistant Professor in the Department of Vocation at St. Vincent Pallotti College of Engineering & Technology, Nagpur (Maharashtra) India. She has more than 21 years of teaching experience. Her research interests Include artificial intelligence, cyber security, deep learning, and AI applications in education and healthcare. She has published research articles and book chapters with international publishers. Email ID:swati.mirlekar@gmail.com ORCID ID: 0009-0005-3921-4588

Sudheer Nandi An internationally seasoned multidisciplinary technocrat and researcher with over 14+ years of international practice across global business strategy, mechanical engineering systems, emerging digital technologies, and corporate treasury operations. PhD in Management and Global Strategy Business Architecture, AI-powered neuroeconomics, CRISP-DM–driven analytics, design thinking, cognitive and ergonomic systems, and decision intelligence, architecting sustainable, scalable, and secure enterprise and future-ready socio-technical ecosystems

P. Selvakumar currently serves as an Associate Professor in the Department of Science and Humanities at Nehru Institute of Technology, Coimbatore, Tamil Nadu, India. With a teaching career spanning over a decade, he previously held positions as an Assistant Professor in the Department of Science and Humanities at various engineering colleges in Coimbatore from 2011 to 2023. Dr. P. Selvakumar's primary area of academic and research interest is phytochemistry, where he has made substantial contributions. His research credentials include 30 journal publications, 14 patents, and 25 conference papers. He has actively promoted faculty and student development by organizing 5 Faculty Development Programs (FDPs) and completing 3 NPTEL courses along with 60 Coursera certifications. His dedication to student success is evident in his role as a committed mentor, consistently guiding and supporting his students academically and personally. Recognized for his excellence in teaching, Dr. P. Selvakumar has received numerous accolades, including Best Teacher Awards. He is also an active member of MISTE (The Indian Society for Technical Education) and continues to play a vital role in both acade

Fares Qtaishat is a fourth-year medical student at the University of Jordan with research experience in oncology and clinical data analysis. He is particularly interested in the applications of artificial intelligence in medicine, including predictive analytics and improving healthcare workflows.

ParthibanR., currently working as an Associate Professor at IFET College of Engineering, with over 13 years of teaching experience. I am a Wipro Certified Faculty and an active TalentNext Trainer under the Digital Skills Readiness Program. I hold the recognition of being an Advanced Technology Certified Faculty and have received a Certificate of Excellence for successfully completing the TalentNext project on Artificial Intelligence. With a strong passion for teaching and technology, I continue to contribute to empowering students with future-ready skills.

MS. S. Saradha completed her Bachelor's degree in Computer Science and Engineering in 2013 and obtained her Master's degree in Computer Science and Engineering in 2015 under Anna University, Chennai. She has a total of seven years of professional experience, including three years in academia and four years in the industry. She is currently working as an Assistant Professor in the Department of Computer Science and Engineering at Thiagarajar College of Engineering, Madurai, Tamil Nadu. Her areas of interest include Natural Language Processing (NLP), Machine Learning (ML), and Conversational AI.

K. Saravanan is an Associate Professor in the Department of Electrical and Electronics Engineering at SRM Institute of Science and Technology (SRMIST), Kattankulathur, Tamil Nadu, India. He is actively involved in teaching, research, and academic development in the field of electrical and electronics engineering. His professional interests include advancing engineering education and contributing to research-driven innovation.

Shelley L. Spessard is an adjunct professor, CORE peer mentor, and faculty fellow at Westcliff University, where she supports faculty development and mentors emerging educators in instructional design and pedagogical innovation. Her scholarly work centers on instructional leadership, artificial intelligence integration in education, and the development of AI-informed pedagogy. Dr. Spessard's research examines how school leaders and educators can effectively implement artificial intelligence tools to enhance teaching and learning while maintaining a commitment to equity, ethics, and learner-centered practices. She is particularly focused on designing professional learning frameworks that prepare teachers to engage with AI critically and creatively in diverse educational environments. With extensive experience in both K–12 education and higher education, Dr. Spessard bridges practice and research through her work on curriculum development, educational leadership, and digital transformation. She contributes to the academic community through scholarly publications, faculty mentoring, and advocacy for future-ready teacher preparation models.

G. Sumathy is an Associate Professor in the Department of CINTEL at SRM Institute of Science and Technology (SRMIST), Kattankulathur, Tamil Nadu, India. She is actively involved in teaching, research, and academic development in interdisciplinary and intelligent technologies. Her professional interests include advancing research, innovation, and higher education in emerging engineering domains.

Vipin Tyagi is a distinguished academician, researcher and author, currently serving as Dean (Academics and Research) at Jaypee University of Engineering and Technology in Guna, Madhya Pradesh. Prof. Tyagi joined JUET, Guna in July 2005. His expertise spans across Image Processing, Cyber Forensics, and Speech Recognition. Prof. Tyagi has a prolific publication record, contributing significantly to his fields of interest. His scholarly work includes numerous journal articles, conference papers, and books. Some of his notable publications are in the areas of image forgery detection, image denoising, and content-based image retrieval. He has authored and edited several books and papers in the field of computing and data sciences, such as "Digital Image Forgery Detection: Techniques, Challenges and Applications", "Predictive Computing and Information Security" and "Content-Based Image Retrieval: Ideas, Influences, and Current Trends" published by Springer Singapore. His scholarly work has earned him a respectable h-index and numerous citations in the academic community. (2020-2022, 2022-2024, 2024-26)

Index

A

C

D

E

F

G

H

I

J

L

www.ingramcontent.com/pod-product-compliance
Lightning Source LLC
LaVergne TN
LVHW062323300926
849161LV00007B/1554